1996
YEAR BOOK OF
NEUROLOGY AND
NEUROSURGERY®

Statement of Purpose

The YEAR BOOK Service

The YEAR BOOK series was devised in 1901 by practicing health professionals who observed that the literature of medicine and related disciplines had become so voluminous that no one individual could read and place in perspective every potential advance in a major specialty. In the final decade of the 20th century, this recognition is more acutely true than it was in 1901.

More than merely a series of books, YEAR BOOK volumes are the tangible results of a unique service designed to accomplish the following:

- to *survey* a wide range of journals of proven value
- to *select* from those journals papers representing significant advances and statements of important clinical principles
- to provide *abstracts* of those articles that are readable, convenient summaries of their key points
- to provide *commentary* about those articles to place them in perspective.
- These publications grow out of a unique process that calls on the talents of outstanding authorities in clinical and fundamental disciplines, trained literature specialists, and professional writers, all supported by the resources of Mosby, the world's preeminent publisher for the health professions.

The Literature Base

Mosby subscribes to nearly 1,000 journals published worldwide, covering the full range of the health professions. On an annual basis, the publisher examines usage patterns and polls its expert authorities to add new journals to the literature base and to delete journals that are no longer useful as potential YEAR BOOK sources.

The Literature Survey

The publisher's team of literature specialists, all of whom are trained and experienced health professionals, examines every original, peer reviewed article in each journal issue. More than 250,000 articles per year are scanned systematically, including title, text, illustrations, tables, and references. Each scan is compared, article by article, to the search strategies that the publisher has developed in consultation with the 270 outside experts who form the pool of YEAR BOOK editors. A given article may be reviewed by any number of editors, from one to a dozen or more, regardless of the discipline for which the paper was originally published. In turn, each editor who receives the article reviews it to determine whether or not the article should be included in the YEAR BOOK. This decision is based on the article's inherent quality, its probable usefulness to readers of that YEAR BOOK, and the editor's goal to represent a balanced picture of a given field in each volume of the YEAR BOOK. In addition, the editor indicates when to include figures and tables from the article to help the YEAR BOOK reader better understand the information.

Of the quarter million articles scanned each year, only 5% are selected for detailed analysis within the YEAR BOOK series, thereby assuring readers of the high value of every selection.

The Abstract

The publisher's abstracting staff is headed by a physician-writer and includes individuals with training in the life sciences, medicine, and other areas, plus extensive experience in writing for the health professions and related industries. Each selected article is assigned to a specific writer on this abstracting staff. The abstracter, guided in many cases by notations supplied by the expert editor, writes a structured, condensed summary designed so that the reader can rapidly acquire the essential information contained in the article.

The Commentary

The YEAR BOOK editorial boards, sometimes assisted by guest commentators, write comments that place each article in perspective for the reader. This provides the reader with the equivalent of a personal consultation with a leading international authority—an opportunity to better understand the value of the article and to benefit from the authority's thought processes in assessing the article.

Additional Editorial Features

The editorial boards of each YEAR BOOK organize the abstracts and comments to provide a logical and satisfying sequence of information. To enhance the organization, editors also provide introductions to sections or individual chapters, comments linking a number of abstracts, citations to additional literature, and other features.

The published YEAR BOOK contains enhanced bibliographic citations for each selected article, including extended listings of multiple authors and identification of author affiliations. Each YEAR BOOK contains a Table of Contents specific to that year's volume. From year to year, the Table of Contents for a given YEAR BOOK will vary depending on developments within the field.

Every YEAR BOOK contains a list of the journals from which papers have been selected. This list represents a subset of the nearly 1,000 journals surveyed by the publisher and occasionally reflects a particularly pertinent article from a journal that is not surveyed on a routine basis.

Finally, each volume contains a comprehensive subject index and an index to authors of each selected paper.

The 1996 Year Book Series

Year Book of Allergy, Asthma, and Clinical Immunology: Drs. Rosenwasser, Borish, Gelfand, Leung, Nelson, and Szefler

Year Book of Anesthesiology and Pain Management: Drs. Tinker, Abram, Chestnut, Roizen, Rothenberg, and Wood

Year Book of Cardiology®: Drs. Schlant, Collins, Engle, Gersh, Kaplan, and Waldo

Year Book of Chiropractic®: Dr. Lawrence

Year Book of Critical Care Medicine®: Drs. Parrillo, Balk, Calvin, Franklin, and Shapiro

Year Book of Dentistry®: Drs. Meskin, Berry, Kennedy, Leinfelder, Roser, Summitt, and Zakariasen

Year Book of Dermatologic Surgery®: Drs. Swanson, Glogau, and Salasche

Year Book of Dermatology®: Drs. Sober and Fitzpatrick

Year Book of Diagnostic Radiology®: Drs. Federle, Clark, Gross, Latchaw, Madewell, Maynard, and Young

Year Book of Digestive Diseases®: Drs. Greenberger and Moody

Year Book of Drug Therapy®: Drs. Lasagna and Weintraub

Year Book of Emergency Medicine®: Drs. Wagner, Dronen, Davidson, King, Niemann, and Roberts

Year Book of Endocrinology®: Drs. Bagdade, Braverman, Horton, Kannan, Landsberg, Molitch, Morley, Nathan, Odell, Poehlman, Rogol, and Ryan

Year Book of Family Practice®: Drs. Berg, Bowman, Davidson, Dexter, and Scherger

Year Book of Geriatrics and Gerontology®: Drs. Beck, Burton, Rabins, Reuben, Roth, Shapiro, and Whitehouse

Year Book of Hand Surgery®: Drs. Amadio and Hentz

Year Book of Hematology®: Drs. Spivak, Bell, Ness, Quesenberry, Wiernik, and Blume

Year Book of Infectious Diseases®: Drs. Keusch, Barza, Bennish, Klempner, Skolnik, and Snydman

Year Book of Infertility and Reproductive Endocrinology: Drs. Mishell, Lobo, and Sokol

Year Book of Medicine®: Drs. Bone, Cline, Epstein, Greenberger, Malawista, Mandell, O'Rourke, and Utiger

Year Book of Neonatal and Perinatal Medicine®: Drs. Fanaroff and Klaus

Year Book of Nephrology®: Drs. Coe, Favus, Henderson, Kashgarian, Luke, and Curtis

Year Book of Neurology and Neurosurgery®: Drs. Bradley and Wilkins

Year Book of Neuroradiology: Drs. Osborn, Eskridge, Grossman, Hudgins, and Ross

Year Book of Nuclear Medicine®: Drs. Gottschalk, Blaufox, McAfee, Wackers, and Zubal

Year Book of Obstetrics and Gynecology®: Drs. Mishell, Kirschbaum, and Herbst

Year Book of Occupational and Environmental Medicine®: Drs. Emmett, Frank, Gochfeld, and Hessl

Year Book of Oncology®: Drs. Simone, Bosl, Cohen, Glatstein, Ozols, and Tallman

Year Book of Ophthalmology®: Drs. Cohen, Augsburger, Eagle, Flanagan, Grossman, Laibson, Maguire, Nelson, Rapuano, Sergott, Tasman, Tipperman, and Wilson

Year Book of Orthopedics®: Drs. Sledge, Cofield, Dobyns, Griffin, Poss, Springfield, Swiontkowski, Wiesel, and Wilson

Year Book of Otolaryngology–Head and Neck Surgery®: Drs. Paparella and Holt

Year Book of Pain: Drs. Gebhart, Haddox, Jacox, Janjan, Marcus, Rudy, and Shapiro

Year Book of Pathology and Laboratory Medicine: Drs. Mills, Bruns, Gaffey, and Stoler

Year Book of Pediatrics®: Dr. Stockman

Year Book of Plastic, Reconstructive, and Aesthetic Surgery®: Drs. Miller, Cohen, McKinney, Robson, Ruberg, and Whitaker

Year Book of Podiatric Medicine and Surgery®: Dr. Kominsky

Year Book of Psychiatry and Applied Mental Health®: Drs. Talbott, Ballanger, Breier, Frances, Meltzer, Schowalter, and Tasman

Year Book of Pulmonary Disease®: Drs. Bone and Petty

Year Book of Rheumatology®: Drs. Sergent, LeRoy, Meenan, Panush, and Reichlin

Year Book of Sports Medicine®: Drs. Shephard, Drinkwater, Eichner, Torg, Col. Anderson, and Mr. George

Year Book of Surgery®: Drs. Copeland, Bland, Deitch, Eberlein, Howard, Luce, Seeger, Souba, and Sugarbaker

Year Book of Thoracic and Cardiovascular Surgery®: Drs. Ginsberg, Williams, and Wechsler

Year Book of Transplantation®: Drs. Sollinger, Eckhoff, Hullett, Knechtle, Longo, Mentzer, and Pirsch

Year Book of Ultrasound®: Drs. Merritt, Babcock, Carroll, Fagan, Finberg, and Fleischer

Year Book of Urology®: Drs. DeKernion and Howards

Year Book of Vascular Surgery®: Dr. Porter

1996
The Year Book of NEUROLOGY AND NEUROSURGERY®

"Published without interruption since 1902"

Neurology

Editor
Walter G. Bradley, D.M., F.R.C.P.
Professor and Chairman, Department of Neurology, University of Miami School of Medicine, Miami, Florida

Neurosurgery

Editor
Robert H. Wilkins, M.D.
Professor and Chief, Division of Neurosurgery, Duke University Medical Center, Durham, North Carolina

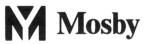 **Mosby**

St. Louis Baltimore Boston Carlsbad Chicago Naples New York Philadelphia Portland
London Madrid Mexico City Singapore Sydney Tokyo Toronto Wiesbaden

Vice President and Publisher, Continuity Publishing: Kenneth H. Killion
Director, Editorial Development: Gretchen C. Murphy
Developmental Editor, Continuity: Kristina Baumgartner, R.N.
Acquisitions Editor: Jennifer Roche
Illustrations and Permissions Coordinator: Lois M. Ruebensam
Manager, Continuity–EDP: Maria Nevinger
Project Manager, Editing: Tamara L. Smith
Senior Project Manager, Production: Max F. Perez
Freelance Staff Supervisor: Barbara M. Kelly
Director, Editorial Services: Edith M. Podrazik, R.N.
Information Specialist: Kathleen Moss, R.N.
Senior Medical Writer: David A. Cramer, M.D.
Vice President, Professional Sales and Marketing: George M. Parker
Senior Marketing Manager: Eileen M. Lynch
Marketing Specialist: Lynn D. Stevenson

1996 EDITION
Copyright © January 1996 by Mosby-Year Book, Inc.

Printed in the United States of America
Composition by Reed Technology and Information Services, Inc.
Printing/binding by Maple-Vail

Mosby–Year Book, Inc.
11830 Westline Industrial Drive
St. Louis, MO 63146

Editorial Office:
Mosby–Year Book, Inc.
200 North LaSalle St.
Chicago, IL 60601

International Standard Serial Number: 0513-5117
International Standard Book Number: 0-8151-2145-8

Contributing Editors

Imaging, *University of Miami School of Medicine, Miami, Florida*

Eugene R. Ramsay, M.D.
Professor of Neurology, Department of Neurology, University of Miami School of Medicine, Miami, Florida

J.R. Sanchez-Ramos, M.D., Ph.D.
Associate Professor, Department of Neurology, University of Miami School of Medicine and Miami Veterans Administration Medical Center, Miami, Florida

Norman J. Schatz, M.D.
Professor of Clinical Neurology and Ophthalmology, Department of Ophthalmology, University of Miami School of Medicine, Miami, Florida

Subramaniam Sriram, M.D.
Professor of Neurology, Department of Neurology, Vanderbilt University Medical Center, Nashville, Tennessee

David A. Stumpf, M.D., Ph.D.
Benjamin and Virginia T. Boshes Professor of Neurology; Chairman, Department of Neurology; Professor of Pediatrics, Northwestern University Medical School, Chicago, Illinois

Ronald J. Tusa, M.D.
Professor of Otolaryngology, University of Miami School of Medicine, Miami, Florida

Table of Contents

Mosby Document Express

Copies of the full text of the original source documents of articles abstracted or referenced in this publication are available by calling Mosby Document Express, toll-free, at 1 (800) 55-MOSBY.

With Mosby Document Express, you have convenient, 24-hour-a-day access to literally every article on which this publication is based. In fact, through Mosby Document Express, virtually any medical or scientific article can be located and delivered by FAX, overnight delivery service, international airmail, electronic transmission of bitmapped images (via Internet), or regular mail. The average cost of a complete, delivered copy of an article, including up to $4 in copyright clearance charges and first-class mail delivery, is $12.

For inquiries and pricing information, please call the toll-free number shown above. To expedite your order for material appearing in this publication, please be prepared with the code shown next to the bibliographic citation for each abstract.

Journals Represented

NEUROLOGY

Walter G. Bradley, D.M., F.R.C.P.

Neurology Health Care Reorganization and Managed Care

WALTER G. BRADLEY, D.M., F.R.C.P.

This volume of the 1996 YEAR BOOK OF NEUROLOGY AND NEUROSURGERY was prepared against the backdrop of significant reorganization of health care in the United States, Canada, and Britain. The reorganization is the response of government and society to the need to contain the rapid inflation in health care costs in all of these countries. In the United States, it is clear that most cost-containment is based on reductions in both the reimbursement to doctors and hospitals, and the provision of services to patients. Although it seems likely that the switch to managed care in the United States is achieving some reduction in the national expenditure on health care, the amount of money going into health insurance companies and administration has increased considerably. This state of affairs is distressing for those of us who are advocates for the patient, research, academic medical centers, and the medical profession.

Most of us have been cognizant that health care costs cannot be allowed to consume an ever-increasing percentage of the gross national product; therefore, many believe that the current reorganization was inevitable. It is, however, important that the medical profession in general and the field of neurology in particular quickly adapt to the changing circumstances. We need to ensure that the highest possible percentage of the health care dollar goes to support the patient and the health care system, and not the insurance industry and administration. We also have to recognize that one detrimental effect of managed care is that it sets one segment of the medical profession, i.e., the generalist, against another segment, i.e., the specialist. In the end, there can be no doubt that this will be detrimental to the care of the patient and to the medical profession as a whole.

How can we avoid what seems to be a never-ending slippery slide into the abyss of managed care? One way would be for the medical profession and its specialties to organize into a *single provider* rather than to be picked off piecemeal by the current format of divide and conquer. This type of organization demonstrates the concept of a *single-payor system,* which some have advocated. Such a move would raise the risk of violation of anti-trust laws, but there are potential ways of approaching this problem that involve the use of labor laws and established procedures for collective bargaining.

In the context of the current climate of managed care, and from the point of view of unity and fiscal stability, it would be advantageous for a specialty like neurology to move into the mainstream of capitation and to avoid staying outside as an item-for-service provider. We should be the ones who determine the most cost-effective way to deliver neurologic care for a defined population, not the generalist or the insurance industry. Two papers reviewed in this volume of the YEAR BOOK OF NEUROLOGY AND NEUROSURGERY give proof to this argument, if proof is needed. The articles (see Abstracts 122-96-2–2 and 122-96-4–13) demonstrate that the care and rehabilitation of stroke patients by neurologists provide a better and more cost-effective outcome than does the care of such patients by generalists.

Another point to remember in the present reorganization of health care is that we do not need to throw out the baby with the bath water. There are many individuals and organizations in the United States that demand the highest level of medical care for themselves and their employees, using the annual executive examination and high-technology screening studies to catch potentially fatal diseases in the early stages. We need to maintain a system that can provide this premium level of care where cost is not a major consideration. Moreover, it is important for everyone that we continue to ride the exciting wave of advances emanating from neuroscience research.

However, social responsibility and self-interest demand that we develop an efficient system that protects the best features of what, until the past few years, has been the best health care system in the world, and avoids the current syphoning of money from patient care into administration and insurance industry profit. The new system must continue to provide medical advances, maintain a high standard of medical care, be cost effective, and maintain patient choice. This can all be achieved if the medical profession is able to take control of the situation and set up a single-provider integrated health care delivery system.

The American Board of Psychiatry and Neurology and Recertification

The American Board of Psychiatry and Neurology held the Part II Examinations in the University of Miami in January 1995.

This prompted me to dwell on matters relating to examinations and certifications. The last group of neurologists to be awarded lifetime Board Certification in Neurology have already taken the Board examinations. Those who graduate in the future will have to be recertified every ten years. The mechanism for recertification has yet to defined, although it will probably be examination. Some neurologists will use the ongoing topic-orientated self-learning program (Continuum) of the American Academy of Neurology to supplement literature review such as that provided by the YEAR BOOK OF NEUROLOGY AND Neurosurgery.

No one *likes* examinations, with the possible exception of the examiners. If the examinees knew how hard examiners strive to pass the candidates, they would be a good deal less anxious. I am aware of this from my own personal experience. As an examiner of medical students in the British system, where there is a final "live" qualifying examination, it was often painfully necessary to help the student to demonstrate knowledge that was obviously in existence but hidden by the stress of the situation. When I took the American Board of Psychiatry and Neurology examination in 1978, the examiners and I realized that I was floundering over questions dealing with the minutiae of pediatric epilepsy and EEG patterns. With a glint in his eye, the senior examiner asked me if perhaps I knew something about peripheral neuropathies!

Apart from generating "war stories," examinations have a definite benefit for the candidate, although this is only perceived from the post-hoc vantage point. Updating the active knowledge base *and* broadening the general scope of understanding of the neurosciences gives the successful candidate a feeling of competence. For those requiring re-certification, it will also ward off the fear of being overtaken by those sharp young doctors who have just finished their residency. I have had the "pleasure" of taking a medical school qualifying examination three times in my career. The first time was to graduate from Oxford University School of Medicine. In the United Kingdom, there is a final examination involving *all* clinical subjects that must be passed *in toto* before the MD degree (which, in the United Kingdom, is termed M.B., B.S., or B.M., B.Ch., depending on the medical school) is awarded. I well remember the Regius Professor of Medicine, in full academic regalia, as is the custom, standing disapprovingly as I tried to convince the Ob-Gyn examiner that I understood the usage of the Hodge pessary, while going through all of its possible positions until I found the correct one.

In 1977, when I moved to the United States, I took the Federation Licensing Examination (FLEX) examination to become licensed to practice medicine in Massachusetts. I did not study for that examination, and it seemed relatively easy at the time. In 1991, I took the FLEX examination again to become licensed in Florida. This time I realized that I had been specializing in neurology for too long and needed to review—at least—the advances in biochemistry, physiology, bacteriology, and pharmacology. I was amazed to find out how many new biochemical pathways had been discovered (and were expected to be learned!) since I had been in medical school. I was also disturbed to find out how many new drugs, particularly antibiotics, had been discovered. I was particularly abashed to discover how much was known about their mechanism of action on bacterial wall biosynthesis and metabolism. For the ingenious examiner, there are many happy questions in that field.! Astoundingly, I passed the FLEX examination the second time, gaining 10 points more than I had achieved 15 years previously.

All of this brings me to the point of this little story: Recertification is undoubtly beneficial, both to the doctor and to the patient. I did not retain for more than a few weeks most of the new biochemical and pharmaceutical information, but I certainly acquired a better stepping-off point for increasing my understanding of new advances. I have been reassured that I can still learn as well a graduating medical student, and I am confident that I have not become so specialized that I cannot remember about breach deliveries, colonic surgery, and congenital heart disease.

Newly certified diplomates of the American Board of Psychiatry and Neurology will likely complain about having to become recertified every ten years. However, they will remain significantly more current than the present group of graybeards that have been grandfathered into lifetime certification. For them, I might transpose the old adage to read: "There is no pain without some gain!"

The Concept of Acute Brain Attack

Thirty years ago, in my internship, I performed internal cardiac massage on a number of patients with cardiac arrest, and I found it to be a bloody and totally unrewarding procedure. When I was doing cardiology as part of my internal medicine training at the Royal Postgraduate Medical School in the Hammersmith Hospital, London, we were just starting to question whether external cardiac massage and emergency cardioversion could improve the mortality of a patient with an acute heart attack. When the code for cardiac arrest was called, the Chairman of the Department, Professor John Goodwin, and I would be the first on the scene, pushing what has now come to be called the "crash cart." At that time, the treatment of myocardial infarction was in its infancy. Over the past 30 years, there have been many discoveries in the field of coronary artery disease. We have proved that we can maintain perfusion with external cardiac massage, and the success of external cardioversion has been demonstrated. Both the acute use of bicarbonate and lidocaine and the value of hyperacute thrombolytics have been demonstrated. Coronary artery by-pass grafts, angioplasty, and the insertion of stents have totally changed the prognosis of patients with an acute heart attack, which, 30 years ago, meant that one third of the patients died, one third recovered but died in the next year with a further heart attack, and one third recovered. The prognosis is now dramatically better. The general public is well aware one should go to the emergency department as rapidly as possible if chest pains develop. As a result, a surprising proportion of patients older than 65 years of age have had some interventional therapy for coronary artery disease.

Can this success be transplanted to the field of cerebrovascular disease? Stroke is still the third major killer of the United States' population, after cancer and heart disease. However, the most individuals' approach to the onset of symptoms of a stroke is to go to bed and hope that the symptoms will be gone by the morning. When the patient wakes with a completed stroke, the horse is out of the barn.

We now have to ask the same questions in the field of stroke that we have answered in the field of myocardial infarction during the past 30 years.

1. *Can we prevent death from an acute stroke?* Postinfarction swelling of the brain can cause generalized cerebral hypoperfusion and death. High-dose corticosteroids and hyperventilation to produce hypocapnia have been used in the therapy of raised intracranial pressure.

2. *Can we save the brain that is ischemic but not yet dead?* The review by Hossmann that is summarized in this issue and the comments by Ginsberg consider this possibility (see Abstract 122-96-1–4). The salvage-able area is termed the *ischemic penumbra*. The results of experimental and some clinical studies suggest that this ischemic penumbra can be

saved. Studies have investigated hypervolemic therapy with low-molecular-weight dextrans, calcium channel blockers, N -methyl- D -aspartate inhibitors, and phenobarbital coma.

3. *Is it worthwhile to dissolve a clot in an intracerebral vessel, using systemic or intra-arterial thrombolytics, such as streptokinase, urokinase, and tPA?* Two papers in this volume of the YEAR BOOK suggest that intra-arterial thrombolytics can bring about revascularization and improved neurologic status (Abstracts 122-96-1–1 and 122-96-1–2).

4. *Is the creation of a bypass around an occlusion beneficial?* The EC-IC (External Carotid–Internal Carotid) Bypass Study failed to demonstrate any such general benefit.

5. *Is removal of an extracranial arterial obstruction with carotid endarterectomy of benefit?* The NASCET trial indicated that symptomatic patients with stenosis greater than 60% who were seen in centers with good records of surgical morbidity and mortality had fewer strokes after endarterectomy than did those treated with medical therapy.

6. *Is balloon angioplasty of intracranial vessels possible and beneficial?* The paper by Tsai et al. that appears in this volume (Abstract 122-96-1–2) indicates that transluminal balloon angioplasty can be beneficial in patients who have had immediate rethrombosis after intra-arterial thrombolytic therapy.

7. *Is insertion of an intra-arterial stent worthwhile?* This procedure is being considered for extracranial and intracranial stenoses that are difficult to treat with angioplasty or endarterectomy.

8. *Are some of the other cardiologic and peripheral vascular interventional techniques, such as the use of endovascular laser and ultrasound probes, of any value?* This remains to be investigated in humans who have arteriosclerotic cerebrovascular disease.

There are enough fruitful areas for research for many years to come. However, answers are needed soon. Each of these individual questions has either been approached or is actively being considered, both clinically and experimentally, in centers in the United States and in other countries. It has become clear to those involved in stroke research that if there is to be much improvement in stroke prognosis, we must learn from the those investigating myocardial infarction. Interventional stroke neurologists should be able to adapt a great deal of the techniques of interventional cardiologists and peripheral vascular specialists. The brain is obviously different from the heart, and the risk of massive hemorrhage resulting from revascularization of ischemic brain is only one example of this. However, it seems likely that hemorhage can be avoided if revascularization is undertaken rapidly, before vascular endothelial damage occurs.

The first lesson from the field of coronary artery disease research is the need to persuade patients urgently to get to an emergency department at the first sign of any symptom that might indicate cerebral ischemia. In centers mounting such programs for the treatment of acute brain attack, there is the need for a widespread publicity campaign to bring to the public the message of urgency that mirrors that related to myocardial ischemia.

Because neurons survive total ischemia even less well than cardiac muscle, there is even more urgency in the stroke arena than in the heart attack arena. The National Institutes of Health (NIH) rPA Pilot Trials incorporated two groups of patients: those able to receive treatment within 90 minutes of the onset of symptoms, and those available to receive treatment between 90 and 180 minutes of symptom onset. This was based on the supposition that the latter time window might be outside the period of benefit. Having patients call 911 and arrive at the hospital rapidly is the key, but developing ultra-rapid in-hospital management from the emergency department to the commencement of interventional therapy is also crucial. I wrote one of the original applications for an NIH tPA Pilot Study while in Vermont, and I became acutely aware of the need to develop an interdisciplinary critical pathway management team. For instance, the neurologist might need to undertake a brief examination while standing on the gurney as it is wheeled toward the CT scanner. Specialized facilities and programs are needed; the spiral ultra-fast CT scanner will be a great help. Eventually, we hope to reach the stage where acute interventional therapy is provided in the ambulance. A great deal of experimentation and delineation of which patients will benefit need to be undertaken before this can be offered. Before we can define the best treatment, there may be many failures, one of which is massive intracerebral hemorrhage resulting from late opening of an occluded carotid artery.

The institution of a publicity campaign that is required for an acute treatment trial *does* bring patients into the hospital more rapidly, as indicated in a paper by Barsan et al. in this volume of the YEAR BOOK (Abstract 122-96-1–3). The paper should be read in detail, because even with the publicity campaign and the best attempts at developing a critical pathway management, only 74 of 1,948 potentially treatable patients (3.5%) actually received tPA. Barsan et al. do not discuss another likely outcome of the publicity campaign for the acute brain attack, i.e., the arrival in the emergency department of many patients with neurologic symptoms not resulting from stroke. We shall see a great number of patients with conditions such as carpal tunnel syndrome, pressure palsies from crossing of the legs, migraine, and anxiety, all of whom think they may be having a stroke. The emergency department will need to be staffed by neurologists on a 24-hour-a-day basis as part of the rapid response team. This is going to be expensive, and such studies are likely to be undertaken only in academic medical centers with research grant funding.

Eventually, the answer for both stroke and myocardial infarction will come from research into the prevention of arteriosclerosis. Until that time, however, many patients with acute thrombotic stroke will require better treatments and better advice on how to receive those treatments. It is now time to develop a network of academic centers able to mount therapeutic trials of hyperacute therapy for acute brain attack.

Neurologic Complication of AIDS

The neurologic section of this 1996 volume of the YEAR BOOK OF NEUROLOGY AND NEUROSURGERY includes ten papers describing some recent findings on the neurologic complications associated with HIV-1 infection. This is appropriate, because HIV-1–associated neurologic complications are becoming an increasing part of the practice of neurology. Those of us who work in larger urban areas have considerable experience with all of these complications. This is not the case in more rural practices; however, as HIV-1 continues to spread into the heterosexual community, we can expect no neurologist to be spared from experience with such cases.

Those who have seen a good deal of the neurology of AIDS come to learn the setting and the presentation, and to make presumptive diagnoses on clinical grounds. Therefore, HIV-1 infection has become similar to that of the various presentations of neurosyphilis 60 years ago. In fact, there are many parallels between HIV-1 and *Treponema pallidum* infection. Syphilis was called the "great imitator" at a time when our neurologic forebears had few diagnostic tools. Now, in a somewhat similar fashion, we find that the neurologic complications of HIV-1 are seen in many ways in virtually every part of the nervous system and neuromuscular apparatus.

It is interesting to look back on how the pattern of neurologic problems associated with HIV-1 infection have changed in the past ten years. Initially, complications were those resulting from the immunosuppression, namely bacterial infections, including meningitis, and *Toxoplasma* abscesses in virtually every area of the brain and even the spinal cord. As these infections were gradually brought under control, frequently by prophylactic therapy, there appeared to be an opportunity for later complications to occur. These included infiltration of the central and peripheral nervous systems by Kaposi's sarcoma and by primary CNS lymphoma. It was recognized relatively early that the peripheral nervous system could be involved in HIV-1-infection, including the Guillain-Barré syndrome (most frequently seen at the time of seroconversion) and chronic inflammatory demyelinating polyneuropathy (seen particularly in the early years of clinical AIDS). Polymyositis is a relatively common association in patients with well-established AIDS, and it has to be separated from the cachetic myopathy seen in the late stages of the disorder. The HIV-1–associated polymyositis responds well to the typical treatment for idiopathic polymyositis. We have seen myasthenia gravis associated with HIV-1 infection, but it is unclear whether this is anything other than a chance association.

The various medications used to treat HIV-1 opportunistic infections can also be neurotoxic. They can produce such problems as the mitochondrial myopathy associated with AZT (zidovudine) therapy, and the sensorimotor polyneuropathy associated with ddI and ddC.

A number of the opportunistic infections, in addition to toxoplasmosis, may give characteristic neurologic complications, such as cytomegalovirus (CMV), ascending polyradiculitis, and herpes zoster-varicella virus (HZV) radiculitis.

Finally, as survival from all of these opportunistic infections and tumors increases, we see what are probably the direct effects of HIV-1 on the nervous system (either directly or through macrophage infiltration and the release of cytotoxic agents, such as cytokines), including the AIDS-dementia complex, HIV-1 vacuolar myelopathy, and the progressive distal, painful sensory polyneuropathy.

When one considers the range of neurologic complictions of HIV-1, it is clear that this infection enters into the differential diagnosis of virtually every disorder of the CNS or the peripheral neuromuscular apparatus. The neurologist needs a high index of suspicion, for one is frequently led to the diagnosis by the presence of risk factors and by the nuances of the clinical picture, rather than by anything which is absolutely diagnostic about the presentation.

Neurologists and Issues Related to Death

Neurologists are inevitably at the forefront of examining issues related to death, because we deal with such matters as coma, brain damage and stroke, persistent vegetative state, brain tumors, and chronic progressive neurologic degenerations (e.g., amyotrophic lateral sclerosis and Alzheimer's disease). The referendum initiative passed in Oregon (1), and the 1994 publication of the book *Ethical Issues in Neurology* (2), by James Bernat, prompts me to think more deeply about our role in such matters.

Criteria are now well established for the declaration of brain death. In most states, it simply requires two physicians, one of whom is usually a neurologist or neurosurgeon, to certify that the patient is brain dead, according to these criteria. In some states, this declaration of brain death may be superseded, and in other states it must be supplemented by a study demonstrating lack of brain function, such as an isoelectric electroencephalogram or absence of cerebral blood flow. On the basis of such a demonstration or the declaration of brain death, most states allow withdrawal of "extraordinary medical treatment and life support," such as respiratory support by a ventilator; however, this has not always been the case. For instance, a number of years ago, in New York State, a group of legislators were able to pass a law containing a provision declaring that withdrawal of life support was illegal in all circumstances and, hence, would constitute murder. This law was eventually struck down as unconsititutional, but for approximately one year it imposed severe difficulties in the care of terminally ill patients in New York State.

The persistent vegetative state is a more difficult situation than brain death for physicians and the lay public to accept. A recent review of the neuropathology of the persistent vegetative state showed that all patients had bilateral lesions that could occur diffusely in the cerebral cortex, the subcortical white matter, or the basal ganglia (3). The essential clinical feature of the persistent vegetative state is the permanent loss of the ability of the brain to sustain the essential human functions of cognition and reactions to others.

However, it is often very difficult to define whether a patient has reached the permanent vegetative state, even for well-experienced neurologists. Patients retain many neurologic reflexes that can convince relatives, nurses, and even physicians that the patient retains intellectual function. These patients have sleep-wake cycles; their eyes may open to stimulation and may often follow people moving around the room; and patients may appear to respond to pain in a semipurposeful fashion. However, such individuals never initiate activity spontaneously, and they show no interactive or intelligent response.

Many, though not all, states accept that the persistent vegetative state is grounds for withdrawal of life support measures. In fact, in Vermont I was involved in a case where the persistent vegetative state was accepted as grounds for withdrawal of parenteral and tube feeding, because these were accepted as being extraordinary means of medical support of life and, hence, were synonymous with support of respiration with a ventilator.

With years of practice, we are all involved in the care of patients who die. I have been involved in the withdrawal of ventilatory support from patients who have amyotrophic lateral sclerosis, have decided that their quality of life is unacceptable, and wish to terminate the extraordinary medical measures used to sustain their lives. Such decisions require a great deal of discussion with—and counseling of—the patient, family, and caregivers. Nevertheless, such patients are fully competent, and with their families, are capable of making an informed decision.

On the last occasion that I turned off the ventilator, the family and the patient wanted to be together at this final event. We therefore collected everyone together for a last goodbye, the patient was sedated with morphine and diazepam, and the family took part in a religious ceremony as the ventilator was turned off. Let no one be deluded into believing that such events are free of stress. However, it is our responsibility to ease the burden for patients and families of that which is inevitable, namely death.

I have also helped many patients with amyotrophic lateral sclerosis and muscular dystrophy achieve a comfortable death when they have decided not to accept ventilatory support. I have also written about the care of patients at this stage of the disease (4). Treatment should be initiated as soon as there is significant respiratory discomfort at rest. Adequate doses of diazepam and nasal oxygen can take away the sympathetic activation and fear that result from hypoxia. The patient can be made comfortable before drifting into a coma and, hence, toward terminal respiratory arrest. That such treatment may hasten the time of death by a few hours or days is inconsequential and is justified by the relief of what otherwise is a very distressing death.

I have been asked by a number of patients and their loved ones how to terminate a life when the quality has become unacceptable. Suicide (i.e., self-killing) is frowned upon by most societies and religions, but it is illegal in few places. Individuals who are bent on committing suicide usually undertake this in private, although infrequently they may be "rescued" by well-meaning individuals who find them comatose but still alive.

To look at a slightly different situation, what can a totally disabled patient do when life becomes intolerable? This situation can occur in amyotrophic lateral sclerosis, severe quadriplegic multiple sclerosis, or high cervical cord trauma. If one accepts that such a patient should be accorded the same rights as a nondisabled patient making the same informed decision, then one can accept that society should allow a relative or physician to assist in the suicide of that patient, with appropriate safeguards, documentation, and restrictions. However, in virtually all jurisdictions, such an act by a layperson or a physician would likely lead to prosecution for a crime related to murder.

In Holland, physician-assisted suicide and voluntary active euthanasia became permissible in 1985 (2). In Holland, the experience has generally been regarded by the public and patients as favorable, although many physicians have found some difficulty with the procedures. Dutch physicians, like their counterparts in the United States, are trained to heal. Some find it difficult to use their skills for the opposite purpose, the termination of a life, even when it is done for all the right reasons, such as saving a patient from an intolerably painful death. There is much debate about physician-assisted suicide (1, 2). In the United States, the Hemlock Society is one of the main proponents of physician-assisted suicide and voluntary active euthanasia, which, despite their efforts, seem unlikely to become legal in more than one or two states for many years to come. Nevertheless, in view of the Oregon initiative, it is important that we all reconsider how we care for the dying patient.

I have always been against euthanasia of all types, for a reason that is personal and perhaps somewhat puritanical. I believe that if euthanasia were readily available to patients with fatal diseases such as cancer and the neurodegenerative disorders, medical scientists would put forth much less effort and the public would provide little support for research to find the cause and cure of these diseases. It would simply be a matter of concluding that a patient had cancer, defining it as being invariably fatal, and offering to the patient that when pain and the quality of life become unacceptable, we, the medical profession, will relieve the situation by "putting the patient to sleep."

As a general matter, I also do not personally favor physician-assisted suicide. I believe that we have at our disposal virtually all of the mechanisms and medications necessary to keep patients comfortable in their preterminal phase. *If these are fully and appropriately applied,* we can keep pain at bay and make the last short period of life acceptable, even in the terminal phases of cancer. Unfortunately, there is clear evidence that, in general, physicians do not provide adequate amounts of such medications to patients in the terminal stages. Often, the reason an inadequate amount of medication is administered stems from a fear that it will shorten life and, hence, result *de facto* in physician-assisted suicide. I believe that this fear is groundless for patients with terminal and distressing diseases. What we, as physicians, need is instruction in the appropriate treatment of the preterminal phase of life and education about the acceptance of death.

Despite this rather conservative view, there are certain situations in which I believe we should permit physician-assisted suicide. One example is the patient who has chronic intractable pain that cannot be controlled and which, therefore, makes life permanently intolerable to the patient. Another example is the patient who is in the terminal phase of a severe dementing process like Alzheimer's disease or has experienced severe and multiple strokes. Many such patients have a syndrome bordering on the persistent vegetative state, but rarely is this diagnosis made and its logical outcome applied.

In addition, there are many patients who do not fulfill the complete criteria for the persistent vegetative state but have no prospect of return of useful brain function. Most of these patients have severe ischemic, hemorrhagic, hypoxic, or traumatic brain damage, and they languish for prolonged periods without any significant return of brain function. Because clinical studies have defined that the prognosis for significant recovery in such patients as zero, it is reasonable to ask why life support ("extraordinary medical measures") should not be terminated. Society, which ultimately foots the bill, should have the right to require the imposition of *DO NOT RESUSCITATE* orders and even the termination of life support for such patients, given adequate safeguards. It is arguable that from society's point of view, such steps should be taken even in those situations in which the patient's family is unable to accept the inevitable bleak prognosis. The Oregon Initiative and its antecedents in Washington (Initiative 119) and California (Proposition 161) require all of us to take a more active role in the debate regarding out patients' diseases and their death.

References

1. Annas GJ: Death by prescription: The Oregon initiative. *New Engl J Med* 331:1240–1243, 1994.
2. Bernat JL: *Ethical Issues in Neurology,* Butterworth Heinemann, Boston, 1994.
3. Kinney HC, Samuels MA: Neuropathology of the persistent vegetative state. *J Neuropathol Exp Neurol* 53:548–558, 1994.
4. Bradley WG: Amyotrophic lateral sclerosis and Duchenne muscular dystrophy: The diseases and the doctor-patient relationship, in Charash LI, Lovelace RE, et al (eds): *Realities in Coping with Progressive Neuromuscular Diseases.* Charles Press Publishers, 1987, pp 3–20.

1 Cerebrovascular Disease

Safety and Efficacy of Delayed Intraarterial Urokinase Therapy With Mechanical Clot Disruption for Thromboembolic Stroke
Barnwell SL, Clark WM, Nguyen TT, O'Neill OR, Wynn ML, Coull BM (Dotter Interventional Inst, Portland, Ore; Oregon Health Sciences Univ, Portland; Portland VA Med Ctr, Ore)
AJNR 15:1817–1822, 1994   122-96-1-1

Objective.—Thirteen patients with acute ischemic stroke who failed to meet inclusion criteria for a systemic recombinant tissue plasminogen activation study were treated with intra-arterial urokinase. The safety and efficacy of intra-arterial delivery of the thrombolytic agent were examined. Previous studies have suggested that this method would carry a decreased risk of systemic hemorrhagic complications relative to IV administration.

Patients and Methods.—The 13 consecutive patients ranged in age from 12 to 81 years. Initial examination of all patients suggested large-vessel occlusion without CT evidence of hemorrhage. Patients were excluded from the systemic recombinant tissue plasminogen activation study because of time from onset of stroke (8 patients), recent surgery (2 patients), or seizure, age, or myocardial infarction (1 patient each). All received catheter-directed intra-arterial urokinase therapy (200,000–900,000 units) with mechanical disruption of the clots. The mean time between thromboembolic stroke and treatment was 12 hours.

Results.—All patients had major neurologic symptoms before treatment. Initial angiographic studies revealed 2 cases of basilar occlusion and 10 cases of occlusion in carotid territory. Repeat angiography 12–24 hours after intra-arterial urokinase showed complete recanalization of the symptomatic vessels in 7 patients, partial opening of the middle cerebral arteries or their branches in 3 patients, and no openings in 3 patients. There were 3 deaths, 1 resulting from an anterior wall cardiac rupture 3 hours after thrombolysis, another from cerebral edema 36 hours after treatment, and the third from pulmonary embolus 1 week after treatment. The patients' average baseline score on the National Institute of Neurologic Disorders and Stroke Scale was 22. At 48 hours, 9 of 13 patients had major neurologic improvement, with an average score of 12. Their average scale value at 3 months was 5, indicating continued improvement.

Conclusion.—Selective catheterization for intra-arterial delivery of urokinase produced a high rate of cerebral vessel recanalization in patients with acute ischemic stroke, especially in those with basilar thrombosis. Clinical benefits were achieved even after the standard 6-hour time window for thrombolytic treatment, with a relatively low rate of adverse side effects.

▶ One must be cautious in drawing any inferences from this optimistic report of 13 patients with acute ischemic stroke treated with intra-arterial urokinase. Remarkably, the time lapse for treatment ranged from 3.5 to 48 hours! This notwithstanding, 7 patients exhibited complete arteriographic recanalization, and in 2 of the 7, time lapses were 36 and 48 hours! The authors report asymptomatic hemorrhagic conversion in 3 patients (only 1 of whom exhibited complete recanalization, with a time lapse to therapy of 36 hours). The main lesson of this interesting, although highly selected and uncontrolled, series is to raise the possibility of a safe and effective outcome even with considerably delayed thrombolysis in certain individuals. No firm conclusions are possible in the absence of a controlled study.—M.D. Ginsberg, M.D.

▶ The authors used an endovascular protocol to treat a series of 13 patients with acute ischemic stroke; in 10 patients stroke occurred in a carotid artery territory and in 3, in the basilar artery territory. The common feature of this endovascular treatment, which resulted in successful arterial recanalization in 10 patients, was the intra-arterial infusion of urokinase, but it also included mechanical disruption of the clot in the larger and more proximal vessels. One would expect that such clot disruption would cause distal embolization, but this phenomenon either did not occur (perhaps as the result of the thrombolytic effect of the urokinase) or was not recognized. Although the authors did not establish scientifically that the angiographic improvement in their patients was the result of the treatment protocol rather than natural thrombolysis, the high incidence of this improvement argues for the former interpretation. Further testing of this approach is necessary to establish whether it can also improve the clinical recovery of patients who have acute ischemic stroke.—R.H. Wilkins, M.D.

Percutaneous Transluminal Angioplasty Adjunct to Thrombolysis for Acute Middle Cerebral Artery Rethrombosis
Tsai FY, Berberian B, Matovich V, Lavin M, Alfieri K (Univ of Missouri, Kansas City)
AJNR 15:1823–1829, 1994   122-96-1-2

Introduction.—The prognosis of middle cerebral artery occlusion or stenosis is not favorable. Although early recanalization can minimize severe complications, some patients experience immediate rethrombosis after complete thrombolysis. Urokinase and adjunctive percutaneous angioplasty were used in 4 patients.

Patients and Methods.—In 7 years, 31 patients with middle cerebral artery occlusion were treated at 1 institution within 6 hours of the onset of symptoms. The maximum dose of urokinase, with 1 exception, was 1.75 million IU. After an initial 250,000-IU bolus, 80,000 IU of urokinase was intermittently injected every 15 minutes. All patients received 3,000 units of heparin with a booster dose of 1,000 units every hour. The average patient age was 54 years. Of the 9 patients with middle cerebral artery stenosis, 3 had acute rethrombosis of the artery distal to the stenosis and required repeat thrombolysis followed by angioplasty. A fourth patient underwent percutaneous transluminal angioplasty immediately after thrombolysis and did not have rethrombosis.

Results.—The patients included a 46-year-old man, a 52-year-old man, a 60-year-old woman, and a 46-year-old woman. All 4 experienced symptoms of stenosis, were treated successfully, and showed signs of improvement. The condition of the first 3 patients deteriorated after initial improvement, necessitating additional urokinase and percutaneous transluminal angioplasty. Two of these patients subsequently recovered without hemorrhage. The third had a high degree of stenosis that prohibited passage of even the smallest Stealth catheter. This patient had persistent speech deficits and right hemiparesis 9 months later. In the fourth patient, percutaneous transluminal angioplasty was performed immediately after the thrombosis was dissolved with urokinase. Rethrombosis was considered very likely when emergency cerebral angiography showed complete thrombosis of the left middle cerebral artery. This patient experienced neither rethrombosis nor recurrent symptoms and recovered with only very minimal right-side sensory deficits.

Discussion.—The middle cerebral artery is the most frequent site of acute thrombosis from thromboembolism. Analysis of this patient group demonstrates that stenosis is also common. Percutaneous transluminal angioplasty may be necessary to prevent rethrombosis when severe stenosis is noted after urokinase therapy.

▶ This is a series of 4 case reports emphasizing the problem of rethrombosis after acute arterial thrombolytic therapy for middle cerebral artery thromboembolic occlusion. The report emphasizes the adjunctive benefit provided by percutaneous transluminal angioplasty in these patients, in whom a stenotic middle cerebral artery was the apparent cause of rethrombosis after initially successful thrombolysis. In the large, controlled, randomized studies currently in progress to assess the efficacy of thrombolytic therapy for acute ischemic stroke, it is conceivable that rethrombosis secondary to underlying stenosis may emerge as a common reason for lack of therapeutic success. If this is the case, it will become necessary to construct a controlled trial to evaluate adjunctive angioplasty in this setting. This procedure has intuitive appeal but, of course, needs to be fully validated.—M.D. Ginsberg, M.D.

Urgent Therapy for Acute Stroke: Effects of a Stroke Trial on Untreated Patients

Barsan WG, Brott TG, Broderick JP, Haley EC Jr, Levy DE, Marler JR (Univ of Michigan, Ann Arbor; Univ of Cincinnati, Ohio; Univ of Virginia, Charlottesville; et al)
Stroke 25:2132–2137, 1994   122-96-1-3

Background.—Interventions aimed at salvaging brain tissue after ischemic stroke must be initiated within a few hours of stroke onset to be effective. The procedures surrounding the process of salvaging heart tissue after acute myocardial infarction can be applied to emergency stroke evaluation and treatment, but there is little public awareness of the need for early hospital arrival after stroke. As part of the National Institutes of Health Tissue Plasminogen Activator (tPA) Pilot Study, a public awareness campaign was conducted to encourage early hospital arrival.

Methods.—Data were gathered on all patients seen at 3 participating centers within 24 hours of the onset of stroke for the period from February 1987 to August 1989. At the start of the study, an educational program was presented to physicians, paramedical personnel, and the public. The public was urged to call 911 if signs and symptoms of stroke occurred, just as they would for acute myocardial infarction. The study period was divided into quartiles to analyze the effect of the educational program on the use of 911 and time to hospital arrival.

Results.—Time data were available for 1,116 of 2,099 patients screened. Of the 1,116 evaluable patients, 39% arrived within 90 minutes, and 77% arrived within 6 hours of the onset of stroke. On average, patients using 911 arrived significantly more quickly than other patients. The mean time from onset of symptoms to hospital arrival decreased significantly during the course of the study, from 3.2 hours to 1.5 hours. Patients arrived for treatment more quickly at community hospitals than at large university/teaching hospitals and when stroke occurred between noon and midnight vs. between midnight and 6 AM. No patients were screened at community hospitals during the first quartile of the study; by the fourth quartile, 38% of the sample came from community hospitals. The use of 911 increased by 55% from the start of the study to its completion. Only 74 of 1,948 patients who met initial study eligibility received tPA.

Conclusion.—Early stroke intervention and treatment are essential to prevent neurologic deficits; however, few stroke trials have emphasized early treatment. Public and professional education and information programs can encourage the use of 911, enabling stroke patients to be admitted within the estimated therapeutic window of 3–4 hours.

▶ The great mass of available evidence suggests that the therapeutic window for the effective treatment of acute stroke is limited to the first 3–4 hours. This very encouraging report demonstrates that vigorous efforts undertaken to educate physicians, paramedical personnel, and the lay public as to the urgent nature of acute stroke can indeed bear great fruit. Particularly encouraging are the observations that community hospitals came to participate in acute stroke management more and more as time progressed. The data presented leave little doubt that the nihilistic view taken by some regarding the logistic ability to treat stroke within a time frame of 3 to 6 hours is unwarranted. As there currently are a great number of acute stroke trials in progress, the medical community will soon be called on to implement rapid stroke therapy in which the time to treatment may be a critical determinant of outcome.—M.D. Ginsberg, M.D.

Viability Thresholds and the Penumbra of Focal Ischemia
Hossmann K-A (Max-Planck Inst for Neurological Research, Cologne, Germany)
Ann Neurol 36:557–565, 1994   122-96-1–4

Background.—The concept of thresholds of tissue viability in states of focal ischemia entails two critical flow rates: one for electrical failure and one for membrane failure. These thresholds denote the upper and lower limits of flow for an ischemic "penumbra," which presumably involves functional but not structural injury. It has been assumed that the penumbral area can be reactivated at any time after vascular occlusion if blood flow becomes greater than the threshold of electrical activity. Nevertheless, most of the interventions that have been tried, including vasoactive drugs and reconstructive surgery, have not substantially improved the outcome of ischemic stroke.

Recent Findings.—Protein synthesis is suppressed at decreasing rates of flow, with a threshold at about .55 mL/g/min. Anaerobic glycolysis is stimulated at a flow rate of .35 mL/g/min. At a rate of about .2 mL/g/min, neurotransmitters are released and energy metabolism begins to be impaired. Anoxic depolarization takes place at flow rates of less than .15 mL/g/min. According to the classic definition, the penumbra does not remain viable for an extended period. However, the penumbra has now been redefined as an area of restricted blood supply within which energy metabolism is preserved. Histologic abnormalities take longer to become manifest than do biochemical and functional changes (Fig 1–1).

Imaging the Penumbra.—Regional blood flow and the energy state may be imaged under experimental conditions by a combination of autoradiography with ^{14}C-iodoantipyrine and adenosine triphosphate–induced bioluminescence (Fig 1–2). Excellent resolution is possible using this approach, but repeat studies are not feasible. Diffusion-weighted nuclear MRI combines high-resolution imaging with the possibility of obtaining repeated measurements.

Pathophysiology.—Expansion of tissue injury into the penumbral zone may reflect spreading depression-like depolarizations in the peri-infarct region. The number of depolarizations correlates closely with infarct vol-

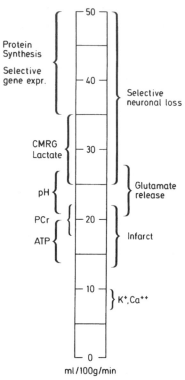

Fig 1–1.—Thresholds of ischemia for the induction of functional, metabolic, and histologic lesions. *Abbreviations: CMRG*, cerebral metabolic rate of glucose; *PCr,* phosphocreatine. (Courtesy of Hossmann K-A: *Ann Neurol* 36:557–565, 1994.)

ume. Spreading depolarizations also may account for the selective neuronal loss seen in the more peripheral zone of an ischemic infarct.

▶ This state-of-the-art review, together with its accompanying editorial (1), emphasizes the concept of the acute ischemic penumbra as a highly dynamic zone of constrained blood flow, in which repeated ischemic depolarizations and their consequent ionic dislocations impose a profound bioenergetic stress on the affected tissue, culminating in irreversible injury over several hours, unless these pathophysiologic events are thwarted. Consistent observations from experimental studies have compellingly established that the life span of the penumbra is limited and that rescue of this metastable zone constitutes the primary goal of metabolic-neuroprotectant therapy of acute stroke. A great variety of ongoing clinical trials during the next decade will surely provide us with a clinically effective neuroprotectant to combat deterioration of the acute ischemic penumbra.—M.D. Ginsberg, M.D.

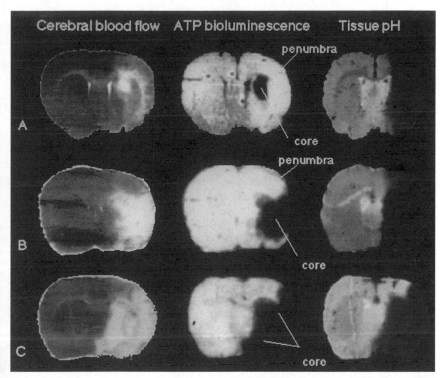

Fig 1–2.—Visualization of the core and penumbra of ischemic infarcts at 2 hours after middle cerebral artery occlusion in a rat. Imaging of regional blood flow is by ^{14}C-iodoantipyrine autoradiography, of adenosine triphosphate (ATP) content is by substrate-induced bioluminescence, and imaging of tissue pH is by umbelliferone. The penumbra is located in the parietal cortex and corresponds to the region of decreased blood flow in which ATP is preserved. Tissue acidosis includes both the core and the penumbra of the ischemic infarct. A–C, coronal brain sections from 3 experiments with different sizes of core and penumbra. (Courtesy of Hossmann K-A: Ann Neurol 36:557–565, 1994.)

Reference

1. Ginsberg MD, Pulsinelli WA: *Ann Neurol* 36:553, 1994.

Glucose Intolerance and 22-Year Stroke Incidence: The Honolulu Heart Program
Burchfiel CM, Curb JD, Rodriguez BL, Abbott RD, Chiu D, Yano K (Natl Heart, Lung, and Blood Inst, Honolulu, Hawaii; Univ of Hawaii at Manoa, Honolulu; Univ of Virginia, Charlottesville; et al)
Stroke 25:951–957, 1994   122-96-1–5

Objective.—Stroke is the third leading cause of death in the United States. Although individuals with diabetes have a higher risk of stroke than individuals without diabetes, little is known about the effect of glucose levels on the risk of stroke. The relationship of glucose intolerance and diabetes to the risk of thromboembolic and hemorrhagic stroke was studied retrospectively in 3,795 men of Japanese ancestry.

Methods.—The men, aged 45–68 years, who were free of coronary heart disease, were classified into 4 glucose tolerance categories on the basis of their 1-hour post-load glucose levels and history of diabetes. Glucose levels of 151 mg/dL or less were termed "low normal," those 151–224 mg/dL were "high normal," and those 225 mg/dL or greater in nontreated men were termed "asymptomatic high." Treated men or men with a history of diabetes and glucose levels of 225 mg/dL or greater were termed "known diabetes." The age-adjusted relative risks for stroke and stroke patterns were determined. Patients were followed for 22 years.

Results.—During the follow-up, there were 374 thromboembolic strokes, 128 hemorrhagic strokes, and 36 unclassified strokes. The age-adjusted relative risk for thromboembolic, but not hemorrhagic, stroke increased with glucose intolerance. After adjusting for other risk factors, the relative risks for the top 2 glucose intolerance groups remained significantly elevated. The relative risk for thromboembolic stroke in younger men, aged 45–54 years, was slightly higher than for older men, aged 55–68 years. There were no significant differences in relative risk for thromboembolic stroke between men who were hypertensive and nonhypertensive.

Conclusion.—Men with diabetes and increased glucose levels appear to be at higher risk of thromboembolic, but not hemorrhagic, stroke. There are no significant differences in relative risk of stroke between men who have hypertension and those without hypertension and between younger and older men.

▶ This careful study, based on the Honolulu Heart Program, followed an impressively large cohort of more than 7,500 Japanese-American men with varying levels of glucose intolerance, for more than 20 years. The subjects were categorized by their baseline plasma level of glucose, measured 1 hour after a 50-g glucose load in the nonfasting state. The salient finding was that the age-adjusted incidence rates of thromboembolic strokes increased with worsening category of glucose intolerance, with a twofold increase in asymptomatic patients with hyperglycemia and a nearly threefold increase in the known diabetes group, when compared with the low-normal category. Thus, this study further substantiates the relationship between glucose intolerance/diabetes and the development of thromboembolic stroke. It does not, however, clarify the mechanisms of this association. In particular, further studies will be needed to differentiate the relative contributory roles of chronic glucose intolerance vs. *acute* elevations of plasma glucose (known from numerous experimental studies to exacerbate ischemic infarction) in worsening ischemic stroke.—M.D. Ginsberg, M.D.

Risk Factors for Intracranial Hemorrhage in Outpatients Taking Warfarin

Hylek EM, Singer DE (Massachusetts Gen Hosp, Boston)
Ann Intern Med 120:897–902, 1994   122-96-1–6

Objective.—To use anticoagulant therapy rationally, particularly in elderly individuals, it is necessary to balance its antithrombotic efficacy with the risk of bleeding. A case-controlled study was planned at a large general hospital to estimate the risk of intracranial hemorrhage in adult outpatients given warfarin therapy.

Study Population.—A review of 1,881 patients admitted with intracranial hemorrhage in 1981–1991 revealed 121 who were taking warfarin at the time. Each of these patients was matched with 3 control outpatients who also received anticoagulant therapy. Seventy-seven of the study patients had intracerebral bleeding, and 44 had subdural hemorrhage. The respective mortality rates were 46% and 20%.

Observations.—The prothrombin time ratio (PTR) was the predominant risk factor for both types of hemorrhage. The risk increased markedly for PTR values above 2.0 (Fig 1–3). Age also was a risk factor, especially for subdural bleeding. The PTR also was the most prominent risk factor for both intracerebral and subdural bleeding on multiple logistic analysis. A history of cerebrovascular disease, the presence of a prosthetic heart valve, and age also were risk factors.

Conclusion.—These findings emphasize the need to closely control anticoagulant therapy at the lowest level that is effective, particularly in older patients. The PTR should be kept below 2.0.

▶ This case-control retrospective analysis of warfarin-related intracranial hemorrhage carries an extremely important message: the PTR in anticoagulated outpatients must be kept under 2.0 to minimize the risk of this potentially lethal complication. Strikingly, the risk of intracerebral hemorrhage doubled for each .5 increase in the PTR; for subdural hematoma, the risk increased for PTR values over 2.0. The conclusions of this study are conso-

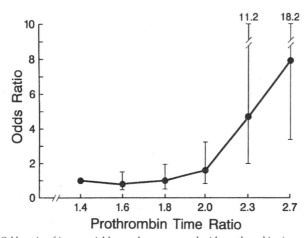

Fig 1–3.—Odds ratio of intracranial hemorrhage compared with prothrombin time ratio. The unadjusted odds ratio for intracranial hemorrhage is shown for different levels of the prothrombin time ratio. The prothrombin time ratios presented are the medians of the following intervals: 1.0–1.5, 1.6–1.7, 1.8–1.9, 2.0–2.1, 2.2–2.3, and 2.4–3.5. (Courtesy of Hylek EM, Singer DE: *Ann Intern Med* 120:897–902, 1994.)

nant with the intuition of experienced practitioners and scrupulously need to be taken to heart.—M.D. Ginsberg, M.D.

Internal Carotid Artery Dissection After Remote Surgery: Iatrogenic Complications of Anesthesia
Gould DB, Cunningham K (St Louis Regional Med Ctr, Mo; Meyer and Williams, Attorneys at Law, Jackson, Wyo)
Stroke 25:1276–1278, 1994   122-96-1-7

Objective.—The cases of 2 patients who were insufficiently anesthetized and had experienced internal carotid artery (ICA) dissection while struggling during surgery were reviewed.

Case 1.—During surgical removal of a thorn from his hand, a man, 44, who was unable to be intubated, began struggling and yelling as a result of receiving light anesthesia. His head was restrained by the anesthetist, and additional anesthesia was given. After surgery the patient woke complaining of pain on the left side of the neck, and he later experienced neurologic problems. Angiography showed that flow ceased at C-2. Despite heparin therapy, CT revealed acute infarction of the left temporal and parietal lobes. The patient requires constant custodial care.

Case 2.—Man, 33, with suspected Klinefelter syndrome, underwent uneventful lumbar laminectomy. The day after surgery he experienced right hemiparesis, and angiography confirmed left internal carotid artery dissection. Computed tomography showed ischemic infarction of the left middle cerebral artery. The patient has permanent aphasia and right hemiparesis.

Discussion.—Internal carotid artery dissection was apparently caused by hyperextension of the neck with axial rotation of the head and neck. Because the damage resulting from the ischemic cerebral infarction was irreversible, care should be taken when positioning the patient and when administering anesthesia by mask.

▶ Extracranial arterial dissection is an uncommon cause of stroke, frequently as a result of trauma or manipulation of the neck. Very few patients have evidence of predisposing disorders of the arterial wall. Dissection secondary to intravascular catheterization is well recognized. Unfortunately, this study also indicates that dissection can arise on an iatrogenic basis during administration of general anesthesia.—W.G. Bradley, D.M., F.R.C.P.

▶ Neurosurgeons are well aware that a general or local anesthetic removes the patient's normal defense mechanisms. This may set the stage for an unrecognized iatrogenic injury, such as a peripheral nerve injury caused by compression of the nerve by a restraining strap or a cervical spinal cord injury caused by excessive flexion of the head and neck in a patient with cervical spondylosis. Gould and Cunningham document that dissection of the internal carotid artery can also occur in the setting of general anesthesia, being caused by direct or positional injury to that vessel.

Patient positioning is an important part of the preparation for an operative procedure. Ideal positioning provides the best exposure of the pathologic lesion with the least impediment to the operating surgeon. It must also minimize the risks to the patient, including the risk of iatrogenic injury. For all of these reasons, it is important that the operating surgeon directly supervise the positioning of the patient in addition to performing the operation.— R.H. Wilkins, M.D.

Atherosclerotic Disease of the Aortic Arch and the Risk of Ischemic Stroke

Amarenco P, Cohen A, Tzourio C, Bertrand B, Hommel M, Besson G, Chauvel C, Touboul P-J, Bousser M-G (Université Pierre et Marie Curie, Paris; Recherches Epidémiologiques en Neurologie et Psychopathologie, Villejuif, France; Centre Hospitalier Universitaire de Grenoble, France)
N Engl J Med 331:1474–1479, 1994   122-96-1-8

Background.—Atherosclerotic disease of the aortic arch may be a source of cerebral emboli. The risk of ischemic stroke associated with atherosclerotic disease of the aortic arch was quantified.

Methods.—Two hundred fifty patients were enrolled in a prospective case-control study of the frequency and thickness of atherosclerotic plaques in the ascending aorta and proximal arch. All of these patients were hospitalized with ischemic stroke. Transesophageal echocardiography was performed in the patients and in an equal number of control subjects. All were older than 60 years of age.

Findings.—Fourteen percent of the patients and 2% of the controls had atherosclerotic plaques of 4 mm or more in thickness. The odds ratio for ischemic stroke among patients with such plaques was 9.1 after adjusting for atherosclerotic risk factors. Among the 78 patients with brain infarcts with no obvious cause, 28.2% had plaques of 4 mm or more in thickness. Among the 172 patients with infarcts of known, possible, or likely causes, this proportion was 8.1%. Plaques of 4 mm or more in the aortic arch were unrelated to the presence of atrial fibrillation or stenosis of the extracranial internal carotid artery, whereas plaques with thicknesses of 1 to 3.9 mm were often associated with carotid stenosis of 70% or more.

Conclusions.—There appears to be a strong, independent relationship between atherosclerotic disease of the aortic arch and the risk of ischemic stroke. This relationship was especially strong when plaques were thick. Thus, atherosclerotic disease of the aortic arch should be considered a risk factor for ischemic stroke and a possible source of cerebral emboli.

▶ This study is valuable in emphasizing that atherosclerotic disease of the aortic arch is associated with increased risk of stroke. Hypertension, hypercholesterolemia, smoking, and diabetes were all more common in the patient group than in controls, however. The odds ratio for cerebral infarction was highest for plaques greater than 4 mm in thickness. The chief questions raised by these tantalizing results are whether these lesions actually *cause* stroke and whether specifically targeted therapy would therefore be warranted. These issues must be further studied.—M.D. Ginsberg, M.D.

Subclavian Steal Phenomenon

Thomassen L, Aarli JA (Univ of Bergen, Norway; Haukeland Hosp, Bergen, Norway)
Acta Neurol Scand 90:241–244, 1994   122-96-1–9

Purpose.—In patients with subclavian steal syndrome, there is no clear relationship between the alterations in vertebrobasilar flow and the clinical symptoms. Surgery or angioplasty to restore normal blood flow does not always lead to symptom relief. The possible association between clinical symptoms and the type of vertebrobasilar steal phenomenon was assessed.

Methods.—The subjects were 58 patients with subclavian artery stenosis. Based on Doppler ultrasound investigation, the vertebral artery flow pattern was graded as no subclavian steal, grade 0; systolic deceleration, grade 1; alternating flow, grade 2; or reversed flow, grade 3. The patients' clinical symptoms were classified as definite or probable vertebral symptoms, carotid symptoms, or no symptoms.

Findings.—Forty-two patients were found to have a subclavian steal phenomenon in the vertebral artery: grade 1, 16 patients; grade 2, 17 patients; and grade 3, 9 patients. Twenty of these 42 patients had signs and symptoms attributable to vertebrobasilar ischemia. This relationship was significant for patients with grades 2 and 3 subclavian steal phenomena: 12 of the 26 patients in these grades had definite vertebrobasilar transient or permanent symptoms compared with just 6 of 32 patients in grades 0 and 1. However, the grade of steal phenomenon was not significantly related to the time course, type, or severity of the clinical symptoms.

Conclusions.—The hemodynamic aspects of subclavian steal phenomena are related to the clinical signs and symptoms. Although the flow disturbance is probably a causal factor in the occurrence of symptoms, it is not the only one. Even patients with reversed vertebral artery flow may be asymptomatic. In symptomatic patients, the subclavian steal phenomenon may represent an unstable hemodynamic system in which transient physiologic flow alterations in hypotension or hypocapnia may lead to transient ischemia as a result of impaired autoregulation.

▶ The initial descriptions of the subclavian steal syndrome required episodes of vertebrobasilar ischemia induced by arm exercise. This study approaches the condition from the opposite direction by reviewing a group of patients with subclavian artery stenosis in whom the pattern of blood flow in the ipsilateral vertebral artery was studied both at rest and with maneuvers to increase subclavian artery blood flow. Although there was some correlation between the extent of retrograde flow in the vertebral artery, it is perhaps striking that this correlation was relatively poor. This suggests that additional factors, such as arm position kinking the blood vessel, may be of equal importance.—W.G. Bradley, D.M., F.R.C.P.

Incidence of Transcranial Doppler-Detected Cerebral Microemboli in Patients Referred for Echocardiography

Tong DC, Bolger A, Albers GW (Stanford Univ, Calif)
Stroke 25:2138–2141, 1994   122-96-1–10

Background.—The ability of transcranial Doppler (TCD) ultrasonography to detect cerebral microemboli might be helpful in screening individuals considered to be at increased risk for embolic stroke. A group of such patients was evaluated with TCD to determine the prevalence of microemboli. An attempt was also made to determine whether the presence of emboli predicted a history of stroke.

Patients and Methods.—Eligible patients were referred for echocardiography from August 1993 to February 1994. Known or potential cardioembolic risk factors were atrial fibrillation (AF), prosthetic cardiac valves, and cardiac thrombus. Also eligible were patients with stroke who were referred to rule out a cardiac source of embolization. The 42 patients who were studied had an average age of 65.2 years; all were men. Fifteen had cardiac valve replacement (group A, considered high risk for cerebral embolism), 13 had AF (group B, moderate risk), and 14 had recent stroke or conditions such as patent foramen ovale and mitral valve prolapse (group C, low risk). Each patient underwent TCD embolus monitoring for a total of 30 minutes.

Results.—Microemboli were detected in 17% of patients and were most common in group A (33%). No patients in group C and 15% of patients in group B had microemboli. Thus, group A and groups A and B (25%) both had significantly more emboli than group C. The number of microemboli varied from 1 to 17 during the 30-minute monitoring period. A patient with AF had the lowest rate, and a patient with a mechanical valve replacement had the highest rate. Patients with a previous stroke had a higher embolization rate than patients without a history of stroke. Among patients with a prosthetic heart valve, those with emboli more commonly had a history of stroke than did those without emboli. No relationship between the acuity of stroke and the presence of microembolism was evident.

Conclusion.—A significant number of these patients referred for echocardiography were found at TCD to have microemboli. Those considered at high risk for cerebral embolism had a greater prevalence of microembolism than those judged to be at low risk. Based on findings in this small series of patients, TCD appears to be a promising method for evaluating embolic stroke.

▶ In this series of patients referred for echocardiography, TCD studies performed for 30 minutes confirmed cerebral microembolization in a substantial proportion of patients, particularly in those with prosthetic cardiac valves. It is interesting that 5 of 7 emboli-positive patients in this series were receiving therapeutic anticoagulation with warfarin, although none were receiving aspirin. It is intriguing that the acuity of stroke in this series was not related to the presence of microemboli, and that emboli-positive and -negative subgroups had similar prevalences of stroke and transient ischemic attack. This study supports the growing impression that microemboli are disturbingly prevalent in patients at risk for stroke, even though that risk may not be high-grade. The pathophysiologic significance of recurrent "asymptomatic" microembolization remains to be elucidated.—M.D. Ginsberg M.D.

Cerebral Microembolism in Symptomatic and Asymptomatic High-Grade Internal Carotid Artery Stenosis

Siebler M, Kleinschmidt A, Sitzer M, Steinmetz H, Freund H-J (Heinrich-Heine-Univ, Düsseldorf, Germany)
Neurology 44:615–618, 1994   122-96-1–11

Background.—Risk of cerebral infarction is increased even for patients with asymptomatic internal carotid artery (ICA) stenosis, which may make some of them candidates for endarterectomy. Long-term transcranial Doppler (TCD) studies of ICA blood flow can demonstrate clinically silent, high-pitched intensity signals suggestive of cerebral formed-element embolism. In a previous study, high rates of such cerebral microemboli were found in patients with symptomatic, high-grade ICA stenosis. The incidence of these microemboli decreases sharply after carotid endarterectomy. Thus, silent microembolism may be a useful measure of the risk of stroke in patients with ICA stenosis.

Methods.—Two groups of patients with ICA stenosis of 70% or greater were studied to determine the relation between silent microembolism of the ipsilateral middle cerebral artery (MCA), as detected by TCD, and a history of ischemic symptoms attributable to the diseased ICA. Thirty-three patients who had had ischemic symptoms within the previous 4 months were defined as symptomatic. Another 56 patients with the same degree of ICA stenosis but no symptoms were also studied. All patients underwent TCD monitoring for at least 1 hour to determine the rate of microembolism of the MCA ipsilateral to the high-grade ICA stenosis.

Results.—Twenty-seven of the symptomatic patients had silent microembolic events at an overall mean rate of 14 per hour. Of the asymptomatic patients, only 9 had silent microemboli at an overall mean rate of 0.35 per hr. None of 20 healthy controls demonstrated microemboli (table). In the patients, a microembolic event rate of 2 or more per hour had a positive predictive value of 0.88 for a history of recent symptoms.

Conclusions.—Transcranial Doppler monitoring can not only differentiate asymptomatic from symptomatic patients with severe ICA stenosis, it may also provide reliable paraclinical evidence of "unstable ICA disease." Larger, prospective follow-up studies are needed to determine how TCD monitoring may be used to refine the therapeutic indications.

▶ This report describes a dramatic difference in the rate of silent microembolism in patients with symptomatic vs. asymptomatic ICA stenosis. The

Age Distribution, Percent Degree of Internal Carotid Artery Stenosis, Transcranial Doppler Monitoring Time of the Ipsilateral Middle Cerebral Artery, and Total Number and Mean Rate of Microemboli of the Latter Vessel in 89 Patients and 20 Controls

	Symptomatic	Asymptomatic	Control
No. of subjects	33	56	20
ICA stenosis (%)			
Range	70–95	70–95	0
(Mean/SD)	(84/7)	(80/8)	(0/0)
Monitoring time (h)			
Sum	82.5	115.5	29
(Mean/SD)	(2.5/1.2)	(2.0/0.5)	(1.3/0.2)
Emboli (no.)			
Sum	893	57	0
(Mean rate/SD)	(14/29)	(0.35/1.4)	(0/0)
Age (years)			
Range	49–78	53–83	24–88
(Mean/SD)	(61/7)	(64/7)	(58/12)

The proportions of microemboli-positive individuals differed significantly between groups ($P < 0.001$), as did the mean rates of microembolism of symptomatic patients vs. asymptomatic patients ($P < 0.008$).
Abbreviations: ICA, internal carotid artery; *SD*, standard deviation.
(Courtesy of Siebler M, Kleinschmidt A, Sitzer M, et al: *Neurology* 44:615–618, 1994.)

effects of this microembolism on brain and vascular structure and function are unknown at this time, but recent experimental studies suggest that such emboli may well lead to endothelial, blood-brain barrier and even parenchymal dysfunction in the absence of frank infarction. Such emboli may also produce microinfarction. These findings need to be taken very seriously and should be the subject of extensive investigation in the future.—M.D. Ginsberg, M.D.

Development of Aspirin Resistance in Persons With Previous Ischemic Stroke

Helgason CM, Bolin KM, Hoff JA, Winkler SR, Mangat A, Tortorice KL, Brace LD (Univ of Illinois, Chicago)
Stroke 25:2331–2336, 1994   122-96-1–12

Purpose.—Aspirin (ASA) is widely used for the prevention of recurrent ischemic stroke. However, unlike other antithrombotic agents, the levels or biological effects of ASA are not routinely measured to ensure adequate dosage or efficacy. Patients require different ASA dosages to achieve complete inhibition of platelet aggregation, the platelet component of thrombosis. Patients taking aspirin for the prevention of recurrent ischemic stroke were studied at repeated intervals to determine the ex vivo effect of ASA on platelet aggregation.

Methods.—Initial platelet aggregation studies were performed in 306 patients who were taking ASA for the prevention of recurrent stroke. Approximately 2 weeks after ASA treatment was started, usually at a dose of 325 mg/day, platelet aggregation was reevaluated; if found to be less than complete, ASA dosage was increased by 325 mg/day. This procedure was repeated until complete inhibition was achieved or a maximum dosage of 1,300 mg/day was reached. Patients continued taking their effective ASA dosage for 6 months and were then tested again.

Results.—At the initial test, 228 patients had complete inhibition of platelet aggregation, and 78 had partial inhibition. Testing was repeated at least once in 119 of those who had complete inhibition and in 52 of those who had partial inhibition. Thirty-three percent of the patients who initially had complete inhibition had lost part of the antiplatelet effect of ASA—they converted from complete to partial inhibition even though their ASA dosage was unchanged. Thirty-five of 52 patients who initially had partial inhibition achieved complete inhibition through either ASA dosage escalation or fluctuation of response at the same dosage. However, when tested again, 8 of these 35 had reverted to partial inhibition. Eight percent of patients ultimately proved resistant to 1,300 mg/day of ASA, including 15% of those with partial inhibition and 5% of those with complete inhibition at their initial test.

Conclusions.—A fixed dose of ASA does not have a constant antiplatelet effect over time in all patients. Therefore, the antithrombotic effect of ASA is presumably inconstant as well. Further study is needed to identify the mechanisms of increased dosage requirement or of ASA resistance, as well as the clinical significance of these phenomena. The therapeutic effects of ASA are more likely to be optimized by adjusting the dosage according to biological effect than by giving a fixed dosage.

▶ This carefully conducted study is unique in charting, over time, the biological efficacy of aspirin in inhibiting patients' platelet aggregation as measured by in vitro tests. Intriguingly, reversion from "complete" to "partial" aspirin effect, or a fluctuating biological effect, was seen in a substantial proportion of patients followed over time. This study thus raises the possibility that an incomplete biological effect of aspirin may underlie aspirin failures in stroke prevention. One hopes that future aspirin studies will be constructed in which an objective biological measure of the aspirin effect, rather than merely the administered dose, will be the guiding principle.— M.D. Ginsberg, M.D.

2 Neurorehabilitation

Where and How Should Elderly Stroke Patients Be Treated?
Kaste M, Palomäki H, Sarna S (Univ of Helsinki, Finland)
Stroke 26:249–253, 1995   122-96-2–1

Background.—Treatment for stroke is highly inconsistent, and elderly patients are at particular risk of receiving suboptimal care. At many hospitals, older stroke patients are generally admitted to medical wards and younger patients to neurologic wards. The effects of receiving care in the medicine department vs. the neurology department were assessed in elderly stroke patients.

Methods.—The controlled trial included 243 consecutive patients, aged 65 years or older, who were admitted to a university hospital with a diagnosis of acute stroke. The patients were randomized to receive care in either the department of medicine or the department of neurology. The department of neurology followed an organized approach to stroke management, including organized diagnosis, acute treatment, and early systematic rehabilitation carried out by special stroke teams. At 1-year follow-up, the 2 groups were compared for mortality, length of hospital stay, ability to live at home after discharge, Barthel Index, and Rankin grades.

Results.—The 2 groups were similar in terms of sex, age, severity or type of stroke, other diseases, and social factors. Both groups had a 1-year mortality of 21%. Those treated in the department of neurology were discharged in an average of 24 days compared with 40 days for those treated in the department of medicine. The difference in length of stay was significant for patients younger than 75 years of age. Seventy-five percent of patients assigned to the department of neurology were able to go directly home after discharge compared with 62% of those assigned to the department of medicine. Functional status, as evaluated by the Barthel Index and Rankin grades, was also significantly better for patients treated in neurologic wards. Treatment in the department of neurology was a significant and independent predictor of a better functional outcome and a shorter hospital stay.

Conclusions.—Organized management in the department of neurology can improve outcomes for elderly stroke patients. A systematic approach to stroke management can shorten hospital stay, reduce the number of patients requiring institutional care, and increase independence in daily life. These improvements have obvious benefits in both human and economic terms. The value of stroke units continues to be underestimated.

▶ The results of this study are of great importance in defining the roles of neurologists and specialized stroke units in the care of patients with stroke. Hospitals and HMOs often provide care for patients with stroke while acting on the principle that the damage has already been done, and that there is little else to be offered other than custodial care and allowing time to heal what it may. Rehabilitation of stroke patients is sometimes seen as being both costly and unlikely to be effective. Neurologists are sometimes at fault in failing to counteract this view when they give their attention to the seemingly more exciting field of acute stroke therapy with its thrombolytics, anti-N-methyl-D-asparate receptor drugs, and similar experimental therapies.

The importance of this study is that it is a randomized trial of neurologic rehabilitation vs. standard medical care in a medicine ward. There was a statistically significant improvement in outcome for the patients treated by the department of neurology compared with those treated by the department of medicine. When somewhat similar data were produced from non-randomized studies in the past, it was suggested that the poor outcome of the medical patients resulted from their having been preselected as having more general medical disorders like diabetes, hypertension, chronic renal failure, and so on. Such an objection cannot be raised against this study, because the patients were identical in the two groups. Hence, the conclusion is clearly demonstrated that neurologic rehabilitation works, both from the patient's point of view and with regard to economic costs.—W.G. Bradley, D.M., F.R.C.P.

The Influence of Stroke Unit Rehabilitation on Functional Recovery From Stroke

Kalra L (King's College School of Medicine, London)
Stroke 25:821–825, 1994   122-96-2-2

Background.—It has been suggested that stroke units may expedite hospital discharge. Shorter hospital stays in these units may be the result of quicker functional recovery or better organization and coordination between caregivers and patients. The rate of functional recovery and therapy input in patients treated in a stroke rehabilitation unit were compared with those of similar patients treated in general wards.

Patients and Methods.—A total of 141 patients with an intermediate prognosis at 2 weeks after stroke were studied. Of these, 73 were randomly assigned to management in a stroke rehabilitation unit, whereas the remaining 68 were managed in general hospital wards. Barthel scores were recorded weekly until hospital discharge. The duration and type of physiotherapy and occupational therapy given to patients in each setting were also documented. The rate of change in Barthel scores, therapy input, and duration of hospitalization were compared between patients in each group.

Results.—Neurologic deficits and median initial Barthel scores were similar between patients in each setting. Patients managed in the stroke rehabilitation unit had a significantly higher median discharge Barthel score compared with those managed in the general ward: 15 vs. 12. In stroke unit patients, median Barthel scores increased rapidly after 2 weeks, reaching a plateau at 6 weeks (Fig 2–1). Patients in general wards had a significantly slower change in median Barthel score, with a plateau seen at 12 weeks. Hospital discharge was also significantly delayed for patients in general wards compared with those in the stroke unit, at 20 weeks vs. 6 weeks, respectively. When the median Barthel scores of patients remaining in the stroke unit and general wards were plotted against time, differences in the speed of functional recovery were also observed, with slower changes noted for patients in the general ward (Fig 2–2). On average, patients in the general wards received significantly more physiotherapy during hospitalization than did those in the stroke unit. The average amount of occupational therapy received did not differ between groups. A trend toward a higher proportion of time in occupational therapy spent on specific needs of individual patients in the stroke unit was noted, although this did not reach statistical significance (table).

Conclusions.—In spite of comparable therapy input, functional recovery is significantly higher and quicker in stroke rehabilitation units compared with general wards. Additional studies may further define how stroke units affect rehabilitation and subsequently facilitate the development of better strategies for stroke management.

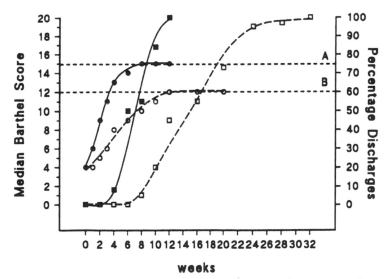

weeks

Fig 2–1.—Line graph showing the weekly median Barthel scores and discharge rates of stroke survivors in the stroke unit ($n = 73$) and general wards ($n = 69$). The *filled circles* indicate the median Barthel score (stroke unit); *filled squares*, percent discharges (stroke unit); *open circles*, median Barthel score (general wards); *open squares*, percent discharges (general wards); A, median discharge Barthel scorce of the stroke unit group; B, median discharge Barthel scorce of the general wards group. (Courtesy of Kalra L: *Stroke* 25:821–825, 1994.)

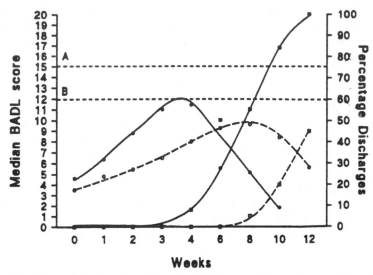

Fig 2–2.—Line graph showing the weekly median Barthel scores of the remaining stroke inpatients in the stroke unit and general wards vs. the rate of discharge. *BADL* indicates Barthel activities of daily living; *open circles,* Barthel score (general wards); *open squares,* discharge rates (general wards); *filled circles,* Barthel score (stroke unit); *filled squares,* discharge rate (stroke unit); *A,* represents the median discharge Barthel score of the stroke unit group; *B,* median discharge Barthel score of the general wards group. (Courtesy of Kalra L: *Stroke* 25:821–825, 1994.)

▶ A major and still controversial question about specialized stroke rehabilitation units is whether they are worth the trouble. This English study reports that they are. Patients who were clinically comparable recovered faster and further in the stroke rehabilitation unit than on the general wards. The

Therapy Input and Type	SU (n=73)	GW (n=68)	P
Therapy Input in Stroke Patients Managed in the Stroke Unit or General Wards			
Physiotherapy			
Mean duration per patient, h*	16.6±4.7	21.5±7.9	<.05
Percent time spent on			
Sitting balance	14.2	14.3	NS
Standing balance	21.1	21.3	NS
Transfers	17.5	19.3	NS
Ambulation	20.0	20.8	NS
Individual rehabilitation†	27.1	24.3	NS
Occupational therapy			
Mean duration per patient, h*	10.2±3.1	10.4±3.2	NS
Percent time spent on			
Personal ADL	57.6	61.8	NS
Kitchen activities	11.1	11.7	NS
Home visits	14.0	14.2	NS
Postdischarge follow-up	4.8	3.4	NS
Individual rehabilitation†	12.5	8.9	NS

* Time spent in face-to-face activities with the patients, excluding administrative time.
† Time spent on activities aimed at addressing the specific needs of individual patients (e.g., specific transfer/washing/dressing techniques, use of aids) identified by the therapist or the patient as to significantly contributing to discharge to the chosen environment.
Abbreviations: SU, stroke unit; *GW,* general wards; *ADL,* activities of daily living.
(Courtesy of Kalra L: *Stroke* 25:821–825, 1994.)

numbers were adequate to allow conclusions ($n = 73$ on the stroke unit and $n = 68$ on the wards), and the differences were statistically significant ($P < 0.01$). These results and others cited by the author indicate that specialized stroke rehabilitation units can have an important role, at least in the British health care system.—J.P. Blass, M.D., Ph.D.

The Influence of Age on Stroke Outcome: The Copenhagen Stroke Study
Nakayama H, Jφrgensen HS, Raaschou HO, Olsen TS (Bispebjerg Hosp, Copenhagen)
Stroke 25:808–813, 1994   122-96-2–3

Background.—Advanced age is frequently considered an impediment to rehabilitation. However, in patients with stroke, the influence of age on patient outcome remains controversial. In a prospective, community-based study, it was determined whether and how age affects stroke outcome.

Patients and Methods.—A total of 515 consecutive patients with acute stroke (mean age, 74.8 ± 11.1 years) were studied. Of these, 79% underwent CT to determine the type and size of the stroke lesion. During the hospital stay, activities of daily living (ADL) and neurologic status were evaluated on a weekly basis using the Barthel Index (BI) and the Scandinavian Stroke Scale (SSS), respectively. Data pertaining to social condition and comorbidity before stroke were also obtained. The independent influence of age on stroke outcome was analyzed using a multiple regression model.

Results.—Elderly patients with stroke were more apt to be widowed or single women. Although age was not related to the type of stroke lesion or infarct size, it did independently influence initial BI, initial SSS, and discharge BI, with a 10-year increase in age resulting in a 4-point, a 2-point, and a 3-point decrease, respectively. Age did not independently influence mortality within 3 months, discharge SSS, length of hospital stay, and discharge placement (table). However, improvement in ADL was influenced independently by age, with a 3-point decrease per 10 year increase in age noted. Age did not affect neurologic improvement and speed of recovery.

Conclusions.—A poorer compensatory ability in elderly patients with stroke is indicated by age independently affecting outcome in ADL-related

---

Mortality Within 3 Months After a Stroke			
Age Group, y	No. of Patients	Dead Within 3 mo	Mortality Within 3 mo, %
≤54	27	2	7.4
55-64	40	4	11.1
65-74	96	23	24.0
75-84	184	53	28.8
≥85	71	28	39.4

(Courtesy of Nakayama H, Jørgensen HS, Raaschou HO, et al: *Stroke* 25:808–813, 1994.)

aspects but not in neurologic aspects. As such, rehabilitation of elderly patients with stroke should be targeted more toward ADL and compensation rather than the recovery of neurological status. Moreover, age itself should not be considered a selection criterion for rehabilitation.

▶ Careful studies of a variety of diseases has shown that age—even advanced age—need not preclude gratifying outcomes of therapy in a high proportion of patients. This Danish study indicates that age itself is not a useful criterion for giving or withholding active stroke rehabilitation. However, because elderly patients are more often widows or widowers and tend to be more impaired in ADLs than do younger patients, stroke rehabilitation may need to focus on recovery of ADLs in the elderly even more so than in younger patients.—J.P. Blass, M.D., Ph.D.

Serum Albumin Level as a Predictor of Geriatric Stroke Rehabilitation Outcome
Aptaker RL, Roth EJ, Reichhardt G, Duerden ME, Levy CE (Kaiser-Permanente Med Ctr, San Francisco, Calif; Northwestern Univ, Chicago; Rocky Mountain Multiple Sclerosis Ctr, Englewood, Colo)
Arch Phys Med Rehabil 75:80–84, 1994   122-96-2–4

Objective.—The serum level of albumin in a critically ill patient is predictive of hospital outcome in a variety of acute care settings, including intensive care. Whether the admission serum level of albumin is useful for predicting complications and outcome in geriatric patients with stroke admitted to a rehabilitation unit was investigated.

Patients.—The patient sample included 46 women and 33 men, aged 65–95 years, who underwent comprehensive inpatient rehabilitation after a first-time, unilateral, thromboembolic stroke. Serum levels of albumin were obtained at admission to the rehabilitation unit. All medical complications that occurred during rehabilitation were recorded. Modified Barthel Index (MBI) Scores were obtained on admission and at the time of discharge to assess changes in functional status. The mean length of stay was 20.7 days in the acute care unit and 33.8 days in the rehabilitation unit.

Results.—Forty-two (53%) of the 79 patients had a total of 69 medical complications; the other 37 (47%) had no medical complications during rehabilitation. The mean admission serum level of albumin for all patients was 3.3 g/dL. Of the 79 patients, 37 had serum albumin levels of 3.5 g/dL or higher, 28 had levels of 3.0–3.4 g/dL, and 14 had levels of 2.9 g/dL or less. Admission serum albumin levels were positively correlated with discharge and improvement MBI Scores for self-care, mobility, and total MBI Scores. Regression analysis of admission serum albumin levels and patient age showed no statistical correlation. The mean age in patients with and without complications was nearly identical.

Conclusions.—Decreased serum albumin levels on admission to rehabilitation units are associated with risk of subsequent medical complications and functional outcome. Protein supplementation in patients with hypoalbuminemia who are undergoing rehabilitation may prevent medical complications and improve functional outcomes.

▶ Low serum levels of albumin have repeatedly been reported to correlate with poorer outcomes in medical and, specifically, in geriatric populations. This report indicates that the same effect can be seen in patients undergoing stroke rehabilitation. A low serum albumin level is, in part, a marker for "poor nutritional state," and it may be a marker for intensity of disease or of "frailty," rather than having primarily a direct mechanistic effect on recovery. However, this study suggests that attention to this commonly available clinical laboratory test may help to direct the physician's attention at admission to patients at high risk for a complicated clinical course during stroke rehabilitation.—J.P. Blass, M.D., Ph.D.

Stroke Rehabilitation Outcome: A Potential Use of Predictive Variables to Establish Levels of Care
Alexander MP (Braintree Hosp, Mass)
Stroke 25:128–134, 1994   122-96-2–5

Background.—Initial stroke severity and patient age are the strongest predictors of functional recovery and eventual home discharge among stroke survivors. A large population was studied to define potentially more efficient patterns of providing rehabilitation.

Methods.—Five hundred twenty consecutive cases were reviewed retrospectively. All patients had been admitted to a rehabilitation center within 1 calendar year with cerebral infarction or hemorrhage.

Findings.—Although overall recovery was most closely associated with severity of stroke on admission and patient age, the relationship between recovery and independent measures were complex. All patients younger than 55 years were discharged home regardless of what their initial disease severity was. Ninety-six percent of patients admitted with modest functional disability were discharged home, whatever their age. In the remainder, admission severity and age interacted to form two groups with very different prospects for home discharge. The groups eventually going home had very different rates of functional improvement directly related to length of hospitalization (Fig 2–3).

Conclusions.—Standard clinical measures available at admission to a rehabilitation hospital have enough predictive power to define management strategies for survivors of stroke. A management algorithm proposed in this study may increase the efficiency of stroke rehabilitation programs and enable comparisons of efficacy among different treatment settings.

▶ This large (*n* = 520), retrospective American study agrees with previous work indicating that the two most powerful predictors of outcome in patients undergoing stroke rehabilitation in a specialized setting are severity of

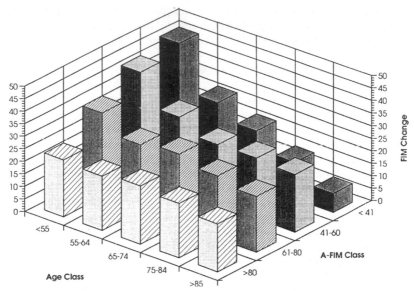

Fig 2–3.—Graph showing the overall relations between admission (*A*) functional independence measure (*FIM*), age, and improvement (*FIM change*). (Courtesy of Alexander MP: *Stroke* 25:128–134, 1994.)

initial stroke and age. However, even among patients aged 75–84 years, more than 75% were discharged home (precisely, 115 of 159). Even among patients aged 84 years or older, more than two thirds went home (33 of 49). The authors point out that social situation (including lack of a living spouse to aid in home care) was one of the reasons for proportionally fewer discharges to home among elderly patients. These data confirm other studies in indicating that age by itself is not a contraindication to intensive stroke rehabilitation.—J.P. Blass, M.D., Ph.D.

Sensory Stimulation Promotes Normalization of Postural Control After Stroke

Magnusson M, Johansson K, Johansson BB (Univ Hosp of Lund, Sweden)
Stroke 25:1176–1180, 1994   122-96-2–6

Background.—A stroke in 1 hemisphere of the brain can cause postural impairment. Two years after a severe stroke, patients who had received standard therapy were compared with those who had received additional sensory and electric stimulation to determine whether improvements in postural control could be maintained during this period.

Methods.—Patients with severe hemiparesis were randomized within 10 days of onset of stroke to either a control group (*n* = 40) that received daily physiotherapy and occupational therapy or a treatment (*n* = 38) group that also received sensory and electric stimulation delivered through acupuncture needles. These treatments continued twice daily for 10 weeks. At 2-year follow-up, 22 patients from the treatment group and 26 patients from the control group were still alive. One patient from the control group did not wish to be included in the study, and 1 patient from the treatment group had an inner ear disturbance and was excluded from the study. The subjects were perturbed by vibrators applied to calf muscles to cause vertical motion or galvanic vestibular stimulation to cause lateral motion. Postural control was assessed by sway variance or sway velocity, and the dynamics of postural control were assessed as a feedback system using a model previously validated for human postural control.

Results.—Significantly more patients in the treatment group than the control group could perform all tests (table). Among the patients who could perform all postural assessment tests, there was no difference between the treatment group, control group, and age-matched healthy subjects in sway velocity, vibration-induced anteroposterior sway, or galvanic-induced sway. However, the control patients were significantly different from the normal and treatment groups in measurements of both stiffness and swiftness.

Conclusions.—Among patients who survived 2 years after severe hemispheric stroke, the treatment group, which had undergone additional sensory and electric stimulation, had better postural control than the control group, which had undergone standard therapy only. The treatment group had postural control values similar to those of healthy age-matched controls, suggesting that they had regained near-normal dynamic postural control. Further studies are required to validate these methods before recommendations can be made on the addition of sensory stimulation to the therapy of stroke patients.

▶ This controlled study from Sweden has the interesting implication that appropriate sensory stimulation after stroke dramatically improves posture. The authors previously reported that sensory stimulation after stroke improves activities of daily living (ADL). Mechanistically, these observations raise the possibility that the remaining (intact) nervous system after a stroke is malleable enough to significantly reorganize functions (presumably synaptic connections) during recovery from the acute event. Therapeutically, they raise the gratifying possibility of active, neurophysiologically based interventions to improve function after stroke. However, as the au-

Status and Ability to Stand Among Survivors of Stroke for 2 Years or More		
	Treatment Group (n=21)	Control Group (n=25)
Age, y (mean ± SD)	74.2 ± 9.9	74.8 ± 9.0
Can perform tests	17	9*
Cannot complete tests	2	3
Cannot stand unaided	2	13

* Two subjects whose recordings were lost because of computer failure are included.
(Courtesy of Magnusson M, Johansson K, Johansson BB: *Stroke* 25:1176–1180, 1994.)

thors emphasize, "further studies are needed before recommendations are made to include...sensory stimulation...in the treatment of stroke patients."—J.P. Blass, M.D., Ph.D.

The Effects of Functional Electrical Stimulation on Shoulder Subluxation, Arm Function Recovery, and Shoulder Pain in Hemiplegic Stroke Patients

Faghri PD, Rodgers MM, Glaser RM, Bors JG, Ho C, Akuthota P (Miami Valley Hosp, Dayton, Ohio; Wright State Univ, Dayton, Ohio; Veteran Affairs Med Ctr, Dayton, Ohio)
Arch Phys Med Rehabil 75:73–79, 1994   122-96-2–7

Background.—Patients with hemiplegia commonly have shoulder subluxation and pain. Traditionally, shoulder subluxation has been treated with some type of sling, which has several disadvantages. The efficacy of a functional electrical stimulation (FES) treatment program designed to prevent glenohumeral joint stretching and subsequent subluxation and shoulder pain in patients with stroke was investigated.

Methods and Findings.—Twenty-six patients recently having hemiplegic stroke and with shoulder muscle flaccidity were randomly assigned to a control group or experimental group. All patients received conventional physical therapy. In addition, the experimental group had FES treatment. Two flaccid/paralyzed shoulder muscles were induced to contract repetitively up to 6 hours per day for 6 weeks. As performance improved, the duration of both the FES session and muscle contraction/relaxation ratio were increased progressively. Compared with the control group, the experimental group had significant improvements in arm function, electromyographic activity of the posterior deltoid, range of motion, and decreased subluxation.

Conclusions.—Functional electrical stimulation treatment appears to effectively reduce the severity of shoulder subluxation and pain, possibly facilitating recovery of arm function. However, pain and subluxation were not completely alleviated in the experimental group. Further research is needed to study the use of longer periods of FES and the FES of additional muscles for improving arm function and accelerating the recovery process.

▶ This pilot study suggests that a relatively simple technique—functional stimulation of muscles of the paretic upper arm—appeared to benefit function of the shoulder joint in the paretic limb in patients undergoing otherwise standard rehabilitation for stroke. The results were statistically significant, although the numbers of patients in the treated (13) and control (13) groups were small. A major fault is the lack of a true blind: Those in the control group did not receive "sham" stimulation. Nevertheless, if confirmed in future studies, this straightforward technique using commercially available equipment could prove to be a valuable adjunct in rehabilitation of appropriate populations of stroke patients.—J.P. Blass, M.D., Ph.D.

Effective Treatment of Poststroke Depression With the Selective Serotonin Reuptake Inhibitor Citalopram
Andersen G, Vestergaard K, Lauritzen L (Aalborg Hosp, Denmark; Frederiksborg General Hosp, Hillerφd, Denmark)
Stroke 25:1099–1104, 1994   122-96-2–8

Introduction.—The incidence of post-stroke depression (PSD) in the first year has been reported to be between 20% and 50%. Initial attempts at medical treatment included the use of tricyclic antidepressants, but the adverse effects of these drugs were too great. Serotonin uptake inhibitors are nonsedative and lack cardiotoxic, anticholinergic, or antihistaminergic effects. The effects of the serotonin reuptake inhibitor citalopram on patients with PSD in the first year after a stroke were determined.

Methods.—The study was a double-blind, placebo-controlled trial of 6 weeks. Of 320 consecutive patients with stroke, depression was diagnosed in 66 based on the outcomes of several tests of mental function. Tests were repeated after 1, 3, and 6 weeks of treatment. Patients were randomly assigned to placebo or treatment groups. Citalopram, 20 mg/day, was given at bedtime in patients younger than 66 years of age, and 10 mg/day was given to older patients. The dosage was doubled in nonresponders.

Results.—The only side effects of treatment were mild and transient. A total of 66 patients participated. There was significant improvement in depression scales at weeks 3 and 6 in the citalopram-treated patients. Half the patients who began the treatment less than 7 weeks after a stroke recovered within 1 month. Recovery was infrequent if treatment began more than 7 weeks after the stroke (table).

Conclusion.—The large number of patients with stroke who improved within a month show that there is a high degree of spontaneous recovery in the early post-stroke phase. The selective serotonin reuptake inhibitor citalopram is a promising new agent in the treatment of PSD that is safe and effective.

▶ This paper indicates that the selective serotonin reuptake inhibitor citalopram, which is relatively free of side effects, can be added to the list of

Intention-to-Treat Analysis of Hamilton Depression Scale Score in Patients With Post-Stroke Depression Treated With Citalopram Starting < 7 or ≥ 7 Weeks After Stroke				
	<7 Weeks (n=28)		≥7 Weeks (n=38)	
Weeks of Treatment	Citalopram (n=15)	Placebo (n=13)	Citalopram (n=18)	Placebo (n=20)
0	20.1 ± 3.2	18.9 ± 3.4	18.9 ± 3.1	18.9 ± 2.5
1	16.7 ± 3.6	14.8 ± 3.8	15.3 ± 2.7	16.4 ± 2.3
3	12.5 ± 4.6	13.0 ± 3.7	12.4 ± 4.0*	16.3 ± 3.2
6	12.7 ± 6.1	11.5 ± 5.0	10.3 ± 3.9*	15.8 ± 3.8
Decrease from week 0 to week 6	7.3 ± 7.4	7.4 ± 4.6	8.6 ± 4.8*	3.1 ± 3.8

Note: Values are mean ± SD, Hamilton Depression Scale score.
* $P < 0.005$, Mann-Whitney U test.
(Courtesy of Andersen G, Vestergaard K, Lauritzen L: *Stroke* 25:1099–1104, 1994.)

medications that are effective treatments for PSD. Other medications include tricyclic antidepressants such as nortriptyline, which has a less attractive side effect profile (1), and trazedone (2). The dexamethasone suppression test has been proposed as a useful biological indicator of response to antidepressant treatment in post-stroke patients, many of whom are aphasic (3). Although about half of all patients with PSD appear to recover spontaneously from their depressive disorder, judicious use of antidepressants can ease their suffering and improve their motivation for rehabilitation.—J.P. Blass, M.D., Ph.D.

References

1. Lipsey JR, Robinson RG, Pearlson GD, et al: Nortriptyline treatment of post-stroke depression: A double-blind study. *Lancet* 1:297–300, 1984.
2. Reding MJ, Orto LA, Winter SW, et al: Antidepressant therapy after stroke. *Arch Neurol* 43:763–765, 1986.
3. Reding MJ, Orto LA, Willensky P, et al: The dexamethasone suppression test: An indicator of depression in stroke but not a predictor of rehabilitation outcome. *Arch Neurol* 42:209–212, 1985.

The Quantitative Measurement of Spasticity: Effect of Cutaneous Electrical Stimulation

Seib TP, Price R, Reyes MR, Lehmann JF (Univ of Washington, Seattle)
Arch Phys Med Rehabil 75:746–750, 1994   122-96-2–9

Background.—Nearly 6 million people each year are affected by spasticity, a debilitating outcome of upper motor neuron lesions. The recently developed Spasticity Measurement System has provided the means to accurately quantify variations in muscle spasticity and thereby more accurately evaluate therapy. The effects of cutaneous electric stimulation on spasticity were evaluated.

Methods.—Five spinal cord–injured and 5 traumatically brain-injured volunteers, all with clinically evident spasticity, received surface electric stimulation over the tibialis anterior muscle. Stiffness around the ankle was measured using the Spasticity Measurement System before, immediately after, and 24 hours after stimulation.

Results.—Immediately after stimulation, 9 of 10 participants had a significant reduction in ipsilateral median path length from 74 mm/rad prestimulation to 50 mm/rad post stimulation. Significant decreases in spasticity were maintained in the ipsilateral path length in 8 of 9 participants at 24 hours post stimulation. Spasticity in the contralateral ankle did not significantly change immediately or 24 hours post stimulation. No significant decrements in spasticity occurred in the same participants under sham conditions. Five of 9 participants reported a perceived decrease in spasticity bilaterally. All of those reporting perceived changes were spinal cord–injured participants.

Conclusions.—Cutaneous electric stimulation applied over the tibialis anterior will decrease gastrocnemius muscle spasticity for 6 or more hours in both head-injured and spinal cord–injured patients. The changes are most notable in the spinal cord–injured patients.

▶ This study documents that small differences in spasticity can be measured in patients with spinal cord injury. It also provides evidence that cutaneous electrical stimulation over the tibialis anterior muscle can reduce spasticity for as much as 24 hours in the stimulated limb. It is important that sham procedures were included in the test protocol and were not effective. The objective findings correlated with subjective patient impressions. This study suggests that a relatively simple procedure may benefit these chronically disabled patients. With appropriate instrumentation, this procedure might be adapted to the home setting—J.P. Blass, M.D., Ph.D.

Cerebral Aetiology of Urinary Urge Incontinence in Elderly People
Griffiths DJ, McCracken PN, Harrison GM, Gormley EA, Moore K, Hooper R, McEwan AJB, Triscott J (Edmonton General Hosp, Alta, Canada)
Age Ageing 23:246–250, 1994   122-96-2–10

Background.—Urge incontinence is the type most often observed in elderly individuals who are institutionalized. Typically, bladder sensation is reduced. The condition is characterized as an uninhibited overactive bladder. It seems possible that cerebral dysfunction in brain regions involved in controlling bladder function is involved.

Study Design.—Seventy-three elderly incontinent patients (mean age, 79 years) were studied, along with 27 continent individuals with a mean age of 78 years. The groups were comparable in cognitive status.

Methods.—Fluid intake was monitored over 24 hours along with urine and bladder volumes. Video-urodynamic studies were done with the subjects supine and sitting. Patients were asked to cough during bladder filling as a stress test. In addition, single-photon emission CT (SPECT) scanning of the brain was done using technetium-labeled hexamethylpropyleneamine oxime to assess regional cerebral perfusion, and cognition was evaluated using the Mini-Mental State Examination (MMSE).

Findings.—Twenty patients were shown to have urge incontinence despite normal bladder sensation. Fourteen others exhibited urge incontinence and reduced sensation of bladder filling. The latter patients had significantly lower MMSE scores than the other groups (table). Impaired perfusion of the right superior frontal lobe was much more frequent in patients with true urge incontinence and reduced bladder sensation than in any other group. The same patients commonly exhibited deficient perfusion of the left side of the cortex. Regional perfusion abnormalities were less marked in patients with urge incontinence who had normal bladder sensation.

Conclusion.—Urge incontinence associated with deficient bladder sensation in elderly persons may result from cortical neuropathy, particularly involving the frontal lobes.

Mini-Mental State Examination (MMSE) Scores for the 4 Patient Groups

	MMSE score
Reference groups:	
Continent	24 (19–26)
Other incontinence	24 (20–28)
Study groups:	
Genuine urge incontinence	
+normal sensation	24 (18–26)
+reduced sensation	17* (15–22)

Note: Values are median and 25th and 75th percentiles. Overall, the differences among the 4 groups are significant ($P = 0.02$ by analysis of variance).
* Significantly different from the continent group ($P = 0.03$), from the nonurge incontinent group ($P = 0.003$), and from the group with urge incontinence and normal sensation ($P = 0.04$), by Mann-Whitney U test.
(Courtesy of Griffiths DJ, McCracken PN, Harrison GM, et al: *Age Ageing* 23:246–250, 1994.)

▶ This paper applies a modern technique of clinical neuroscience—namely, imaging of cerebral blood flow in humans—to the common problem of urge incontinence in elderly individuals. Genuine urge incontinence with reduced sensation of bladder filling was associated with underperfusion of the right superior frontal lobe. This observation is in accord with current thinking about CNS control of voluntary voiding. Although this finding does not now lead to any obvious therapeutic interventions for this common problem, it does help to explain the association of urge incontinence with diseases causing cognitive impairment, specifically in older men. A possible difference in the frequency of urge incontinence between elderly men with Alzheimer's disease and elderly women with the same illness requires further documentation and, if real, mechanistic explanation.—J.P. Blass, M.D., Ph.D.

Physiotherapy for Young People With Movement Disorders: Factors Influencing Commencement and Duration
Ekenberg L, Erikson A (College of Health and Caring Sciences, Boden, Sweden; County Hosp, Boden)
Dev Med Child Neurol 36:253–262, 1994   122-96-2–11

Introduction.—The most common intervention for children with movement disorders is physiotherapy. Recently, however, the efficacy of this therapy has been questioned. Whether factors such as family composition, age, gender, diagnosis, mobility, communication, age at diagnosis, parent participation and belief in the efficacy of therapy have influenced the duration of physiotherapy was investigated.

Patients.—The patient group consisted of 2 previously studied groups of children with motor disorders. One group included all children with motor disorders born between 1975 and 1981 in Norrbotten, Sweden and the other group consisted of all children with motor disorders born between 1969 and 1974 in this area. The total number of children included in the

TABLE 1.—Distribution of Diagnosis and Age Group With Continuing or Discontinued Physiotherapy

Diagnosis	9–14 years (n=31) Physiotherapy		15–20 years (n = 49) Physiotherapy	
	Continuing	Discontinued	Continuing	Discontinued
Cerebral palsy	14	7	12	14
Developmental disorder	3	2	2	5
Spina bifida	2	0	2	1
Muscular dystrophy	0	0	3	0
Neuropathy	0	0	1	3
Malformation	0	0	0	4
Other	1	2	1	1
Total	20 (65%)	11 (35%)	21 (43%)	28 (57%)

(Courtesy of Ekenberg L, Erikson A: *Dev Med Child Neurol* 36:253–262, 1994.)

follow-up questionnaire was 105, with the majority being given a diagnosis of cerebral palsy. The children's age ranged from 9 to 20 years; 63% were boys.

Results.—Of the 105 questionnaires, 81 were returned. One was eliminated because of a failure to state whether physiotherapy was continuing. More younger children than older children were continuing therapy (Table 1). More boys than girls were continuing therapy. The mean mobility scores were lower among those continuing therapy (Table 2). Participation of both parents was associated with a higher rate of therapy continuation. The majority of parents who responded believed that physiotherapy was

TABLE 2.—Mean Mobility Scores for Children With Continuing or Discontinued Physiotherapy With Regard to Gender and Age Group

	Physiotherapy		p
	Continuing Mean (SD)	Discontinued Mean (SD)	
Whole sample	n = 41 3·1 (1·3)	n = 39 4·2 (1·4)	<0·01
9- to 14-year group	n = 20 3·0 (1·1)	n = 11 4·5 (1·6)	<0·01
15- to 20-year group	n = 21 3·2 (1·4)	n = 28 4·0 (1·4)	NS
Boys	n = 27 3·2 (1·3)	n = 24 4·2 (1·3)	<0·01
Girls	n = 14 3·0 (1·1)	n = 15 4·1 (1·6)	NS
Boys 9- to 14-year group	n = 11 2·8 (1·2)	n = 5 4·6 (1·5)	<0·05
Girls 9- to 14-year group	n = 9 3·2 (1·1)	n = 6 4·5 (1·8)	NS
Males 15- to 20-year group	n = 16 3·4 (1·4)	n = 19 4·1 (1·3)	NS
Females 15- to 20-year group	n = 5 2·6 (1·1)	n = 9 3·9 (1·6)	NS

(Courtesy of Ekenberg L, Erikson A; *Dev Med Child Neurol* 36:253–262, 1994.)

effective. All 5 sets of parents of children with spina bifida believed that physiotherapy had had a positive effect on their children. However, parental belief in physiotherapy did not appear to effect therapy continuation or discontinuation.

Conclusions.—Children with lower mobility scores and with the participation of both parents in physiotherapy were more likely to continue with therapy. As the demands for parent participation are increasing and the benefits of physiotherapy are being questioned, research on the efficacy and duration of such therapy is increasingly important.

▶ This careful Swedish questionnaire study indicates that, on the whole, parents of children with cerebral palsy believed that physiotherapy helped their children. Not surprisingly, the more parent participation was involved and the more immobilized the child became, the longer the duration of therapy. The authors conclude "It is questionable whether physiotherapy should continue for as long as it has in many of the cases in this study [for more than 10 years]. Research about criteria for continuation of physiotherapy for children with movement disorders is of increasing importance..." In addition to the intrinsic interest of this study, it documents the continuing reevaluation of established procedures which can be part of a prepaid system of health care.—J.P. Blass, M.D., Ph.D.

3 Movement Disorders

Longitudinal Fluorodopa Positron Emission Tomographic Studies of the Evolution of Idiopathic Parkinsonism
Vingerhoets FJG, Snow BJ, Lee CS, Schulzer M, Mak E, Calne DB (Univ of British Columbia, Vancouver, Canada)
Ann Neurol 36:759–764, 1994   122-96-3–1

Purpose.—The rate of progression of the nigral lesion underlying idiopathic parkinsonism has been determined primarily from pathologic studies. However, little information is available regarding the longitudinal development of these lesions. In vivo measurements from positron emission tomography (PET) with [^{18}F]fluorodopa (FD) of nigrostriatal function have been shown to correlate linearly with nigral cell count. To assess the rate of nigrostriatal lesion progression and to determine the reliability of the measurement of change, FD PET and quantitative evaluations were performed over 7 years on patients with idiopathic parkinsonism.

Subjects.—The FD PET was performed twice on 16 patients given a diagnosis of idiopathic parkinsonism, at a mean interval of 7.4 ± 0.6 years. Patients were evaluated clinically and assigned a modified Columbia Score (MCS). Scans and examinations also were performed on 10 normal subjects to serve as controls. Eight patients underwent 3 scans and were also assessed at 3.8 ± 0.72 years after the first scan; 6 of the control subjects were also assessed at 3.89 ± 0.52 years. The annual rate of lesion progression and the reliability of change were calculated.

Results.—A significant decrease in the (striatum–background)/ background ratio was observed in 15 of 16 patients with idiopathic parkinsonism, from 0.49 ± 0.08 to 0.43 ± 0.08; a nonsignificant decrease was observed in control subjects. These figures represented a decrease of 1.7% per year in the PET index in patients as compared with .31% for control subjects (Fig 3–1), marking a statistically significant difference between the 2 groups. Treatment with deprenyl did not result in a significant difference in the slope of progression as compared with results in those who did not receive the drug. Based on clinical examination, progression of disease was noted in all patients, requiring increases in antiparkinsonism drug treatment. The MCSs correlated significantly with FD PET ratios for patients with parkinsonism. A reliability of 98% for patients and 96% for controls was calculated for the measurements of change.

Conclusions.—Nigrostriatal function decreases more rapidly in patients with idiopathic parkinsonism than does that seen with the progression of

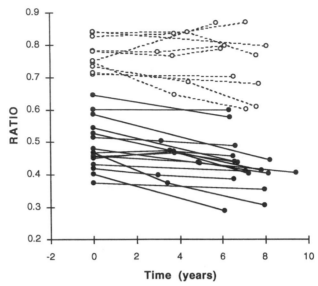

Fig 3-1.—Striatal FD accumulation in patients with idiopathic parkinsonism (*filled circle*) and normal individuals (*open circle*). The results are expressed as the ratio (striatum − background)/background. Time 0 is at the first scan. (Courtesy of Vingerhoets FJG, Snow BJ, Lee CS, et al: *Ann Neurol* 36:759–764, 1994.)

normal aging in control subjects. These results are consistent with findings from pathologic studies. However, in contrast to pathologic studies that showed a rate of nigrostriatal neuron loss of 6–10 times the rate of normal aging, a rate 2.5 times that of normal aging was found in these patients with idiopathic parkinsonism. This discrepancy in the magnitude of neuron loss may result from a selection bias inherent to pathologic studies, in which patients with a more rapidly progressing disease are chosen for postmortem study. The FD PET is a reliable method for measuring change of neuron concentration, with a reliability-of-change coefficient calculated at 98% and 96% for patients and controls, respectively.

▶ Striatal FD activity reflects the transport of levodopa into the brain, its decarboxylation, and its entrapment (as [^{18}F]fluoro-dopamine) in nigrostriatal dopaminergic terminals. Although striatal FD activity in the striatum is used as an index of dopamine neuron functional integrity, one wonders whether the chronic administration of increasing doses of levodopa/carbidopa results in compensatory changes in the nigrostriatal system that confound the interpretation of the rate of decline of striatal FD activity. It is known that dopamine receptors and dopamine transporters are regulated in response to dopaminergic therapies. For obvious ethical reasons, a completely untreated cohort of patients with Parkinson's disease has never been, and may never be, studied longitudinally and compared with age-matched controls. Ligands that bind to the monoamine vesicular transporter may, in the future, be used for assessing dopamine terminal integrity, because they tend not to be influenced by dopaminergic agents. Despite these caveats, longitudinal FD

PET scanning may be useful in assessing "neuroprotective" pharmacotherapies.—J.R. Sanchez-Ramos, M.D., Ph.D.

The Sydney Multicentre Study of Parkinson's Disease: A Randomised, Prospective Five Year Study Comparing Low Dose Bromocriptine With Low Dose Levodopa-Carbidopa
Hely MA, Morris JGL, Reid WGJ, O'Sullivan DJ, Williamson PM, Rail D, Broe GA, Margrie S (Westmead Hosp, Sydney, Australia; Univ of Sydney, Australia; St Vincent's Hosp, Sydney, Australia; et al)
J Neurol Neurosurg Psychiatry 57:903–910, 1994   122-96-3-2

Objective.—Although bromocriptine has been used extensively in Parkinson's disease, its role in treatment has not been fully defined. A 5-year follow-up was reported for a randomized study comparing low-dose levodopa-carbidopa with low-dose bromocriptine in the treatment of newly diagnosed Parkinson's disease.

Patients and Methods.—The initial study group consisted of 149 patients, aged 37–79 years, who were recruited between 1984 and 1987. Twenty-six had to be excluded from follow-up analysis, leaving 126 patients who completed the titration phase and have not shown atypical features of Parkinson's disease. Sixty-four were randomized to receive levodopa-carbidopa ($\leq$ 600/150 mg/day) and 62 to bromocriptine ($\leq$ 30 mg/day). During the titration phase, the dose of each drug was gradually increased until a satisfactory response was reported. A neurologist assessed the patients for clinical signs and Columbia score (Fig 3–2). Additional data recorded were activities of daily living, severity of disease, severity of dyskinesia, and fluctuations.

Results.—The 2 treatment groups were comparable at study entry in age, duration of disease, and disability scores. The bromocriptine group, however, contained more patients with both dementia and gait disorder. No patient could continue receiving bromocriptine only for the full 5 years, and few were able to be managed solely with the drug for 2 years. The median time for use of bromocriptine as monotherapy was 12.1 months; in contrast, the median time of use of levodopa-carbidopa therapy alone was 52.3 months. There was a lower prevalence of dyskinesia in the bromocriptine group, and this drug alone was not associated with end-of-dose failure. Use of low-dose levodopa-carbidopa sufficiently controlled symptoms in most patients and reduced both dyskinesia and end-of-dose failure, particularly in the first 3 years, compared with conventional doses of the drug. Figure 3–3 indicates the time to dyskinesia according to randomization group.

Conclusions.—Although low-dose bromocriptine monotherapy did not cause dyskinesia and only rarely led to mild end-of-dose failure, the drug was not very effective. Levodopa-carbidopa was helpful in controlling symptoms of Parkinson's disease, and the low dosage delayed the appearance of dyskinesia and end-of-dose failure. The prevalence of levodopa-

Group	Time(y)					
	0·5	1	2	3	4	5
B	−2·41**	−0·42	+3·47**	+5·20	+4·0	—
	(0·67)	(0·80)	(1·04)	(3·22)	(−)	
LD	−3·69***	−3·96***	−3·19***	−1·67	+0·10	+2·31
	(0·72)	(0·74)	(0·87)	(1·06)	(1·28)	(1·80)
B → B + LD	—	−5·75	−5·36	−3·81	−1·44	−1·94
		(3·08)	(2·60)	(1·80)	(2·27)	(1·92)
B → LD	—	−5·44*	−2·64	+0·27	+5·86*	+9·73*
		(1·86)	(2·51)	(1·66)	(2·41)	(3·18)

*p < 0·05; **p < 0·01;
***p < 0·001.
Values are means (SEM).

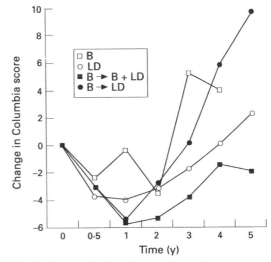

Fig 3–2.—Mean change in modified Columbia score for the patient groups over 5 years, expressed as the score for each patient compared with his or her score at baseline (patients taking anticholinergic drugs excluded). *Asterisk* indicates P < 0.05; **P < 0.01; ***P < 0.001. Values are means (SEM). *Abbreviations:* B, bromocriptine alone; B → B + LD, bromocriptine to bromocriptine and levodopa-carbidopa combined; LD, levodopa-carbidopa alone; B → LD, bromocriptine to levodopa-carbidopa. (Courtesy of Hely MA, Morris JGL, Reid WGJ, et al: *J Neurol Neurosurg Psychiatry* 57:903–910, 1994.)

induced dyskinesia was reduced when patients had started on bromocriptine and then had levodopa-carbidopa added to their treatment regimen. Bromocriptine is most effective for mild Parkinson's disease at an early stage and should not be given to patients with dementia. Those receiving the drug on a long-term basis need to be monitored for retroperitoneal fibrosis.

▶ This study confirms what most neurologists know: bromocriptine monotherapy is less efficacious than levodopa monotherapy. Moreover, the study supports the concept that levodopa-sparing agents (or the use of low doses of levodopa) decrease the incidence of drug-induced dyskinesia. The important lesson to be learned from this study is that combination therapies with low doses of levodopa and dopamine agonists, albeit more difficult to manage than monotherapy, serve the patient better in the long run.—J.R. Sanchez-Ramos, M.D., Ph.D.

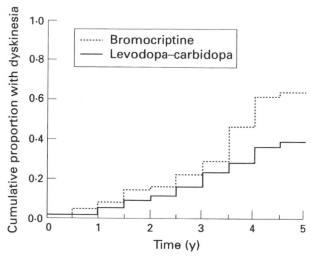

Fig 3–3.—Kaplan-Meier plot showing the time to dyskinesia according to randomized treatment groups. The 5 patients who did not receive levodopa-carbidopa are excluded. (Courtesy of Hely MA, Morris JGL, Reid WGJ, et al: *J Neurol Neurosurg Psychiatry* 57:903–910, 1994.)

Increased Risk of Parkinson's Disease in Parents and Siblings of Patients

Payami H, Larsen K, Bernard S, Nutt J (Oregon Health Sciences Univ, Portland, Ore)
Ann Neurol 36:659–661, 1994   122-96-3-3

Introduction.—The etiologic role of genes in Parkinson's disease (PD) was first proposed in 1949 but has yet to be documented. Although an autosomal dominant inheritance pattern exists in some families, studies of risk to relatives have been inconclusive. The familial aggregation of PD was examined in a large group of patients and controls, using analytical methods that were lacking in previous studies.

Patients and Methods.—Patients were recruited by mail or telephone from those receiving a medical diagnosis of idiopathic PD at a single clinic between 1991 and 1993. The patients were asked to invite their spouse or a friend of similar age to serve as controls. Family histories were obtained by questionnaire, and data on affected relatives were confirmed by phone interviews and available medical records. Information on symptoms suggestive of PD was obtained for the parents and full siblings of patients and controls. Not included in the analysis were asymptomatic individuals and those with tremor only.

Results.—The study group consisted of 586 first-degree parents and siblings of 114 white patients with PD and 522 first-degree relatives of 114 age-matched white controls. Patients were significantly more likely than controls to have a family history of PD (16% vs. 4%). The age-specific cumulative incidence of PD was significantly higher in first-degree relatives of patients than in the first-degree relatives of controls. The mean age at onset did not differ significantly for the parents and siblings of patients vs. controls.

Conclusion.—With an age-adjusted odds ratio of 3.5, the risk of PD was found to increase more than threefold for parents and siblings of patients. Therefore, genes do appear to play a role in the etiology of the disease, although the mode of inheritance and other questions remain unanswered. Isolated tremor, which was not included in the overall analysis, was also more common in parents and siblings of patients (4.4%) than among parents and siblings of controls (1%).

▶ The strongest evidence for a genetic etiology for PD is the autosomal inheritance pattern in rare families. The search for genetically determined factors is hampered because most PD appears sporadically with absolutely no family history, and because, if there are affected family members, the pattern of inheritance does not fit mendelian genetics. This paper provides epidemiologic evidence for familial aggregation of PD, and it should stimulate the search for markers that may eventually lead to identification of the PD gene(s).—J.R. Sanchez-Ramos, M.D., Ph.D.

Clozapine: A 2-Year Open Trial in Parkinson's Disease Patients With Psychosis
Factor SA, Brown D, Molho ES, Podskalny GD (Albany Med College, NY)
Neurology 44:544–546, 1994   122-96-3–4

Background.—Advanced Parkinson's disease (PD) is characterized by psychosis, including paranoid delusions, hallucinations, and confusion. These complications are usually attributable to antiparkinsonian medications and, often, an underlying dementia. Clozapine is an atypical antipsychotic medication that is effective in the treatment of psychotic symptoms in PD. Its long-term safety and efficacy were investigated.

Methods.—Seventeen patients with PD complicated by psychosis were treated for 6 to 24 months in an open-label, prospective trial. The patients were assessed every 3 months.

Findings.—Mean Psychiatric Rating Scale scores were significantly improved over 1 year compared with baseline. In the second year, the mean score was nonsignificantly improved. Doses of levodopa were maintained at levels 17% to 68% higher than baseline. The mean motor examination score improved by 11% to 22% in the first 15 months. The clozapine dosage used ranged from 6.25 mg every other day to 150 mg/day. Adverse effects, such as sedation and confusion, were common (Figs 3–4 and 3–5).

Conclusions.—Clozapine can be effective in treating psychosis in patients with PD over 1–2 years. The reduction in efficacy seen in the second year in this series was probably associated with an increase in the daily dose of levodopa, progression of dementia, and the inability of the patients to tolerate higher doses of clozapine.

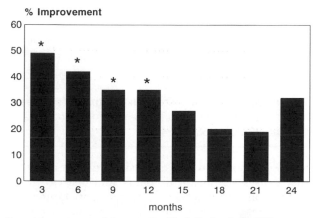

Fig 3–4.—Percent improvement of the mean Psychiatric Rating Scale (PRS) score at each 3-month interval compared with baseline. Significant improvement occurred over the first 12 months, but the decrease in response occurred in the second year. *Asterisk* indicates significant improvement over the baseline score ($P < 0.01$). (Courtesy of Factor SA, Brown D, Molho ES, et al: *Neurology* 44:544–546, 1994.)

▶ Clozapine, developed as an antipsychotic drug with minimal extrapyramidal side effects, has been proven useful in the treatment of 3 difficult problems associated with advancing PD. The benefits of treating medication-induced psychosis in PD with clozapine were to be expected, based on its atypical neuroleptic pharmacologic profile. Its usefulness in alleviating resting tremor came as a small surprise, and even more astonishing was its capacity to control levodopa-induced dyskinesias, albeit at much higher doses than those used for controlling tremor (1). Of course, the benefits must be weighed against the costliness of close monitoring of potential blood dyscrasias.—J.R. Sanchez-Ramos, M.D., Ph.D.

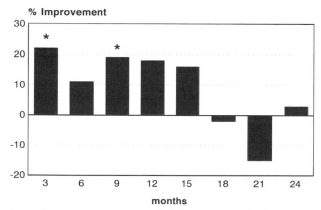

Fig 3–5.—Percent improvement (or worsening) of the motor examination score at each 3-month interval compared with baseline. An improvement of 11% to 22% occurred in the first 15 months, followed by a decrease in motor function in the last 9 months. The *asterisk* indicates significant improvement over baseline ($P < 0.03$). (Courtesy of Factor SA, Brown D, Molho ES, et al: *Neurology* 44:544–546, 1994.)

Reference

1. Bennett JP Jr, Landow ER, Dietrich S, et al: Suppression of dsykinesias in advanced Parkinson's Disease: Moderate daily clozapine does provide long-term dyskinesia reduction. *Mov Disord* 9:409–414, 1994.

Clozapine in the Treatment of Tremor in Parkinson's Disease

Jansen ENH (Hosp Medisch Spectrum Twente, Enschede, The Netherlands)
Acta Neurol Scand 89:262–265, 1994   122-96-3–5

Background.—Tremor at rest is a classic symptom of Parkinson's disease (PD) that causes significant disability and distress. It generally responds poorly to conventional therapy such as anticholinergic and dopaminergic medication. The value of using clozapine in the treatment of tremor in patients with PD was investigated.

Methods.—Twenty-three patients with PD and a troublesome tremor despite optimal antiparkinson therapy were studied. Because agranulocytosis has been associated with clozapine, all patients underwent blood testing several times a month.

Findings.—Clozapine substantially alleviated parkinsonian tremor in 73% of the patients. The beneficial response was achieved with a relatively low dose of the drug: 18 mg/day. Previous antiparkinson medication was unchanged. The improvement of tremor at rest generally was noticeable within 2 weeks of the initiation of treatment. There was no tolerance to the antitremor efficacy of clozapine during the 6-month or longer study. Leukopenia developed in 1 patient. Hypersalivation and daytime drowsiness were the other major adverse effects (Fig 3–6; table).

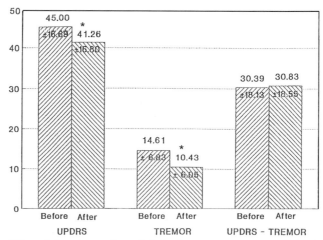

Fig 3–6.—Effect of clozapine on the unified PDRS score, tremor score, and the difference score (PDRS−Tremor). The mean score is given above each *bar*. The standard deviation ± is given in each bar. An *asterisk* indicates a significant difference (*P* < 0.001), as shown by a paired *t*-test. (Courtesy of Jansen ENH: *Acta Neurol Scand* 89:262–265, 1994.)

Side Effects in 23 Clozapine-Treated Patients

	Total number of patients
Agranulocytosis	1*
Sedation	8†
Hypersalivation	6
Epilepsy	1
Decrease of Nausea	5
Sleep Benefit	11
Weight Gain	3
Improvement of Dyskinesias	1

* Lowest value of leukopenia 2.3.
† Two of 8 patients requiring treatment with naloxone.
(Courtesy of Jansen ENH: *Acta Neurol Scand* 89:262–265, 1994.)

Conclusions.—Clozapine has substantial antitremor efficacy in PD. It appears to be indicated in patients with PD who have severe disabling tremor that is not controlled by conventional therapy.

▶ When given in low doses, clozapine appears to be effective in controlling the resting tremor of PD, and although this is another useful aspect of the drug, the pharmacologic mechanism for ameliorating tremor is far from clear. Unlike the typical neuroleptics, clozapine functions as a D1 antagonist more than as a D2 antagonist. Clozapine also preferentially binds to mesolimbic, mesocortical, and hippocampal D2 receptors, which accounts for its minimal extrapyramidal side effects. Clozapine is a potent serotonin antagonist at the 5 HT2 and 5HT-1C receptors, and it also has strong antinoradrenergic, antihistaminergic, and anticholinergic properties. Precisely how this complex symphony of pharmacologic actions of clozapine results in an antitremor effect requires further research.—J.R. Sanchez-Ramos, M.D., Ph.D.

Initial and Follow-up Brain MRI Findings and Correlation With the Clinical Course in Wilson's Disease
Roh JK, Lee TG, Wie BA, Lee SB, Park SH, Chang KH (Seoul National Univ, Republic of Korea; Boramae City Hosp, Seoul, Republic of Korea)
Neurology 44:1064–1068, 1994   122-96-3–6

Introduction.—Wilson's disease shows CNS sequelae such as brain atrophy and areas of low density in the basal ganglia, thalami, cerebellum, and the white matter of the cerebrum. High-signal intensities in the lenticular nucleus of the basal ganglia have been reported in MRI studies. A series of 25 patients had MRI, and 16 were followed up with subsequent MRI.

Methods.—The patients had dysarthria as well as intention tremor, dystonia, drooling, and behavioral changes. The duration of symptoms ranged from 1 month to 8 years, averaging 25 months. The average patient age was 23 years. A "Functional Disability Score" was derived, with 0 indicating minimal neurologic disability and 3, severe neurologic disability/patient confined to a wheelchair. Brain MRIs were performed on all patients. Sixteen of the patients had repeat MRI at follow-up. All patients were being treated with D-penicillamine.

Findings.—Just more than half of the patients had a functional disability score of 1 (mild disability/patient competent for usual job). The MRIs revealed brain lesions in all patients and diffuse brain atrophy in 22 of 25 patients. The most common location of lesions were the bilateral thalami (92%), brain stem (84%, mostly midbrain), and basal ganglia (72%). Some lesions were seen in the cerebellum, resulting in posterior fossa atrophy. Follow-up studies of 16 patients showed no change in brain atrophy. Fourteen of the 16 showed improvement in the Functional Disability Score. There was some resolution of the lesions in the thalami, brain stem, or basal ganglia.

Conclusion.—There was no change in brain atrophy during the course of the 5- to 24-month follow-up. The nature of the brain lesions is speculative. Gliosis or neuronal loss are possible explanations; the reversible lesions may originate from edema or gliosis.

▶ Visualization of brain lesions with MRI and watching some of them disappear with treatment would be a simple means of documenting the neurologic effects of penicillamine chelation therapy. Unfortunately, MR imaging was not done frequently enough to document what happens to the lesions when some patients' condition worsens after initiation of therapy. Careful clinical observations and meticulous monitoring of copper balance during chelation therapy is the best strategy for producing an optimal neurologic outcome. Even under the most vigilant care, penicillamine may produce a transient worsening, which may be obviated in the near future by the use of tetrathiomolybdate (see Abstract 122-96-3-7).—J.R. Sanchez-Ramos, M.D., Ph.D.

Treatment of Wilson's Disease With Ammonium Tetrathiomolybdate: I. Initial Therapy in 17 Neurologically Affected Patients

Brewer GJ, Dick RD, Johnson V, Wang Y, Yuzbasiyan-Gurkan V, Kluin K, Fink JK, Aisen A (Univ of Michigan, Ann Arbor)
Arch Neurol 51:545–554, 1994   122-96-3–7

Introduction.—In patients with Wilson's disease, the use of penicillamine can exacerbate the acute neurologic symptoms and can even lead to sustained neurologic disability. The mechanism may be the redistribution of hepatic copper to or within the brain. Another drug, the chelator trientine, has a similar mechanism of action, but its effect on patients with Wilson's disease is unknown.

Methods.—Twelve male and 5 female patients, aged 14–36 years at diagnosis, were generally treated with ammonium tetrathiomolybdate (trientine) over 8 weeks, followed by zinc maintenance therapy. Several copper-related variables as well as a large number of biochemical and clinical variables were studied. Patients were followed up for 1–5 years.

Findings.—There was no loss of neurologic function over the course of the study. The copper status and potential further toxic effects were generally well controlled quickly. There were no other side effects. The neurologic recovery over the follow-up was good to excellent.

Discussion.—Ammonium tetrathiomolybdate appears to be an excellent form of initial treatment for patients with Wilson's disease. When used for 8 weeks, it is free of side effects. In animals, the toxic effects of the drug are the result of copper deficiency.

▶ Fifty percent of patients with Wilson's disease who are seen with neurologic signs and symptoms deteriorate initially while receiving penicillamine chelation therapy, and 25% of these never recover to their pre-penicillamine neurologic status. The use of tetrathiomolybdate did not appear to produce an initial worsening, was not toxic to liver or bone marrow, and was well tolerated. Most importantly, the drug was effective in promoting neurologic recovery, as documented by improvement or stabilization of neurologic rating scores. However, the drug tends to deteriorate when stored in the presence of oxygen, but with appropriate precautions it should be stable enough for clinical use. The excellent results obtained by the investigators were not simply a consequence of the chelating activity of the drug, but were, in part, the result of the meticulous monitoring of copper balance, a chore that is clearly explained by the authors.—J.R. Sanchez-Ramos, M.D., Ph.D.

Multiple System Atrophy: Natural History, MRI Morphology, and Dopamine Receptor Imaging With [123]IBZM-SPECT

Schulz JB, Klockgether T, Petersen D, Jauch M, Müller-Schauenburg W, Spieker S, Voigt K, Dichgans J (Univ of Tübingen, Germany)
J Neurol Neurosurg Psychiatry 57:1047–1056, 1994   122-96-3–8

Background.—Multiple system atrophy (MSA) is a sporadically occurring adult-onset neurodegenerative disease. Neurologically, it is characterized by olivopontocerebellar atrophy, striatonigral degeneration, and degeneration of the intermediolateral cell columns of the spinal cord. Patients may initially be seen with parkinsonism, a cerebellar syndrome, progressive autonomic failure, or some combinations of these. Clinical, MRI, and ^{123}I-iodobenzamide (IBZM) single-photon emission CT (SPECT) data were gathered from a series of patients with probable MSA of parkinsonian (MSA-P) or cerebellar (MSA-C) type.

Patients.—Sixteen patients were studied prospectively, and 16 were studied retrospectively. Eleven had prominent MSA-P, and 21 had prominent MSA-C.

Findings.—All patients had autonomic symptoms. In 63%, these symptoms preceded the onset of motor symptoms. The calculated median lifetime and median time to becoming wheelchair bound after the onset of disease were significantly shorter in the MSA-P group than in the MSA-C group. In 63% of the patients, a significant loss of striatal dopamine receptors was detected by IBZM-SPECT. The MSA-C group did not differ from the MSA-P group in the proportion of patients with significant receptor loss or the extent of dopamine receptor loss. Planimetric MRI demonstrated cerebellar and brainstem atrophy in both groups. Atrophy was more marked in patients with MSA-C than in those with MSA-P. Both groups had pontocerebellar hyperintensities and putaminal hypointensities on T2-weighted MRI. Pontocerebellar signal abnormalities were more marked in MSA-C than in MSA-P. The rating scores for area, but not intensity, of putaminal abnormalities were greater in the MSA-P group.

Conclusions.—In almost all the patients, MRI and IBZM-SPECT provide in vivo evidence for combined basal ganglia and pontocerebellar involvement. The combination of clinical criteria for the diagnosis of MSA with imaging criteria that help to distinguish MSA from other movement disorders would be beneficial.

▶ Multiple system atrophy is really a neuropathologically defined entity, and this paper summarizes the clinical and neuroimaging criteria that are useful for making the diagnosis in life. It was the intent of the authors to use neuroimaging techniques to complement clinical criteria for the diagnosis of MSA. Unfortunately, imaging techniques to visualize spinal cord involvement in MSA have not yet been developed. The authors caution that single imaging criteria, such as pronounced putaminal hypointensity, decreased IBZM binding, or cerebellar atrophy, are insufficient because they lack specificity and sensitivity. Additional studies are needed to determine which combination of imaging criteria will improve diagnostic accuracy.—J.R. Sanchez-Ramos, M.D., Ph.D.

The Syndrome of 'Pure Akinesia' and Its Relationship to Progressive Supranuclear Palsy
Riley DE, Fogt N, Leigh RJ (Case Western Reserve Univ, Cleveland, Ohio; Veterans Affairs Med Ctr, Cleveland)
Neurology 44:1025–1029, 1994   122-96-3–9

Introduction.—Patients with "pure akinesia" have a remarkably consistent clinical picture, which includes akinesia of handwriting, gait, and speech with no rigidity in the extremities, tremors, dementia, or response to levodopa. Data on 5 cases were reviewed.

Case Report.—Man, 59 in 1978, had progressive deterioration in his handwriting. Four years later, he had trouble with his gait and he stuttered. Parkinson's disease was diagnosed in 1984, and treatment with carbidopa/levodopa (CD/LD) was begun with little effect. His gait continued to worsen over the next 6 years. By 10 years, his speech was unintelligible and his handwriting illegible. He had to type to communicate with his wife. Falls were more frequent, and involuntary eyelid closure was corrected with repeated injections of botulinum toxin. His gait freezing became worse; once, in 1992 (14 years after the onset of illness), he actually stood up all night until his wife found him the next morning. The toxin injections were providing relief of shorter duration. There was no change in his status when the dose of CD/LD was tapered and discontinued. The MRI studies were normal, even after 14 years of illness.

Discussion.—The evidence suggests that pure akinesia is a preocular motor, or even ocular motor–sparing, form of progressive supranuclear palsy (PSP). Gaze palsy was not evident in these patients. Among 4 patients who had eye movement recordings, slow or small vertical saccades were seen in the 2 with the longest history of the disease.

Conclusions.—Patients with pure akinesia may have a vertical gaze palsy late in the natural progression of the disease. Akinesia and rigidity are separate phenomena of the basal ganglia. Knowing the syndrome of pure akinesia may, before the development of ocular abnormalities, suggest the diagnosis of PSP.

▶ The 5 cases presented in this paper would have been big puzzles for most neurologists. The meticulous clinical description of this syndrome is useful to the practitioner who is confronting atypical cases of parkinsonism that are unresponsive even to high doses of levodopa. The authors review the relationship of "pure akinesia" to PSP; however, the best evidence for this—neuropathologic examination—can be found in earlier studies. Post-mortem studies of patients with PSP who were seen with "pure akinesia" revealed neuronal depletion, gliosis, and neurofibrillary tangles in the globus pallidus, subthalamic nucleus, and substantia nigra (1, 2). The authors do not fail to mention other conditions that produce clinical syndromes similar to "pure akinesia," including hypoxic-ischemic pallidal lesions, pallidonigroluysian atrophy, striatonigral degeneration, olivopontocerebellar atrophy and others.—J.R. Sanchez-Ramos, M.D., Ph.D.

References

1. Mizusawa H, Mochizuki A, Ohkoshi N, et al: Progressive supranuclear palsy presenting with pure akinesia. *Adv Neurol* 60:618–621, 1993.
2. Imai H, Nakamura T, Kondo T, et al: Dopa-unresponsive pure akinesia or freezing: A condition within a wide spectrum of PSP? *Adv Neurol* 60:622–625, 1993.

Dopa-responsive Dystonia: Pathological and Biochemical Observations in a Case
Rajput AH, Gibb WRG, Zhong XH, Shannak KS, Kish S, Chang LG, Horny-kiewicz O (Univ of Saskatchewan, Saskatoon; Clarke Inst of Psychiatry, Toronto; Inst of Psychiatry, London; et al)
Ann Neurol 35:396–402, 1994   122-96-3–10

Background.—Several findings implicate the nigrostriatal dopamine system as the pathogenic focus in dopa-responsive dystonia (DRD): dramatic symptomatic response to low-dose levodopa; the absence of levodopa-related motor fluctuations; low CSF levels of homovanillic acid and tetrahydrobiopterin; and reduced striatal fluorodopa uptake. The histologic and biochemical findings of the nigrostriatal system in a patient with DRD who achieved complete symptomatic improvement with levodopa, 750 mg/day, and who maintained these improvements for 11 years, were reported.

Methods.—Autopsy was performed 16 hours after death, which was caused by abdominal and chest injuries sustained in an automobile accident. Sections of frozen brain were compared with sections from controls. Striatal slices were taken from the right hemisphere and analyzed. Dopamine, homovanillic acid, tyrosine hydroxylase (TH) activity, and hydroxylase protein levels were measured. Presynaptic dopamine reuptake sites were measured by GBR 12935 binding assay.

Results.—Histology revealed normal numbers of hypopigmented substantia nigra neurons, normal TH immunoreactivity, and TH protein in the substantia nigra. Neither inclusion bodies nor gliosis were seen; nor was there evidence of striatal degeneration. Nigrostriatal dopamine was reduced to 8% of control values in the putamen; the dopamine level was only 18% of control values in the caudate. The subregional dopamine distribution was similar but not identical to that associated with idiopathic Parkinson's disease. Striatal TH protein and TH activity were reduced to a greater extent in the putamen than in the caudate. The GBR 12935 binding to the dopamine transporter was normal in the caudate and at the low end of control range in the putamen.

Conclusion.—The major disturbance in DRD appears to be either altered dopamine synthetic capacity or reduced arborization of striatal dopamine terminals.

▶ Clinically, juvenile-onset Parkinson's disease (PD) with dystonia and DRD may be difficult to distinguish because of similar age and mode of onset. There are clues that help, such as the development of severe clinical fluctuations in response to levodopa in juvenile PD, and decreased ^{18}F-dopa uptake in the range seen in adult PD, but not in DRD. Even these assessments can be ambiguous, so we rely on the neuropathologic confirmation that the two disorders are definitely distinct. The scarcity of clinical-neuropathologic material from cases of both juvenile-onset PD and DRD leaves the issue open for further study.—J.R. Sanchez-Ramos, M.D., Ph.D.

Botulinum Toxin in the Management of the Lower Limb in Cerebral Palsy
Cosgrove AP, Corry IS, Graham HK (Queen's Univ of Belfast, Northern Ireland; Musgrave Park Hosp, Belfast, Northern Ireland; Royal Belfast Hosp for Sick Children, Northern Ireland)
Dev Med Child Neurol 36:386–396, 1994   122-96-3–11

Introduction.—Botulinum toxin A has become a routine form of therapy in a variety of localized neurologic conditions during the past decade. The botulinum toxins are selectively taken up by endocytosis at the cholinergic nerve terminals, blocking the release of the synaptic vesicles

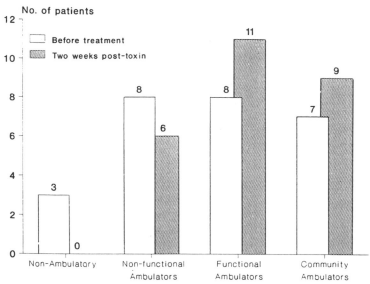

Fig 3–7.—Ambulatory status of all patients before and 2 weeks after injection of hamstrings and/or calfs with botulinum toxic A. Nonambulatory patients were unable to walk with or without assistance. Nonfunctional ambulators were able to walk with assistance or supervision. Functional ambulators could walk independently indoors with or without aids, and community ambulators elected to walk indoors and outdoors at all times. Eight subjects had a 1-level improvement in ambulatory status, and 1 subject had a 2-level improvement in ambulatory status. (Courtesy of Cosgrove AP, Corry IS, Graham HK: *Dev Med Child Neurol* 36:386–396, 1994.)

until the nerves generate new neuromuscular junctions. To determine whether the action of botulinum toxins might benefit patients with cerebral palsy, injections were given to 26 children with dynamic contracture of lower limb muscles.

Patients and Methods.—All of the children had an abnormal increase in muscular activity in the calf and/or the hamstring muscle groups. Indications for injection were determined by clinical assessments; patients who were ambulatory also underwent gait analysis. The mean age of the children at the time of injection was 6 years. Eleven had quadriplegia and 3 were nonambulatory. Botulinum toxin type A was dissolved in normal saline and given at a concentration of 200 units/mL. Total dosages per patient ranged from 100 to 400 units of toxin. The percutaneous injections were administered with the limb positioned to achieve the greatest stretching of the target muscles.

Results.—Patients were evaluated after 5 days and at 2, 4, 6, 10, 16, and 26 weeks after injections of botulinum toxin. Tone was clinically decreased in all patients, starting at 1 to 4 days after the injections and reaching a maximum at 2 weeks. There was a static period for 6 to 16 weeks, then a gradual return to baseline tone during the subsequent 2 months. Parents reported that 14 children had marked functional improvement, 10 had moderate improvement, 1 was unchanged, and 1 showed moderate deterioration. Nine of 19 children with potential for ambulatory improvement showed such improvement after the injections (Fig 3–7), and 6 still had an enhanced ambulatory status after 6 months. The response to injections was more lasting in the hamstring muscles than in the calf muscles.

Conclusion.—The increase in the tone of various muscle groups in patients with cerebral palsy produces functional problems and probably contributes to the decrease in longitudinal muscle growth. No systemic drugs have been useful in reducing tone. The injections of botulinum toxin given to these patients yielded promising results, objectively reducing spasticity without toxicity or systemic side effects. Improvements were also seen in ambulatory status and in sagittal plane kinematics at the knee and ankle.

▶ This interesting study from Northern Ireland reports that focal injections of botulinum toxin benefitted most children with spasticity caused by "cerebral palsy." In 6 of 25 children studied, improvements were reported to be maintained for 6 months. Although further studies are needed to define the appropriate role of this treatment, it is a simple procedure that may prove to be a valuable addition to the armamentarium of treatments for these unfortunate children.—J.P. Blass, M.D., Ph.D.

Hemiballism: Report of 25 Cases
Vidaković A, Dragašević N, Kostić VS (School of Medicine, Belgrade, Serbia)
J Neurol Neurosurg Psychiatry 57:945–949, 1994   122-96-3–12

Background.—Hemiballism is a relatively infrequent hyperkinetic disorder characterized by vigorous and irregular limb movements mainly caused by involuntary activity of the proximal muscles of the extremity and the associated axial muscles. The most common neuropathology is a lesion—usually vascular in nature—in the contralateral subthalamic nucleus.

Objective.—The findings and course of the disorder were studied in 23 patients with hemiballism and 2 with biballism who were followed for 2½ years on average.

Clinical Aspects.—Only 2 patients had "pure" hemiballism without other types of involuntary movements. Sixteen patients had ipsilateral hemichorea, and 11 had facial and oromandibular-lingual dyskinesias that sometimes interfered with speaking and swallowing. Two patients had parkinsonism develop. Two thirds of the patients were severely disabled by their involuntary movements. An ischemic stroke was responsible for the movements in 10 patients. Seven patients had diabetes and 12 were hypertensive. Imaging demonstrated lesions in the basal ganglia, pons, and midbrain as well as in the subthalamic nucleus.

Course.—Ballistic movements resolved in 9 patients, 5 of whom received only haloperidol in a daily dose not greater than 15 mg. Drugs used in the other patients included diazepam, clonazepam, tetrabenazine, and reserpine. Seven other patients gained considerable relief from ballistic movements. Four patients did not respond at all.

Conclusion.—The prognosis for patients with hemiballism who receive appropriate treatment is generally good.

Radiologic-Clinical Correlation: Hemiballismus
Provenzale JM, Schwarzschild MA (Duke Univ Med Ctr, Durham, NC; Massachusetts Gen Hosp, Boston)
AJNR 15:1377–1382, 1994   122-96-3–13

Clinical Features.—Hemiballismus is a rare disorder of involuntary large-amplitude movements of the extremities on 1 side of the body. Typically, the movements resemble throwing motions. Usually there is some volitional control over the affected extremities, but only for a few moments. The affected extremities may be injured if they forcefully contact nearby objects. Movements are most evident during rest and are increased by stress. Most patients are affected in middle age or later.

Causes and Pathogenesis.—Vascular causes are prominent in elderly patients; they often involve the contralateral subthalamic nucleus. Nonvascular causes include primary and secondary tumors, multiple sclerosis, tuberculous meningitis, encephalitis, lupus, and nonketotic hyperglycemia. A destructive lesion in the subthalamic nucleus may disinhibit excitatory thalamocortical pathways, thereby producing hemiballistic movements.

Imaging.—Infarctions usually appear as small areas of low attentiation in the subthalamic nucleus on cranial CT or as foci of hyperintense signal on T2-weighted MR images. A ring-enhancing mass lesion may represent a neoplasm—most often a metastasis—or an abscess.

Management.—Many patients with hemiballismus secondary to stroke will improve spontaneously. Streotactic ventrolateral thalamotomy is still performed in selected patients, but drug treatment is now the rule and is based on the use of dopamine antagonists such as haloperidol and the phenothiazines to inhibit the firing of neurons in the subthalamic nucleus. Dopamine-depleting drugs such as reserpine are also used. A majority of patients either improve spontaneously or respond to drug treatment.

▶ The link between hemiballismus and subthalamic lesions represents a well-known pathologic correlation in hyperkinetic movement disorders. As the connectivity and circuitry of motor loops within the basal ganglia become better understood, it is not surprising to realize that this "classical" association is present in only one fourth of patients in this and other series. Moreover, approximately one fourth of the cases of hemiballismus/chorea do not reveal any lesions at all, using current neuro-imaging techniques. It can be inferred that these cases of hemiballismus represent alterations of neurotransmitter activities in motor circuits involving striatum, globus pallidus, and thalamus as well as the subthalamic nucleus.—J.R. Sanchez-Ramos, M.D., Ph.D.

Pseudochoreoathetosis: Movements Associated With Loss of Proprioception

Sharp FR, Rando TA, Greenberg SA, Brown L, Sagar SM (Univ of California, San Francisco; Veterans Affairs Med Ctr, San Francisco; Albert Einstein School of Medicine, Bronx, NY)
Arch Neurol 51:1103–1109, 1994   122-96-3–14

Purpose.—Proprioceptive sensory loss may manifest as choreoathetoid movements. However, the movement disorder frequently is not considered true chorea and has been described as pseudochorea. The development of choreoathetoid movements, similar to true choreoathetosis, in 7 patients with proprioceptive and other sensory losses was described.

Patients.—Patient 1, who had a history of craniotomy after head trauma, had continuous choreoathetotic movements of the hands and fingers develop with sensory loss. A right-sided parietal lesion was detected from an MRI scan of the brain. Patient 2 had sudden numbness of the right side develop, with involuntary movements and proprioceptive loss of the

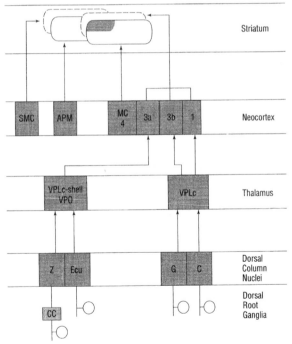

Fig 3–8.—Schematic diagram of the pathways that mediate proprioceptive sensation. Note the parallel pathways from the dorsal root ganglia to the cortex and the convergence of cortical inputs in the striatum. The *lightly shaded area* in the striatum represents the region of overlap of cortical inputs from the supplementary motor cortex (SMC), the arcuate premotor area (APM), the primary motor cortex (MC), and areas 3a, 3b, and 1, subdivisions of the somatosensory cortex. *Abbreviations:* VPLc, ventral posterolateral nucleus of the thalamus, pars caudalis; VPO, ventral posterior nucleus of the thalamus, pars oralis; G, gracilis; C, cuneatus; Z, nucleus Z; Ecu, external cuneate; and CC, Clarke's column. (Courtesy of Sharp FR, Rando TA, Greenberg SA, et al: *Arch Neurol* 51:1103–1109, 1994.)

right hand and foot. A left-sided thalamic lesion was noted upon MRI scanning. Patients 3, 4, and 5 also exhibited proprioceptive loss of the extremities, with choreoathetoid movements of the arms and legs. Spinal cord lesions were found in patient 3, who had a history of systemic lupus erythematosus, and in patient 4. Patient 5 was presumed to have an acute sensory neuronopathy with a dorsal root ganglia lesion. In patient 6, position and vibration senses were absent in the arms and legs, as were pinprick sensations and deep tendon reflexes. Choreoathetosis was present in the extremities. Lesions were found in the dorsal root ganglia and limbic structures. Patient 7 exhibited chorea of 1 finger on the left hand with left ulnar pain, tingling, and weakness. An ulnar neuropathy with degeneration of sensory and motor neurons was presumed.

Discussion.—The abnormal movements described included chorea, athetosis, and dystonia. The abnormal movements were unnoticed by the patients when their eyes were closed. Abnormal movements were noted only in areas of the body which had proprioceptive sensory loss and were found to correlate with the duration of sensory loss. Sensory loss occurred in conjunction with lesions along the proprioceptive sensory pathways. These pathways are illustrated in Figure 3–8. The etiology of pseudo-choreoathetosis may aid in determining the pathogenesis of true choreoathetosis.

▶ The phenomenonologic similarity between true choreoathetosis (caused by lesions of the basal ganglia), and pseudochoreoathetosis (caused by deficits anywhere along proprioceptive sensory pathways) is quite striking. The essential difference is that true choreoathetosis occurs in the absence of sensory deficits. The pathologic substrates are, of course, also very different. This paper suggests that pseudochoreoathetosis results from failure of the striatum to properly integrate limb proprioceptive information with motor commands in the striatum.—J.R. Sanchez-Ramos, M.D., Ph.D.

The "Jerky Dystonic Unsteady Hand": A Delayed Motor Syndrome in Posterior Thalamic Infarctions
Ghika J, Bogousslavsky J, Henderson J, Maeder P, Regli F (Service de Neurologie, CHUV, Lausanne, Switzerland; Service de Radiologie, CHUV, Lausanne, Switzerland)
J Neurol 241:537–542, 1994   122-96-3–15

Introduction.—Three patients who had a thalamic infarct in the territory of the posterior choroidal artery (Fig 3–9) involving the posterior thalamic nuclei were described. In all cases, delayed myoclonic complex hyperkinetic syndromes that developed had not been observed in other topographic forms of thalamic infarcts. This previously unreported disorder is termed "the jerky dystonic unsteady hand."

Patients.—The first patient, a 90-year-old woman with hypertension and atrial fibrillation associated with mitral valve disease, had a 20-year history of ischemic events resulting in tremor and various sensory deficits.

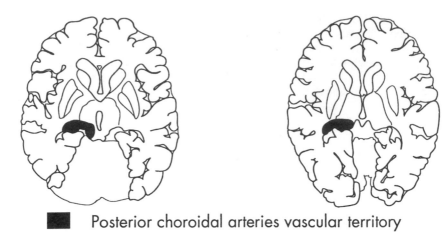

Posterior choroidal arteries vascular territory

Fig 3–9.—Territory of the posterior choroidal artery (*blackened area*) (Modified from Bogousslavsky J, Regli F, Uske A: *Neurology* 39:837–848, 1988. Courtesy of Ghika J, Bogousslavsky J, Henderson J, et al: *J Neurol* 241:537–542, 1994.)

She eventually became wheelchair-bound and was unable to control her left arm. In 1992, a CT scan (Fig 3–10) showed an infarction in the territory of the posterior cerebral artery involving the territory of the posterior choroidal artery, with no evidence of subthalamic nucleus involvement.

The second patient, a 61-year-old man, had a painful Déjerine-Roussy syndrome in the right hand and upper extremity several months after experiencing an abrupt headache and a coma of several days' duration. More than 20 years later, this patient was found to have a rubral tremor—myoclonic ataxia with resting, action, and wing-beating tremor. The third patient, a 32-year-old man, had a history of migraine without aura. Right sensorimotor deficit developed in the patient shortly after the onset of an abrupt headache. About 4 years later, he was found to have a dystonic and ataxic hand with intermittent mild action myoclonus.

Discussion.—All 3 patients had mild and almost totally regressive corticospinal syndrome with normal or even increased uncontrollable strength. Other common findings were a sensory thalamic syndrome and a superior homonymous quadrantanopia. Most striking was that the syndrome was delayed, appearing months or even years after the stroke. This syndrome was not observed in a series of 54 patients with a thalamic infarct in the other topographical vascular territories of the thalamus. Because of the common clinical feature of hyperkinetic movement, the term "jerky unsteady dystonic hand" was coined.

▶ There is some similarity between the "jerky dystonic unsteady hand" syndrome described in this study and pseudochoreoathetosis (see the comment that follows Abstract 122-96-3–14). The elements common to both entities relate to the presence of sensory deficits in the limbs exhibiting involuntary movements, and a hypothesized failure of integration of sensory

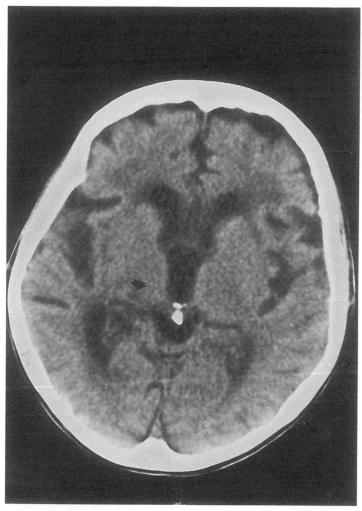

Fig 3–10.—A CT scan of the first patient. Small infarct in the right posterior thalamic nuclei corresponding to the territory of the posterior choroidal artery; enlargement of the occipital horn in relation to an old superficial posterior cerebral infarct. (Courtesy of Ghika J, Bogousslavsky J, Henderson J, et al: *J Neurol* 241:537–542, 1994.)

and motor influences at the level of the thalamus or the striatum. Unlike pseudochoreoathetosis, the involuntary movements of the "jerky dystonic unsteady hand" are more complex (combinations of resting and action tremor, myoclonus, ataxia, dystonia, and chorea) and have a variable latency after the neurologic insult.—J.R. Sanchez-Ramos, M.D., Ph.D.

Symptomatic and Essential Palatal Tremor: I. Clinical, Physiological and MRI Analysis

Deuschl G, Toro C, Valls-Solé J, Zeffiro T, Zee DS, Hallet M (Natl Inst of Neurological Disorders and Stroke, Bethesda, Md; Johns Hopkins Hosp, Baltimore, Md)
Brain 117:775–788, 1994   122-96-3–16

Background.—Two different nosologic entities—essential palatal tremor (EPT) and symptomatic palatal tremor (SPT)—apparently comprise palatal tremor. The site of the abnormality in EPT is unknown. It is believed that SPT arises from a lesion of the brain stem or cerebellum.

Methods and Findings.—A group of 4 patients with EPT and a group of 6 with SPT were studied to determine the clinical and physiologic properties of these conditions. Patients with EPT had normal cerebellar function, whereas those with SPT had clinical signs of cerebellar dysfunction. The palatal motions in patients with EPT were consistent with the activation of the tensor veli palatini muscle, whereas those with SPT appeared to have activation of the levator veli palatini muscle. Essential palatal tremor stopped during sleep, but SPT continued with only slight variations in the rate of tremor. In both groups, the cycle of palatal tremor could not be reset by stimulation of trigeminal afferents. The rhythm of the tremor in patients of either group was not consistently affected by Valsalva's maneuver. In patients with SPT only, the palatal tremor cycle had remote effects on the tonic electromyographic activity of the upper and lower extremities; these effects were present only on the side of the cerebellar signs in patients with a unilateral syndrome. Patients with EPT had only polysynaptic brain stem reflex abnormalities. Patients with SPT had abnormalities of monosynaptic, oligosynaptic, and polysynaptic brain stem reflexes. There was no evidence of structural abnormalities on MRI in patients with EPT. However, patients with SPT had a hyperdense signal of the ventral upper medulla on T2-weighted images.

Conclusions.—These data support the notion that EPT and SPT are 2 different diseases. In patients with SPT, cerebellar dysfunction ipsilateral to the palatal tremor may be partly caused by abnormal function of the contralateral hypertrophic inferior olive. The basis of SPT is proposed to be a disturbance in electronic coupling between the cells of the inferior olive induced by a lesion of the dentato-olivary pathway. In general, similar mechanisms may be responsible for postural tremors. The pathophysiologic basis of EPT has yet to be discovered.

▶ This thorough and thoughtful study of palatal tremor (previously bearing the misnomer "palatal myoclonus") clarifies concepts related to the only tremor linked to a distinct anatomical abnormality: hypertrophic degeneration of the inferior olive. For a long time it was thought that the rhythm in palatal tremor was highly resistant to external and internal influences, and this study confirms this view for those patients with SPT. Neither sleep nor stimulation of trigeminal afferents had much effect on the rhythmic proper-

ties of the tremor, and so the presumed oscillator (the inferior olive) functions as an autonomous pacemaker. However, in EPT, sleep had a profound
attenuating effect, casting doubt on the idea of independent functioning of
this biological oscillator. Another fascinating facet of this study is the description of the strong influence of the pacemaking rhythm of the inferior
olive on distant motor neuron pools, a phenomenon that is discussed in the
context of postural tremor.—J.R. Sanchez-Ramos, M.D., Ph.D.

4 Neuromuscular Disorders

Development of Central Nervous System Pathology in a Murine Transgenic Model of Human Amyotrophic Lateral Sclerosis
Dal Canto MC, Gurney ME (Northwestern Univ Med School, Chicago)
Am J Pathol 145:1271–1280, 1994   122-96-4–1

Background.—Approximately 1 in every 10 cases of amyotrophic lateral sclerosis (ALS) is familial, and approximately one fourth of these have mutations in the gene encoding Cu,Zn superoxide dismutase (SOD), which catalyzes the conversion of the superoxide ion to hydrogen peroxide. A disease involving mainly the motor neurons develops in transgenic mice expressing a mutant human SOD containing a substitution of glycine by alanine at position 93. Affected animals have paralysis of 1 or more extremities develop, secondary to a loss of cholinergic motor neurons in the spinal cord, and they die by 5–6 months of age.

Objective.—The pathologic characteristics of this disorder were examined in 10 affected transgenic mice, 73–188 days old.

Observations.—The earliest pathology was the presence of microvesiculations in large anterior horn neurons. The vacuoles appeared to derive from dilated rough endoplasmic reticulum and degenerating mitochondria. Vacuolar changes also were present in several brain-stem nuclei. Subsequently, the anterior horns became markedly depleted of neurons, and some surviving neurons contained hyaline, filamentous inclusions. The posterior horns and dorsal root ganglia were not affected. The anterior and lateral columns became moderately degenerated as disease progressed, and mild degenerative changes were noted in the posterior columns and roots. The cerebrum and cerebellum remained normal.

Conclusion.—These changes are very similar to those seen in natural familial ALS.

▶ The first real breakthrough in our understanding of the causes of ALS came with the recognition that some cases of familial ALS are due to a mutation of SOD-1. This mutation is responsible for only a minor proportion of ALS, but it may be a way of allowing us to understand the pathogenetic mechanisms in the more frequent sporadic ALS. This paper describes motor neuron degeneration in transgenic mice overexpressing one of the mutant forms of human SOD-1 derived from familial ALS. The authors clearly demonstrate that there is a motor neuron degeneration in these mice.

The way in which the mutant SOD-1 produces degeneration is still unclear. Studies suggest that there is some reduction in the specific activity of SOD-1 and a decrease in the half-life of the enzyme in some of the cells of the patients bearing the mutant SOD-1 gene. However, these changes are unlikely to be sufficient to explain the degeneration. An alternative hypothesis suggests that there is some "toxic gain of function," but the exact way in which this is produced still remains to be determined. This paper provides, however, a very exciting demonstration of the way in which molecular neurogenetics is helping to reveal the underlying pathogenetic mechanisms of these inherited diseases.—W.G. Bradley, D.M., F.R.C.P.

Intravenous Immunoglobulin Treatment in Patients With Motor Neuron Syndromes Associated With Anti-GM₁ Antibodies: A Double-Blind, Placebo-Controlled Study

Azulay J-P, Blin O, Pouget J, Boucraut J, Billé-Turc F, Carles G, Serratrice G
(Univ Hosp Timone, Marseilles, France)

Neurology 44:429–432, 1994   122-96-4-2

Objective.—Motor neuron syndromes, associated with anti-GM₁ antibodies, can be treated with cyclophosphamide. Because cyclophosphamide has serious long-term side effects, the result of high-dose intravenous immunoglobulin (IVIg) therapy in patients with motor neuron syndromes was evaluated in a double-blind, placebo-controlled, crossover study.

Methods.—Patients had either multifocal motor neuropathy (MMN) or lower motor neuron syndrome. Each of the 12 patients aged 19–63 years received each of 2 treatments. Saline or IVIg, .4g/kg/day, was administered for 5 days. The second trial treatment was administered 8 weeks later. Patients were evaluated for muscle strength; disability, using the Norris scale; motor nerve conduction velocities; and measurements of immunologic markers before, and at 5, 28, and 56 days after treatment.

Results.—All 5 patients with MMN benefited from IVIg therapy. The differences in strength between the MMN group and the placebo group were significant only at day 28. Some deterioration was observed at day 56. No significant differences between the 2 groups were observed for change in disability, conduction, or immunologic markers. The 7 patients with lower motor neuron syndrome did not respond to treatment.

Conclusion.—Therapy with IVIg improved muscle strength in patients with conduction disorders. Additional studies need to be conducted to determine the long-term effects of IVIg therapy for patients with motor neuron syndromes.

▶ The role of anti-GM₁ antibodies in patients with motor neuron syndromes remains controversial. However, this paper goes a long way toward reassuring many of us that these antibodies may be pathophysiologically significant. A double-blind controlled trial of IVIg demonstrated improvement in 5 patients with multifocal motor neuropathy as demonstrated by the presence of multifocal conduction block. Those patients with anti-GM_1 antibodies but no evidence of multifocal conduction block failed to show any improvement.—W.G. Bradley, D.M., F.R.C.P.

Excessive Muscular Fatigue in the Postpoliomyelitis Syndrome

Sharma KR, Kent-Braun J, Mynhier MA, Weiner MW, Miller RG (Univ of California, San Francisco; VA Med Ctr, San Francisco)
Neurology 44:642–646, 1994   122-96-4–3

Background.—Patients with postpoliomyelitis syndrome (PPS) typically exhibit weakness, fatigue, and decreased endurance. The underlying pathophysiology of PPS is unclear, and there is still some question as to whether excessive muscular fatigue is actually involved. Anterior tibial muscle fatigability and metabolism were assessed in patients with PPS vs. normal controls.

Methods.—Seven patients (mean age, 63 years) with PPS were studied. All had moderate weakness of the anterior tibial muscle; their functional status ranged from normal ambulation to wheelchair dependence. Five sedentary controls were also studied. Both groups underwent measurement of force and relaxation time of the anterior tibial muscle, as well as ^{31}P magnetic resonance spectroscopy during intermittent, low-intensity, isometric, voluntary exercise.

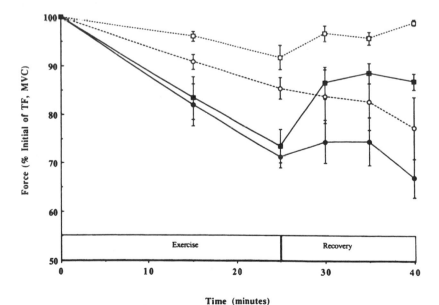

Time (minutes)

Fig 4–1.—Changes in maximum voluntary contraction (*MVC*) and tetanic force (*TF*) during intermittent isometric exercise and recovery in 7 patients and 5 controls (controls' MVC, *open square with dotted line*; patients' MVC, *filled square with solid line*; controls' TF, *open circle with dotted line*; patients' TF, *filled circle with solid line*). All data are expressed as the mean ± SE percent of the initial value. (Courtesy of Sharma KR, Kent-Braun J, Mynhier MA, et al: *Neurology* 44:642–646, 1994.)

Results.—The patients exhibited greater fatigue, with greater declines in both maximum voluntary contraction and tetanic force during exercise. Subsequent recovery was also lower in patients (Fig 4–1). The groups were no different in intracellular pH or phosphocreatine at rest or during exercise or recovery; therefore, the patients' higher levels of fatigue did not result from excessive metabolite exchange. The patients demonstrated a prolonged pre-exercise half-relaxation time of tetanus. Furthermore, the decrease in tetanic force during exercise showed a linear relation to the half-relaxation time of tetanus, indicating an impairment of calcium kinetics.

Conclusions.—Compared with normal controls, patients with PPS show increased muscular fatigability, delayed recovery, and prolonged half-relaxation, with no differences in metabolites. The fatigue of PPS may therefore result from impaired activation beyond the muscle membrane, at the level of excitation-contraction coupling.

▶ One of the major complaints of patients with the postpolio syndromes is fatigue. Patients describe this as "like running in wet sand." Sometimes this is part of the syndrome of progressive postpolio muscular atrophy, but at other times it may be the only manifestation. The fatigue has been suggested to originate at many levels of the neuraxis. It seems such a reproducible phenomenon that a psychogenic origin seems unlikely. Spinal cord, neuromuscular junction and muscle seem the most likely origin. Miller and Sharma show convincingly that there is an intrinsic skeletal muscle abnormality leading to fatigue in these patients. Somewhat similar changes have also been seen by this group to underlie fatigue in multiple sclerosis and amyotrophic lateral sclerosis. Exactly what is the common denominator in these different diseases remains to be determined.—W.G. Bradley, D.M., F.R.C.P.

Treatment of Guillain-Barré Syndrome With High-Dose Immune Globulins Combined With Methylprednisolone: A Pilot Study
The Dutch Guillain-Barré Study Group (Erasmus Univ, Rotterdam, The Netherlands; Canisius-Wilhelmina Ziekehuis, Nijmegen, The Netherlands; St. Clara Ziekehuis, Rotterdam, The Netherlands; et al)
Ann Neurol 35:749–752, 1994   122-96-4–4

Objective.—A previous study found that high-dose immunoglobulins given intravenously (IVIg) are at least as effective as plasma exchange in patients with Guillain-Barré syndrome (GBS). Although IVIg is safer, morbidity is still a problem. The combination of IVIg and methylprednisolone was evaluated for safety and efficacy.

Methods.—The open pilot study included 25 patients with acute GBS. The patients were unable to walk 10 miles without assistance and were entered into the study within 2 weeks of the onset of weakness. All were treated for 5 days with IVIg, .4 g/kg/day, and IV methylprednisolone, .5 g/day. The results were compared with those of 74 patients from a previous trial, who were treated with IVIg only.

Distribution of Factors Shown to Have Prognostic Importance in Previous
Studies, According to Treatment Group

Baseline Characteristics	MG-IVIg	IVIg
No. of patients	25	74
Age (mean, yr)*	47.2	46.2
Duration of disease	84	76
≤7 days at entry (%)		
Functional score at entry (%)		
3 (ambulant with support)	20	18
4 (bedridden)	68	66
5 (artificial respiration)	12	16
Amplitude of compound	15/27	63/27
muscle action potential		
≤ 3 mV (no. tested/%)		
Anti-GM$_1$ antibodies (%)	40	30
Positive *Campylobacter*	25/24	63/25
jejuni serology		
(no. tested/%)		

Comparison with the χ^2 test.
* Age was tested with the unpaired rank sum test of Wilcoxon.
Abbreviations: MP, methylprednisolone; *IVIg*, intravenous immunoglobulin.
(Courtesy of The Dutch Guillain-Barré Study Group: *Ann Neurol* 35:749–752, 1994.)

Results.—Improvement of at least 1 functional grade occurred in 76% of the patients receiving IVIg plus methylprednisolone, compared with 53% of those treated with IVIg alone. The difference remained significant after adjustment for variables of possible prognostic value (table). The median time to recovery of independent locomotion was 27 days for patients receiving the combined treatment compared with 55 days for those receiving IVIg only.

Conclusions.—The combination of IVIg with methylprednisolone may be more effective than IVIg alone in patients with GBS. The combined treatment appears to be safe, although the usual side effects of corticosteroids can be expected. A multicenter, randomized study of this treatment is being prepared.

▶ The Dutch Guillain-Barré Study Group showed that high-dose IVIg produced a slightly better response than plasmapheresis in patients with GBS (1). Lately, there has been some suggestion that relapses may be more frequent in patients with GBS treated with IVIg than in those treated with plasmapheresis. However, relapses undoubtedly occur after plasmapheresis, and the question of the frequency of relapses associated with the 2 treatments has yet to be answered. This study is interesting, because the role of corticosteroids in GBS has been debated for many years. Although historical controls are notoriously suspect for a treatment trial such as this, there is sufficient evidence to warrant the undertaking of a large multicenter randomized clinical trial. Until the results of such a trial are available, it is my practice to recommend monotherapy with IVIg, with plasmapheresis being done if improvement is not observed after 10 days.—W.G. Bradley, D.M., F.R.C.P.

Reference

1. Dutch Guillain-Barré Study Group: Plasmapheresis and acute Guillain-Barré syndrome. *Neurology* 35:1096–1104, 1985.

Pure Motor Demyelinating Neuropathy: Deterioration After Steroid Treatment and Improvement With Intravenous Immunoglobulin

Donaghy M, Mills KR, Boniface SJ, Simmons J, Wright I, Gregson N, Jacobs J (Radcliffe Infirmary, Oxford, England; Guy's Hosp, London; Inst of Neurology, London)

J Neurol Neurosurg Psychiatry 57:778–783, 1994   122-96-4–5

Background.—Unexpected differences in the response to steroid treatment of various types of acquired chronic demyelinating neuropathy were reported. These differences have significant clinical applications concerning the selection of proper therapy for patients with chronic inflammatory demyelinating sensorimotor neuropathy (CIDP) compared with those with diagnosed motor demyelinating neuropathy or multifocal motor neuropathy (MFMN).

Patients and Methods.—Twelve patients with diagnosed CIDP and 4 with MFMN were included in a retrospective study. Patient age ranged from 10 to 75 years in those with CIDP and from 34 to 75 years in those with MFMN. All patients underwent daily treatment with 60 mg of oral prednisone for 2 to 4 weeks, which was then reduced to 45 mg/day until the symptoms stabilized or improved. Maintenance treatment, consisting of 25 to 45 mg of prednisone given on alternate days, was then initiated. Ten of the patients with CIDP and all 4 of those with MFMN also received azathioprine, 2.5 mg/kg/day. In addition, 2 of the 4 patients with MFMN received IV immunoglobulin; .4 g/kg/day for 5 days, at 33 and 26 months after they had last received any other immunodulatory treatment. Before and after treatment, these 2 patients were evaluated with myometry, a timed walk over a fixed distance, stamina tests of upper and lower limbs, and electrophysiology.

Results.—Four weeks after treatment with oral prednisone was initiated, an unexpected weakness was noted in all 4 patients with MFMN. In contrast, the expected improvement was observed in patients with CIDP after steroid therapy was begun. Two of the 4 patients who were given IV immunoglobulin experienced rapid improvements in strength measurements and motor nerve conduction.

Conclusions.—Intravenous immunoglobulin appears to be the preferred treatment in patients with MFMN. Steroids should be used with extreme caution, if at all, in patients given a diagnosis of purely motor forms of acquired demyelinating polyneuropathy.

▶ This paper describes deterioration with high-dose oral corticosteroid therapy in 4 patients with MFMN of the demyelinating type. This is not a well-recognized complication, and widespread dissemination of this information is important. I saw such a patient 13 years ago, before the description of MFMN appeared. The middle-aged man appeared to have progressive motor neuron disease, except that the reflexes were depressed, and there was some patchy slowing of nerve conduction. He deteriorated with oral prednisone treatment but eventually made a quite dramatic improvement with repeated plasmapheresis.

Although Donaghy and colleagues found no patients with more typical CIDP who showed deterioration after receiving corticosteroid therapy, I have also seen deterioration in this disease. The middle-aged woman had moderate proximal and distal muscle weakness and sensory impairment with somewhat slowed nerve conduction, which are typical of CIDP. On 2 occasions she became quadriplegic with IM adrenocorticotropic hormone therapy. The second episode lasted for more than 2 years, and some degree of improvement was eventually shown with repeated plasmapheresis and azathioprine therapy. Such corticosterioid-induced relapses can be easily put down to spontaneous relapses that would have occurred without therapy.—W.G. Bradley, D.M., F.R.C.P.

What Is the Best Diagnostic Index of Conduction Block and Temporal Dispersion?

Oh SJ, Kim DE, Kuruoglu HR (Univ of Alabama, Birmingham)
Muscle Nerve 17:489–493, 1994   122-96-4–6

Background.—Two of the main electrophysiologic indicators of demyelination are conduction block and abnormal temporal dispersion. A number of different criteria have been proposed to define these parameters. Patients with acquired chronic demyelinating neuropathies were compared with normal controls in an attempt to identify the best diagnostic index of conduction block and abnormal temporal dispersion.

Methods.—The subjects were 28 patients with acquired demyelinating neuropathies, mainly chronic inflammatory demyelinating polyneuropathy, and 40 normal controls. All patients underwent motor nerve conduction studies of the median ulnar, peroneal, and posterior tibial nerves. The investigators compared the amplitude, duration, and area of the compound muscle action potentials (CMAP) in the 2 groups (Fig 4–2).

Results.—Controls showed significant variation between nerves in the degree of CMAP amplitude reduction and CMAP duration prolongation with proximal stimulation. In the patients, 28% of nerve segments tested demonstrated nerve conduction velocity reduction as evidence of demyelination. The best criterion to detect conduction block in these segments was the total area method in 71% of cases. The best criterion for abnormal temporal dispersion was the negative-peak duration method.

Conclusions.—The best diagnostic indices for conduction block and abnormal temporal dispersion in patients with chronic demyelinating neuropathies were identified. The findings in normal controls show significant variation between nerves in CMAP amplitude reduction and prolongation

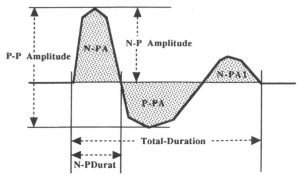

Fig 4–2.—Various parameters of the compound muscle action potentials. *Abbreviations: P-P Ampli-tude* represents peak-to-peak amplitude; *N-P Durat*, negative-peak duration; *N-PA*, negative-peak area; *P-PA*, positive-peak area; *N-PA1*, negative peak area 1. Total area = (N-PA) + (P-PA) + (N-PA1). (Courtesy of Oh SJ, Kim DE, Kuruoglu HR: *Muscle Nerve* 17:489–493, 1994.)

of CMAP duration. When it is not possible to measure the area, amplitude measurement is reasonably sensitive for the detection of conduction block.

▶ Patients with chronic demyelinating neuropathies show markedly slow maximum motor conduction velocity and dispersion (prolonged duration) of CMAP. These changes are sufficient to make the diagnosis. Also, patients with acquired demyelinating polyneuropathies, but not those with inherited demyelinating neuropathies, have conduction block, with reduction in the amplitude of the CMAP evoked by maximum nerve stimulation in proximal sites compared with distal stimulation sites. This is of great relevance to the current controversy about the possibility of an underlying demyelinating neuropathy in patients with motor neuron disease–like syndromes. Of the 28 cases studied by Oh et al., 22 had typical chronic inflammatory demyelinating polyneuropathy. These results helped clarify the techniques to be used when looking for evidence of multifocal block in those with motor neuron disease–like syndromes.—W.G. Bradley, D.M., F.R.C.P.

Peripheral Neuropathy Associated With Primary Sjögren's Syndrome

Gemignani F, Marbini A, Pavesi G, Di Vittorio S, Managanelli P, Cenacchi G, Mancia D (Univ of Parma, Italy; Univ of Bologna, Italy)
J Neurol Neurosurg Psychiatry 57:983–986, 1994   122-96-4–7

Background.—Various forms of peripheral neuropathy have been documented in primary and secondary Sjögren's syndrome. The prevalence of clinically significant peripheral neuropathy and its range in a group of patients with well-characterized primary Sjögren's syndrome were investigated. Possible factors relating to its occurrence were also evaluated.

Method.—An evaluation of 46 patients with primary Sjögren's syndrome was done to assess the symptoms and signs of peripheral neuropathy. The diagnosis was made according to the Copenhagen criteria with minor modifications, when at least 2 of 4 criteria were met for both xerophthalmia and xerostomia. Sural nerve biopsy was done in 7 patients with peripheral neuropathy according to previously reported methods.

Results.—Clinical and electrophysiologic signs of peripheral neuropathy were found in 10 of the 46 patients with Sjögren's syndrome (21.7%). One patient had multiple mononeuropathy, 7 had symmetric polyneuropathy with mainly sensory or autonomic features, and 2 patients had sensory neuronopathy. Peripheral neuropathy was the presenting manifestation in 5 patients (10.9%) and the most common onset of the disease in neuropathic patients (50%), followed by sicca syndrome (30%), which was, conversely, the most common sign at onset in non-neuropathic patients (55.5%). Onset of the disease after the age of 50 was significantly more common in the polyneuropathy group (6 of 7) than in non-neuropathic patients (14 of 36). This was the only difference in clinical or laboratory variables between the 2 groups. Neurophysiologic study showed variable abnormalities usually suggesting axonopathy in patients with distal symmetric polyneuropathy. Nerve biopsy revealed moderate changes consisting of thinly myelinated fibers isolated or in clusters suggesting remyelination and regeneration in patients with symmetric polyneuropathy. Electron microscopy showed prominent alterations of the endoneurial microvessels, with thickening and reduplication of the basal laminae in all patients.

Conclusion.—A prevalence of 21.7% of peripheral neuropathy in primary Sjögren's syndrome, similar to other studies, was revealed. Patients in this group had Sjögren's syndrome develop at a significantly older age than did patients without neuropathy. Aging may therefore be a critical factor for polyneuropathy in Sjögren's syndrome, and it may favor microangiopathic changes in the endoneurial vessels.

▶ Sjögren's syndrome is sometimes considered a possible cause of otherwise idiopathic peripheral neuropathy, and this review delineates the type of neuropathy that most frequently occurs in this disorder. The most common pattern was a distal symmetrical polyneuropathy, sometimes being restricted to the small fibers with pain and autonomic involvement, and sometimes being a large fiber neuropathy with ataxia and numbness. A mononeuropathic presentation is uncommon. The most commonly applied diagnostic procedures are Schirmer's test and biopsy of the lower lip. A nerve biopsy is insufficiently specific for diagnosis.—W.G. Bradley, D.M., F.R.C.P.

Application of OpSite Film: A New and Effective Treatment of Painful Diabetic Neuropathy
Foster AVM, Eaton C, McConville DO, Edmonds ME (King's College Hosp, London)
Diabetic Med 11:768–772, 1994   122-96-4–8

Background.—Patients with diabetes may experience painful neuropathy, an unpleasant complication that is difficult to treat. OpSite, an adherent polyurethane film, has proven effective in relieving painful neuropathy

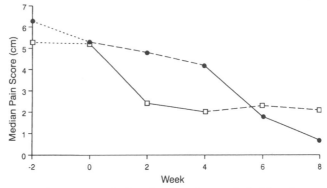

Fig 4–3.—Leg pain by treatment order. Plot of median pain scores for both legs. *Open squares,* OpSite starter legs; *filled circles,* non-OpSite starter legs; *solid lines,* periods in which OpSite was worn; *broken lines,* periods in which no OpSite was worn. (Courtesy of Foster AVM, Eaton C, McConville DO, et al: *Diabetic Med* 11:768–772, 1994.)

when used to dress diabetic feet complicated by ulcers. However, evidence for its effect on unbroken skin in diabetic patients is anecdotal. The effect of OpSite dressings on the painful feet and legs of patients with diabetic neuropathy was investigated.

Patients and Methods.—Thirty-three patients (mean age, 57 years) were studied. All patients had a symmetrical painful neuropathy of the lower limbs for at least 3 months. After a 2-week run-in period, OpSite was applied to 1 of the painful legs for 4 weeks. The OpSite dressing was then applied to the opposite leg for another 4-week period. Pain was evaluated using a visual analogue scale. The treatment effect was defined as within-patient difference in pain between the OpSite leg and the no-treatment leg at week 4, corrected for baseline. Secondary variables, including ingestion of an acetaminophen pill and quality-of-life factors (sleep, mobility, contact discomfort, appetite, and mood) were also assessed from baseline to weeks 4 and 8.

Results.—A significantly greater reduction in pain was noted in the OpSite-treated limbs as compared with the control limbs (Fig 4–3). Acet-aminophen intake was also significantly decreased by week 4, and patients reported significant improvements in sleep, mobility, contact discomfort, mood, and appetite.

Conclusions.—Application of OpSite dressings relieves the pain associated with diabetic neuropathy. The treatment is safe and should be used before resorting to pharmacologic management, which may lead to adverse side effects.

▶ Painful sensory neuropathies, including those caused by diabetes, are difficult to treat. Double-blind, controlled trials have demonstrated that the tricyclic antidepressants mexiletine and sertraline are better than placebo for controlling the pain. Nevertheless, the degree of improvement is often insufficient for patient satisfaction, and the side effects are often significant. In my experience, a combination of sertraline, 50 mg each morning, and amitriptyline, 20–50 mg each night, produces the best control of pain. I have not seen a significant benefit from mexiletine. This paper offers a more direct and mechanical approach to painful neuropathies affecting the feet. The "artificial skin" probably acts as a simple barrier, limiting the access of stimuli to the hyperesthetic sensory endings in the feet. I doubt whether this will do more than partially relieve the symptoms, but with painful neuropathies even a little benefit is worthwhile.—W.G. Bradley, D.M., F.R.C.P.

▶ A painful peripheral neuropathy is difficult for both patient and physician. It is difficult for the patient to tolerate and for the physician to treat. Because tactile stimuli typically will precipitate or aggravate the pain of peripheral neuropathy, various maneuvers (such as the use of a small frame to keep the covers elevated off the patient's legs and feet at night) have been used to minimize this aspect of the problem. In this study, Foster and colleagues show the value of the simple application of an adhesive barrier to the painful areas.—R.H. Wilkins, M.D.

Exacerbation of Myasthenia Gravis After Removal of Thymomas

Somnier FE (Natl Hosp (Rigshospitalet), Copenhagen)
Acta Neurol Scand 90:56–66, 1994   122-96-4-9

Background.—There is a well-recognized association between thymoma and myasthenia gravis (MG). Thymectomy has traditionally been viewed as having a favorable effect on the long-term prognosis of MG; however, several case reports have described the onset or exacerbation of MG in patients after removal of thymomas. The short- and long-term immunologic effects of thymectomy in patients with MG were prospectively studied.

Methods.—The study included 34 patients with generalized MG who were offered thymectomy. Twenty-eight patients underwent the operation; 5 declined and 1 died. Histologic examination of the thymectomy specimens revealed 6 thymomas, 20 cases of hyperplasia, and 2 cases of involution. The patients were followed up by means of a modified Oosterhuis scale and by anti-acetylcholine receptor (AChR) antibody status.

Results.—Patients who underwent removal of thymomas had rapid clinical exacerbation of the clinical severity of their MG and of their anti-AChR antibody titers, which peaked at about 300 days postoperatively and continued for up to 2 years. At a mean follow-up of 5.5 years, these patients had returned to their presurgical immunologic and clinical state, but with no apparent long-term benefit of the surgery. In contrast, the patients without thymoma who underwent thymectomy showed significant improvement in clinical status and decreasing anti-AChR antibody titers. Both of these changes were significant by the end of the first postoperative year, with further improvement at a mean follow-up of 4 years. The patients with MG who did not undergo surgery also had a good prognosis.

Conclusions.—Neoplasia of the thymus may be part of immunoregulation, with a predominantly inhibitory effect. If this is so, it suggests that thymomas should be managed conservatively as long as possible. The current results suggest that the diagnosis of MG is not, in itself, sufficient reason for thymoma removal.

▶ It is the generally accepted practice that thymectomy should be undertaken in otherwise healthy young individuals who have severe generalized myasthenia. It is also generally accepted practice that suspected thymomas should be removed, regardless of whether there is myasthenia, in all individuals in whom the general condition and age would warrant a thoracotomy, which can be curative of a tumor of the thymus. There are examples in the literature of the appearance of MG after removal of a thymoma, and of improvement of MG in the same situation. The literature and my own experience do not suggest that it is a general rule, as reported in this paper, that MG deteriorates for months or years after removal of a thymoma and then returns to preoperative levels of severity. Different patients behave differently. Unfortunately, there is no way of determining whether the thymoma is behaving as an invasive tumor or is remaining well encapsulated and, therefore, is likely to be prognostically benign. In these circumstances, one should proceed to remove the thymoma while fearing the exacerbation but hoping for the remission.—W.G. Bradley, D.M., F.R.C.P.

Familial Autoimmune Myasthenia Gravis

Bergoffen J, Zmijewski CM, Fischbeck KH (The Children's Hosp of Philadelphia; Univ of Pennsylvania, Philadelphia)
Neurology 44:551–554, 1994   122-96-4–10

Objective.—Myasthenia gravis (MG) can be associated with a genetically predisposing factor such as human leukocyte antigen (HLA) type, or it can be caused by a hereditary defect in neuromuscular transmission with or without acetylcholine receptor (AChR). The generation of autoantibodies was studied in a family with parental consanguinity and 5 of 10 siblings with late-onset MG to elucidate the predisposing genetic factor responsible for the disease.

Methods.—Two sisters and 3 brothers, 52 years of age and older, had neurologic symptoms and concomitant conditions such as coronary artery disease, diabetes, arthritis, gall bladder disease, hyperthyroidism, hearing loss, carcinoma of the nasopharynx, and retinal disease. Their DNA was isolated and analyzed for major histocompatibility complex, the β-subunit of the AChR, and the T-cell receptor α- and β-subunits.

Results.—No association was found between HLA haplotype and MG. Whereas the symptoms of the disease in these patients were typical, no genetic predisposing factor was found. No homozygosity or linkage with other markers was detected.

Conclusion.—Although this family appears to have inheritable MG, the cause of autoimmune disease is still obscure.

▶ This is a very interesting and puzzling report of a family with late-onset autoimmune MG. The consanguinity of the parents and the presence of the disease in half the siblings suggest that this is an autosomal recessive disorder; however, restriction fragment-length polymorphisms fail to show linkage to the β-subunit of AChR. The presence of anti-AChR antibodies suggests that there is a specific inherited abnormality of factors predisposing to autoimmune diseases, and yet no linkage is found with the T-cell receptor α- and β-subunits. It is possible that some inherited conformational or change of another subunit of AChR predisposed to the development of autoantibodies. Further investigation of this family might lead to a greater understanding of classic autoimmune MG.—W.G. Bradley, D.M., F.R.C.P.

Congenital Myasthenic Syndrome Caused by Prolonged Acetylcholine Receptor Channel Openings Due to a Mutation in the M2 Domain of the ε Subunit

Ohno K, Hutchinson DO, Milone M, Brengman JM, Bouzat C, Sine SM, Engel AG (Mayo Clinic and Found, Rochester, Minn)

Proc Natl Acad Sci U S A 92:758–762, 1995   122-96-4–11

Introduction.—In the inherited congenital myasthenic syndromes (CMSs), the safety margin of neuromuscular transmission is compromised by one or more specific mechanisms. Clinical, morphological, and electrophysiologic studies have identified 3 types of CMSs: end plate acetylcholinesterase deficiency, presynaptic abnormalities effecting the release or size of transmitter quanta, and acetylcholine receptor (AChR) deficiency with or without an associated AChR kinetic abnormality. The discovery of a spontaneous mutation in the human AChR that leads to significantly prolonged AChR channel openings and causes a CMS was reported.

Findings.—A woman, who was 20 years old at the time of the study, had a CMS with a severe end plate myopathy. None of her relatives had myasthenic symptoms. On patch-clamp studies, she was found to have markedly prolonged AChR channel openings. Molecular genetic analysis of AChR subunit genes was performed, revealing a heterozygous adenosine-to-cytosine transversion at nucleotide 790 in exon 8 of the ε-subunit gene. This mutation predicted substitution of proline for threonine at codon 264. The entire coding sequences of genes encoding the α-, β-, δ-, and ε-subunits revealed no additional mutations.

Expressed in a human embryonic kidney fibroblast cell line, genetically engineered mutant AChR also showed markedly prolonged openings in the presence of agonist. Even in the absence of agonist, opening was observed. The mutation in the ε-subunit involved a highly conserved residue in the M2 domain lining the channel pore. As such, it was thought likely to disrupt the putative M2 α-helix.

Conclusions.—An εT264P mutation in the nicotinic AChR at the end plate associated with CMS suggests that mutations involving subunits of neuronal AChRs and other central ligand-gated channels may also exist. These mutations could serve as the basis of a variety of other neurologic or psychiatric disorders.

▶ The CMSs comprise a number of rare conditions that are all seen with fatigue with onset in the neonatal period. Some have the same distribution of weakness as myasthenia gravis, particularly involving the eye and bulbar muscles, but others have diffuse weakness with fatigue. Dr. Andrew Engel and his colleagues have played a major role in analyzing the various disorders that underlie these syndromes. This paper is a brilliant example of that type of work. The exact molecular genetic defect has been identified, and its pathophysiologic effect characterized. The possibility that similar mutations of central nervous system AChR receptors may exist opens a potential insight into a number of central neurologic disorders.—W.G. Bradley, D.M., F.R.C.P.

Cardiac Involvement in Myotonic Dystrophy

Fragola PV, Luzi M, Calò L, Antonini G, Borzi M, Frongillo D, Cannata D (Univ of Rome Tor Vergata, Italy; Univ of Rome La Sapienza, Italy)
Am J Cardiol 74:1070–1072, 1994   122-96-4–12

Background.—Heart involvement in myotonic dystrophy is common and has been investigated extensively. There seldom are overt signs or symptoms of heart failure; the most prominent features are a range of conduction disturbances that become worse with time and may be life threatening. Atrial and ventricular arrhythmias may occur and be symptomatic. An experience with 56 patients with various degrees of myotonic dystrophy followed for a mean of 52 months was evaluated.

Methods.—Subjects were 56 consecutive patients with mild to severe myotonic dystrophy who were referred for cardiovascular evaluation. No patient had known cardiac disease or other systemic disease able to involve the heart. Most had not been treated for myotonic dystrophy with the usual drugs.

Results.—Of the 56 patients, 20 had at least one of the following conduction disturbances: first-degree atrioventricular block, nonspecific intraventricular conduction delay, bundle branch block, and hemiblocks. One patient had received a pacemaker before the study. Seven patients had a variety of atrial or complex ventricular arrhythmias, or both. Other ECG abnormalities included abnormal Q waves, right ventricular hypertrophy, and left ventricular hypertrophy. Echocardiography showed mitral valve prolapse in 2 patients with mild disease and normal ECGs. Echocardiography showed signs of mildly depressed left ventricular systolic function in 3 patients with severe disease. Of 20 patients with conduction disturbances, 14 had a range of additional defects during the study, suggesting progression of conducting system disease. At the last observation, 6 patients with previously normal ECGs had serious conduction disturbances. Nine patients required permanent pacemaker insertion and were alive in

April 1994, when the study was submitted. At final study, no patient had new echocardiographic abnormalities.

Conclusions.—Conduction disturbances are a major problem in considering heart involvement in myotonic dystrophy and may influence prognosis. The appearance or progression of cardiac involvement in myotonic dystrophy cannot be predicted. All patients should have close cardiologic observation. Invasive evaluation of cardiac conduction and vulnerability should be performed on recognition of serious conduction defects or complex ventricular arrhythmias.

▶ This study shows a surprisingly large number of patients with myotonic dystrophy requiring permanent pacemakers. Half of these had severe neuromuscular disease (criteria not defined), and half had moderate disease. All had episodes of recurrent vertigo and at least one episode of syncope. The strength of this paper is the considerable number of patients with a moderately long follow-up. The incidence of major cardiac symptoms is higher than what I've seen in my experience, but it justifies the conclusion that yearly electrocardiograms and review of cardiac symptomatology should be undertaken in patients with myotonic dystrophy.—W.G. Bradley, D.M., F.R.C.P.

Proximal Myotonic Myopathy: A New Dominant Disorder With Myotonia, Muscle Weakness, and Cataracts
Ricker K, Koch MC, Lehmann-Horn F, Pongratz D, Otto M, Heine R, Moxley RT III (Univ of Würzburg, Germany; Univ of Marburg, Germany; Univ of Ulm, Germany; et al)
Neurology 44:1448–1452, 1994   122-96-4-13

Objective.—The clinical and neurophysiologic findings in 3 families exhibited a dominantly inherited disorder that resembled a mild type of myotonic dystrophy (DM) or an unusual form of myotonia congenita. None of those who were affected had expansion of the CTG repeat in the DM gene.

Clinical Findings.—The 15 affected individuals had an onset of myotonic symptoms at age 20–40 years. They initially had myotonic symptoms in the hands and, later, in the proximal leg muscles. Most of them were infrequently symptomatic. Six patients had cataracts. None had cardiac symptoms, and the resting ECG was consistently normal.

Investigations.—The results of nerve conduction studies were normal. Quadriceps biopsy specimens from 2 of the 6 patients with proximal leg weakness demonstrated a mild, nonspecific myopathy with increased central nuclei in the muscle fibers and hypertrophied type 2 fibers. The in vitro studies of muscle fiber bundles showed normal resting membrane potentials. Impaling the fibers produced prolonged runs of repetitive action potentials that were abolished by tetrodotoxin. Force recordings revealed intense spontaneous twitch activity that was abolished by a potassium channel activator. The DNA analysis ruled out DM.

Conclusions.—This form of myotonia appears to arise in the muscle fibers. Subsequent studies may clarify the pathogenesis of myotonia in patients with proximal muscle weakness and cataracts.

▶ Proximal myotonic myopathy is a newly described disorder that may encompass a number of the earlier reports in the literature of patients with atypical myotonic dystrophy. As always, when a condition is well described, additional cases become immediately obvious. Soon after the publication of this paper, I saw my first patient! Such patients have significant myotonia of the hands, a progressive proximal myopathy like limb girdle muscular dystrophy, but none of the dysmorphic features of myotonic dystrophy. We await the localization of the gene in this disorder.—W.G. Bradley, D.M., F.R.C.P.

Autosomal Recessive, Fatal Infantile Hypertonic Muscular Dystrophy Among Canadian Natives
Lacson AG, Seshia SS, Sarnat HB, Anderson J, DeGroot WR, Chudley A, Adams C, Darwish HZ, Lowry RB, Kuhn S, Lowry NJ, Ang LC, Gibbings E, Trevenen CL, Johnson ES, Hoogstraten J (All Children's Hosp, St Petersburg, Fla)
Can J Neurol Sci 21:203–212, 1994   122-96-4–14

Introduction.—Eleven infants, all Canadian natives from northern regions of several midwestern provinces, were given a diagnosis of a fatal, autosomal recessive muscular dystrophy. The clinical features, pathologic findings, and course of the disorder were described.

Clinical Features.—The age at onset of infantile hypertonic muscular dystrophy ranged from 3 to 8 weeks in 10 of the infants; the remaining infant exhibited symptoms of rigidity from birth. Other symptoms included respiratory distress, apneic spells, chest and lung infiltrates, and seizures. Progressive stiffness was described as a board-like rigidity, although cognition appeared to be preserved. The serum level of creatine kinase (CK) was elevated in all cases, often 10 times that of normal values. Electromyography showed increased insertion activity and profuse fibrillation potentials. The infants were all of Cree ancestry, and consanguinity existed in 3 families. Three affected infants were known to have had siblings who died in infancy. Nine patients died during the first year, and 2 survived to 18 months. Death was generally the result of infection, inadequate gas exchange because of poor chest wall compliance, or cardiac arrest.

Pathological Findings.—Light microscopy examination of muscle biopsy specimens showed single to multiple hyalin inclusions resembling cytoplasmic bodies within the central area of the sarcoplasm. Muscle fibers had eosinophilic, homogeneous, dense bodies interrupting the myofibrils. There was considerable variation in fiber size, and some fibers had enlarged nuclei with prominent nucleoli (Figs 4–4 and 4–5). In 1 muscle sample, SDS-gel electrophoresis revealed increased 54-kDa and reduced 80-kDa protein frac-

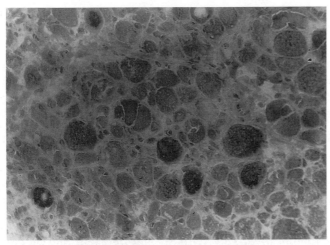

Fig 4–4.—(Patient 6, postmortem muscle) Notice the marked variation in fiber size; many small basophilic fibers have large nuclei suggesting regenerative activity. Endomysial fibrosis with "myopathic grouping" is evident as well (Hematoxylin and eosin; original magnification, ×250). (Courtesy of Lacson AG, Seshia SS, Sarnat HB, et al: *Can J Neurol Sci* 21:203–212, 1994.)

tions. Progressive, granular to powdery Z-band transformation was observed, as were myofibrillar loss and muscle regeneration.

Conclusion.—The muscle disorder described appears to represent a previously unreported myopathy. Its progressive nature, consistently marked elevation of serum CK, and pathologic features qualify it as a dystrophy. Motor unit potentials are normal until late in the course, and

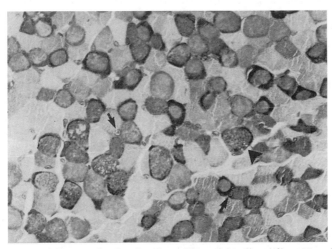

Fig 4–5.—Increased desmin is distributed at the periphery of the affected fibers. Note the apparent selectivity in staining; some apparently normal fibers show an insignificant amount of desmin. Some fibers have enlarged nuclei with prominent nucleoli (*arrows*), whereas others have pronounced sarcoplasmic vacuolation (*arrowheads*). (Desmin MAb, ABC technique; original magnification ×100). (Courtesy of Lacson AG, Seshia SS, Sarnat HB, et al: *Can J Neurol Sci* 21:203–212, 1994.)

systemic metabolic disturbances are not present. The most likely mode of transmission is autosomal recessive inheritance.

▶ The 11 infants presented in this paper, some of whom had affected siblings, all had a similar syndrome of early-onset progressive stiffness, muscle fiber degeneration, and eventual death. The muscle fibers showed a variety of degenerative features. The electrophysiologic studies clearly showed that the disorder arose primarily in the muscle fibers and not as a result of excessive neural activity, such as in the stiff-man syndrome. The hypercontraction of the muscle fibers is somewhat similar to that seen in malignant hyperthermia, although there is no comment about fever being a feature of this disorder. The degenerative features in the muscle are probably secondary to excessive muscle contraction, the cause of which remains undetermined.—W.G. Bradley, D.M., F.R.C.P.

Rapidly Evolving Myopathy With Myosin-Deficient Muscle Fibers
Al-Lozi MT, Pestronk A, Yee WC, Flaris N, Cooper J (Washington Univ, St Louis, Mo)
Ann Neurol 35:273–279, 1994   122-96-4–15

Background.—Rapidly evolving myopathy with myosin-deficient fibers seems to be a recognizable clinical syndrome. Five patients with rapidly evolving, severe weakness, all of whom demonstrated an almost compete loss of myosin in 5% to 40% of muscle fibers, were described.

Patients and Findings.—A history of corticosteroid therapy was noted for each patient. In 3 of the 5 patients, the onset of weakness occurred 1 to 2 weeks after lung transplantation. The fourth patient had weakness develop after a febrile illness, whereas the fifth was seen with diabetic ketoacidosis and weakness. In each instance, the weakness was progressive and resulted in severe disability. No underlying cause for this disability was noted after initial diagnostic testing. Guillain-Barré was a significant diagnostic concern in each patient, although electrodiagnostic assessment, CSF analysis, and various other serum tests failed to confirm this syndrome or any other neuropathic process. In addition, no evidence of a neuromuscular transmission disorder was noted. In all patients, creatinine kinase was normal or slightly elevated, whereas electromyography generally revealed minimal myopathic or nondiagnostic changes. However, muscle biopsy showed multiple small angular fibers with no myosis ATPase staining at any pH. A severe loss of myosin in numerous fibers was verified after immunocytochemical staining and ultrastructural studies (Fig 4–6). Sarcomeres were absent, and clear vacuoles and phagolysosomes were observed in the most severely involved fibers, whereas others showed disorganized sarcomeres with chaotic Z bands.

Conclusions.—This rapidly evolving myopathy with myosin-deficient muscle fibers seems to differ both clinically and pathologically from previously reported syndromes involving rapidly progressive weakness (table). Gradual recovery over months is the most common outcome, as

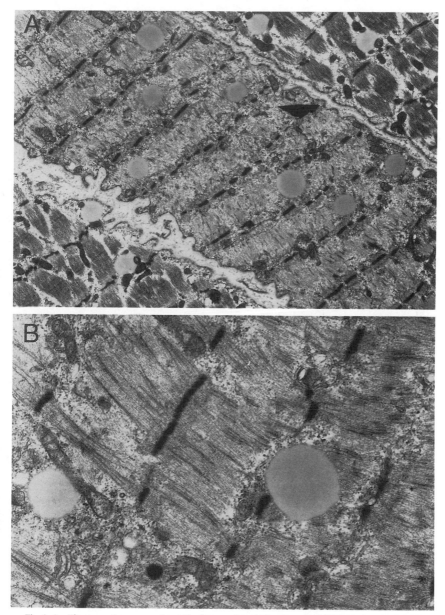

Fig 4–6.—Electron microscopy of muscle from patient 2 showing thick filament loss with relative preservation of thin filaments. **A,** muscle fiber (*center*) with loss of thick (myosin) filaments (×5,000 before 52% reduction). In contrast, the neighboring fibers (*top right* and *bottom left*) have clearly visible thick filaments. **B,** loss of thick filaments, shown with higher magnification (×13,000 before 52% reduction). (Courtesy of Al-Lozi MT, Pestronk A, Yee WC, et al: *Ann Neurol* 35:273–279, 1994.)

Comparison of Rapidly Evolving Myopathy With Myosin-Deficient Fibers and Weakness Associated With Corticosteroids and Neuromuscular Blocking Agents

Feature	Rapidly Evolving Myopathy With Myosin-Deficient Fibers	Weakness Associated With Corticosteroids and Neuromuscular Blocking Agents
Clinical course	Progression over 1–2 weeks; patients are usually ambulant at the onset of weakness	Weakness is usually in immobile, artificially ventilated patients with corticosteroid and nondepolarizing blocking agent therapy
Medication history	Corticosteroids; minimal or no exposure to neuromuscular blocking agents	Corticosteroids; prolonged exposure to neuromuscular blocking agents
Electrophysiology	Nondiagnostic	Nondiagnostic or decrement in CMAP amplitude with RNS, early in the course of the disease [26]
Typical patterns of myosin loss	Diffuse, predominantly in the atrophic muscle fibers	None or focal regions within normal sized or atrophic muscle fibers
Prognosis	Gradual recovery	Gradual recovery

Abbreviations: CMAP, compound muscle action potential; *RNS,* repetitive nerve stimulation.
(Courtesy of Al-Lozi MT, Pestronk A, Yee WC, et al: *Ann Neurol* 35:273–279, 1994.)

noted in 3 of the 5 patients without additional disorders. A muscle biopsy with histochemistry, including myosin ATPase staining, seems to be the only useful test for diagnosing this disorder in patients.

▶ There are increasing numbers of reports of patients with severe muscle weakness after receiving ventilatory support and high-dose corticosteroid therapy. Some of the patients have had asthma and have received neuro-muscular blocking drugs such as pancuronium. The neuropathy of critical illness and corticosteroid myopathy enter into the differential diagnosis. This paper is important, because neuromuscular blocking drugs were not responsible in these 5 patients. Loss of the thick filaments of skeletal muscle and of myosin appears to be the hallmark of these cases. The mechanism by which this loss occurs remains to be determined.—W.G. Bradley, D.M., F.R.C.P.

Andersen's Syndrome: Potassium-Sensitive Periodic Paralysis, Ventricular Ectopy, and Dysmorphic Features

Tawil R, Ptacek LJ, Pavlakis SG, DeVivo DC, Penn AS, Özdemir C, Griggs RC (Univ of Rochester, NY; Univ of Utah, Salt Lake City; The New York Hosp, Cornell Med Ctr, NY; et al)
Ann Neurol 35:326–330, 1994   122-96-4–16

Purpose.—Andersen's syndrome is an uncommon, potentially fatal, inherited disorder characterized by potassium-sensitive periodic paralysis, ventricular ectopy, and dysmorphic features. A gene lesion in the sodium channel locus on chromosome 17 was recently demonstrated for hyperkalemic periodic paralysis (HyperKPP), paramyotonia congenita, and potassium-sensitive myotonia congenita. A genetic linkage study was performed to determine whether Andersen's syndrome is allelic to HyperKPP or to the long QT syndrome (LQT).

Methods.—Four patients from 3 kindreds were studied. All underwent neurologic examinations, electrophysiologic studies, needle muscle biopsy, hypokalemic and hyperkalemic challenges, serum electrolyte measurements, and cardiac evaluation, including Holter monitoring. The relatives of 2 index patients were not available for genetic studies. The other 2 patients belonged to a 3-generation kindred that was available for investigation. The genetic studies were done with markers tightly linked to the HyperKPP gene and the LQT syndrome locus.

Results.—All 4 patients had potassium-sensitive periodic paralysis without myotonia. The clinical symptoms of Andersen's syndrome were indistinguishable from those of other forms of HyperKPP. All 4 index patients had dysmorphic features of varying severity, including low-set ears, a hypoplastic mandible, or clinodactyly. In 2 cases, the diagnosis was made only after repeated evaluations when the dysmorphic features were recognized. Muscle biopsy specimens showed tubular aggregates. Holter monitoring of 3 patients showed ventricular ectopy with periods of bigeminal rhythm. Genetic evaluation of the 3-generation kindred revealed that the gene defect in Andersen's syndrome is not genetically linked to the other forms of HyperKPP, and is probably distinct from the long QT syndrome locus.

▶ Andersen's syndrome is an uncommon cause of hypokalemic periodic paralysis, with associated dysmorphic features and cardiac problems. This review of 4 such cases is one of the larger series to be reported. In 1 kindred, genetic linkage appeared to exclude the gene for the α-subunit of the sodium channel on chromosome 17q. However, a paper by Baquero et al. (1) reported the presence of a valine 783 to isoleucine substitution in the skeletal muscle sodium channel gene. It is possible that Andersen's syndrome may prove to be genetically heterogeneous.—W.G. Bradley, D.M., F.R.C.P.

Reference

1. Baquero JL, Ayala RA, Wang J, et al: Hyperkalemic periodic paralysis with cardiac dysrhythmia: A novel sodium channel mutation? *Ann Neurol* 37:408–411, 1995.

Indications for Intravenous Gammaglobulin Therapy in Inflammatory Myopathies

Cherin P, Herson S (Hôpital Salpétriere, Paris)
J Neurol Neurosurg Psychiatry 57:50–54, 1994   122-96-4–17

Introduction.—Polymyositis (PM) and dermatomyositis (DM), inflammatory muscular diseases that may result from disordered immunoregulation, are usually treated with corticosteroids. The therapies available to patients who are resistant to corticosteroids are not always effective and may have serious side effects. In an uncontrolled trial, the value of immunomodulatory therapy with IV immunoglobulins (IVIg) was examined in patients with chronic refractory PM/DM.

Patients and Methods.—Thirty-five white patients, 25 women and 10 men with a mean age of 42.5 years, who had an average duration of disease of 3.6 years were studied. Twenty-two had PM, 10 had DM, and 3 had PM associated with connective tissue disease. All had at least 3 of 4 typical disease features: proximal muscle weakness, elevated serum muscle enzymes, myopathic changes on electromyography, and muscle biopsy changes. An esophageal disorder was present in 16 patients, and Raynaud's phenomenon was seen in 5. All had failed to respond to standard therapies. In 30 of 35 patients, IVIg was added to other treatments, including methotrexate, azathioprine, and plasma exchange. Patients received IVIg, 1 g/kg/day during 2 days (26 cases) or .4 g/kg/day during 5 days (9 cases). Outcome was determined by clinical and biochemical assessment.

Results.—No patient had to withdraw from therapy because of side effects. Twenty-four patients (70%) showed clinical improvement, 10 were unchanged, and 1 had a worsening of clinical status. In chronic refractory myopathy (Fig 4–7), clinical and biochemical improvement always occurred after the first 2 infusions. Patients who improved with IVIg infusions gained at least 18 points on the initial muscular testing and showed a statistically significant improvement in muscle power. Twenty of 29 patients receiving steroids could significantly reduce their doses. Immunosuppressive treatment was discontinued in 3 patients, and plasma exchange in 1 patient. Twenty-eight of 32 patients with elevated creatine kinase levels before IVIg treatment showed biochemical improvement, with changes considered major in 22 and moderate in 6.

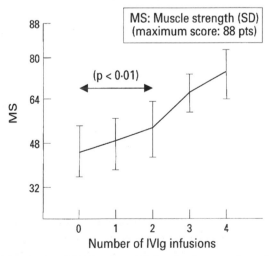

Fig 4–7.—Clinical evaluation of the 35 patients with chronic refractory polymyositis/dermatomyositis who were given IV immunoglobulin (*IVIg*). (Courtesy of Cherin P, Herson S: *J Neurol Neurosurg Psychiatry* 57:50–54, 1994.)

Conclusions.—Patients with a variety of immune disorders have benefitted from IVIg. The IVIg plays an important role in patients with refractory PM/DM. The 2 protocols were equivalent in efficacy, and disease duration was unrelated to response to IVIg therapy. Although IVIg appears to be less effective as a first-line therapy in PM/DM, it brings improvement when added to corticosteroids, allowing these drugs and their potential side effects to be reduced.

▶ Intravenous immunoglobulin is being used for an increasing number of autoimmune disorders, including the inflammatory myopathies. This article presents a valuable analysis of its use in 35 such patients. Almost three quarters of the patients improved, whereas previously they had proved refractory to standard treatment regimens, including corticosteroids and cytotoxic immunosuppressants. This was an uncontrolled trial, however, and the need for a double-blind, randomized, controlled study remains. It is impossible in a paper such as this to provide full clinical details on every patient, and it is well known that response to immunosuppressive therapy in PM/DM is quite slow. Hence, as in previous uncontrolled studies of plasmapheresis, there is always a possibility that the slow improvement is going to occur in response to prior immunosuppressant therapy rather than to the new therapy under consideration. Despite that reservation, it appears likely that IVIg is likely to be of significant benefit in some patients with refractory inflammatory myopathies.—W.G. Bradley, D.M., F.R.C.P.

Abnormal Accumulation of Prion Protein mRNA in Muscle Fibers of Patients With Sporadic Inclusion-Body Myositis and Hereditary Inclusion-Body Myopathy
Sarkozi E, Askanas V, Engel WK (Univ of Southern California, Los Angeles)
Am J Pathol 145:1280–1284, 1994   122-96-4–18

Background.—The most common progressive muscle disease in older adults is sporadic inclusion-body myositis (s-IBM). The muscle biopsy specimen is characterized by mononuclear cell inflammation and vacuolated muscle fibers containing paired helical filaments and fibrils of 6–10 nm (which resemble those found in the brain of patients with Alzheimer's disease) as well as Congo-red stain positivity. Hereditary inclusion-body myopathy (h-IBM) is similar cytopathologically but is not associated with inflammation. In both diseases, prion, several proteins characteristic of Alzheimer brain, and apolipoprotein E accumulate abnormally in vacuolated muscle fibers. The mechanisms underlying this accumulation are unknown.

Methods and Findings.—Diagnostic muscle biopsy specimens from 31 patients aged 34–79 years were studied. In normal muscle fibers, accumulated PrP^c mRNA was found at 20% to 30% of the neuromuscular junctions. Nonjunctional regions expressed no detectable PrP^c mRNA signal. About 80% of the PrP immunopositive vacuolated muscle fibers expressed very strong PrP^c messenger RNA (mRNA) signal in s-IBM and h-IBM. The strong signal in those fibers was typically distributed unevenly, commonly in the form of hot spots. Occasionally, it corresponded to the uneven deposits of PrP immunoreactivity in them. An interesting, although non–disease-specific, finding was that of slightly to moderately increased, evenly distributed PrP^c mRNA and PrP immunoreactivity in small regenerating muscle fibers in IBM, polymyositis, and other myopathies. This suggests that PrP^c may play a role in normal muscle-fiber development.

Conclusions.—In both s-IBM and h-IBM, prion mRNA is strongly expressed in the vacuolated muscle fibers, suggesting that their accumulated prion protein at least partially results from increased gene expression. This is the first demonstration of abnormally increased prion mRNA in human disease.

▶ We appear to be seeing increasing numbers of patients with inclusion-body myositis. Whether this is simply a result of better recognition or whether there is a true "epidemic" remains uncertain. The work of Drs. Askanas and Engel has raised the possibility that the accumulation of fibrils in the intranuclear inclusion bodies and in the cytoplasm of muscle fibers might be the result of an abnormal prion protein. We are still a long way from a complete understanding of the prion diseases and, hence, this paper must be regarded as a step along the way of our understanding of this strange disease. To my knowledge, no one has yet reported studies that transmit the disease into host animals, but this remains the gold standard for proof of a prion disease.—W.G. Bradley, D.M., F.R.C.P.

5 Demyelinating Diseases

Tonic "Seizures" in a Patient With Brainstem Demyelination: MRI Study of Brain and Spinal Cord
Libenson MH, Stafstrom CE, Rosman NP (The Floating Hosp for Children, Boston; New England Med Ctr, Boston)
Pediatr Neurol 11:258–262, 1994   122-96-5-1

Background.—Tonic seizures, first reported in 4 patients with multiple sclerosis, remain an uncommon and inadequately understood manifestation of demyelinating disease. A patient was described whose first manifestation of demyelinating disease was tonic extension of the left limbs caused by a right-sided brain stem lesion.

Case Report.—Male, 19, was evaluated for a 4-month history of spontaneous mild paresthesias of the left arm and leg followed by 15–45 seconds of rigid extension of the left limbs. These episodes occurred up to 25 times per day. Two months after onset, MRI showed areas of T2 abnormality in the lateral right cerebral peduncle and deep frontal white matter. The electroencephalogram was normal and remained so during hyperventilation, which produced a typical episode. Treatment with carbamazepine, phenytoin, and valproate monotherapy successfully suppressed the attacks. Serologic testing was negative for toxoplasmosis, cytomegalovirus, Epstein-Barr virus, Lyme disease, and HIV. Cerebrospinal fluid oligoclonal bands were not noted, although CSF IgG was mildly raised, at 4.2 mg/dL. Serial MRIs performed during the next 30 months showed a normal spinal cord and persistence of the midbrain lesion. Resolution of some of the white matter lesions was also observed, although others reappeared. The midbrain lesion had resolved at 46 months, as demonstrated via MRI. Attacks no longer occurred spontaneously and could not be induced by hyperventilation at 46 months.

Conclusions.—Although 2 previous reports have suggested that internal capsule lesions underlie the tonic spasms in demyelinating disease, this is the first report in which a brain stem lesion has been the causal factor.

▶ Transient neurologic phenomena of brief duration in multiple sclerosis have been recognized for many years. The best characterized of these is trigeminal neuralgia. Other transient sensory and, occasionally, motor phenomena have been reported, including clonic contractions or spasms, as in this case. "Seizure" probably is not the correct description but, nevertheless, the picture can certainly be confused with an epileptic seizure. This paper is of interest because it increases our knowledge of these unusual phenomena and because the patient readily responded to a number of anticonvulsants.—W.G. Bradley, D.M., F.R.C.P.

Chronic Systemic High-Dose Recombinant Interferon Alfa-2a Reduces Exacerbation Rate, MRI Signs of Disease Activity, and Lymphocyte Interferon Gamma Production in Relapsing-Remitting Multiple Sclerosis
Durelli L, Bongioanni MR, Cavallo R, Ferrero B, Ferri R, Ferrio MF, Bradac GB, Riva A, Vai S, Geuna M, Bergamini L, Bergamasco B (Universitá di Torino, Italy)
Neurology 44:406–413, 1994   122-96-5-2

Introduction.—Multiple sclerosis (MS) now is considered likely to be an immune-mediated disorder characterized by increased production of IgG in the CNS, decreased suppressor activity of blood lymphocytes, and the accumulation of T cells in active lesions. Interferon (IFN)-γ appears to upregulate immune responses and disease activity in MS, whereas IFN-α (IFNA) and IFN-β may have an opposite effect.

Objective.—In a randomized, double-blind, placebo-controlled trial, the use of systemic high-dose recombinant IFNA (rIFNA) was assessed in 20 patients with clinically definite MS who had followed a relapsing-remitting course.

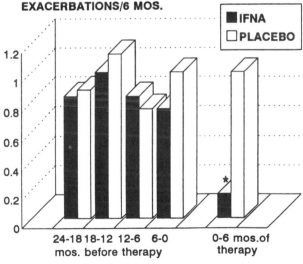

Fig 5–1.—Exacerbation rate (calculated on a 6-month basis) in the 2 years before and during treatment for patients receiving high-dose systemic recombinant interferon-α2a (*IFNA*) or placebo. *Significantly different from prestudy (*P* < 0.03) and from placebo (*P* < 0.03) groups. (Courtesy of Durelli L, Bongioanni MR, Cavallo R, et al: *Neurology* 44:406–413, 1994.)

IFNA GROUP

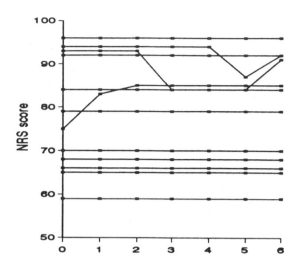

PLACEBO GROUP

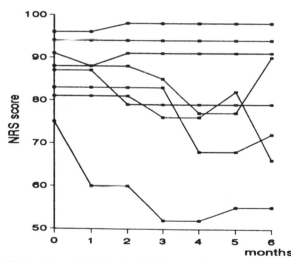

months

Fig 5–2.—Serial Scripps Neurologic Rating Scale (*NRS*) scores for patients receiving high-dose systemic recombinant interferon-α2a (*IFNA*) or placebo. (Courtesy of Durelli L, Bongioanni MR, Cavallo R, et al: *Neurology* 44:406–413, 1994.)

Study Plan.—Twelve patients received IM rIFNA in a dose of 9 million IU given on alternate days for 6 months. Eight patients received a placebo. The patients were admitted to the hospital for 3–5 days at the start of treatment. Acetaminophen, 1 g, was given 2 hours before rIFNA or placebo was administered and 2 and 8 hours afterward.

Results.—There were 2 exacerbations in patients who were given active treatment and 8 in placebo recipients, yielding a significant difference in exacerbation rates (Fig 5–1). Severe exacerbations occurred only in the placebo group. Significantly more patients given placebo had evidence of activity on MRI. There were no significant group differences in either Scripps Neurologic Rating Scale (NRS) scores (Fig 5–2) or in Kurtzke Expanded Disability Status Scale scores. None of the actively treated patients had side-effects necessitating withdrawal from the trial. Only fever occurred significantly more frequently than in the placebo group.

Conclusions.—Systemic administration of a high dose of rIFNA reduces the rate of exacerbations as well as MRI evidence of disease activity in patients with relapsing-remitting MS, and serious side effects do not occur. A large multicenter study is now warranted.

▶ An approach to the management of MS by targeting the inflammatory cytokines has shown to be of promise. Both IFN-α and IFN-β use the same cell surface receptor and have similar in vitro biological functions. Therefore, it is not surprising that treatment with IFN-α has produced results similar to those seen with IFN-β. The next series of studies will have to assess whether arresting relapses prevents or delays the development of secondary progressive MS.—S. Sriram, M.D.

Cladribine in Treatment of Chronic Progressive Multiple Sclerosis
Sipe JC, Romine JS, Koziol JA, McMillan R, Zyroff J, Beutler E (Scripps Research Inst, La Jolla, Calif)
Lancet 344:9–13, 1994   122-96-5–3

Background.—Although the cause of multiple sclerosis (MS) has not been fully elucidated, autoimmune processes appear to play an important role. The efficacy and safety of cladribine, a nucleoside agent that has proven effective in treating lymphoid leukemias, was evaluated in a randomized double-blind trial of patients given a diagnosis of MS.

Patients and Methods.—Fifty-one patients, 48 of whom entered the study as matched pairs, were included in this study. Of these, 24 were assigned to receive 4 monthly courses of cladribine, .7 mg/kg, and 24 were given placebo. Neurologists blinded to the treatment regimens examined each of the patients on a monthly basis. Two neurologic evaluations, including the Scripps Neurologic Rating Scale and the Kurtzke Expanded Disability Status Scale, were scored at every visit. Cerebrospinal fluid and brain MRI were performed at 6 and 12 months.

Results.—In patients who were given cladribine, stable or improved average neurologic scores, demyelinated volumes on MRI, and concentrations of oligoclonal bands in CSF were noted. However, those receiving placebo showed continued deterioration in each of the above measures. The mean paired differences at 12 months (placebo minus matched cladribine) in relation to baseline were 1.0 for Kurtzke scores and -13.9

for Scripps scores, 4.57 mL for demyelinated volumes, and 7.3 arbitrary units for concentrations of oligoclonal bands. Cladribine was well tolerated overall, although one patient experienced clinically significant toxicity. Severe marrow suppression developed in this patient, but a full recovery was noted after several months. One patient acquired hepatitis B and subsequently died, although this event was most likely unrelated to cladribine.

Conclusions.—In patients with chronic progressive MS, the administration of cladribine positively influences the course of the disease.

▶ In this well-conducted study, cladribine, a potent antilymphocytic agent, was shown to be useful in retarding the progression of—and improving the clinical scores of—disability in patients with chronic progressive MS. The improvement observed both clinically and on MRI scans further attests to underlying immune abnormalities as a cause of MS. An easier means of administration (the study used a central venous access) is needed before the drug can be widely used in practice.—S. Sriram, M.D.

Cerebrospinal Fluid in the Diagnosis of Multiple Sclerosis: A Consensus Report

Andersson M, Alvarez-Cermeño J, Bernardi G, Cogato I, Fredman P, Frederiksen J, Fredrikson S, Gallo P, Grimaldi LM, Grønning M, Keir G, Lamers K, Link H, Magalhães A, Massaro AR, Öhman S, Reiber H, Rönnbäck L, Schluep M, Schuller E, Sindic CJM, Thompson F.I, Trojano N, Wurster U (Sahlgrenska Hosp, Gothenburg, Sweden; Hospital Ramon y Cajal, Madrid; Instituto Nazionale Neurologico "C Besta," Milan, Italy; et al)
J Neurol Neurosurg Psychiatry 57:897–902, 1994   122-96-5-4

Introduction.—Five workshops organized by the Committee of the European Concerted Action for Multiple Sclerosis examined CSF analytical standards in the diagnosis of multiple sclerosis. Delegates to the workshops were to reach a consensus that would guide neurologists in the use of various tests.

Methods.—The delegates represented 12 European countries and were selected from among those who had provided a laboratory diagnostic service by CSF analysis. Three categories of tests were identified: essential, complementary, and optional. When results of several tests with parallel information were available, an integrated report with a quantitative graphical representation was recommended.

Results.—A clinical diagnosis of multiple sclerosis is supported by analysis of CNS fluid, specifically determination of oligoclonal bands or increased CNS production of IgG. Isoelectric focusing was decidedly the most sensitive method for detection of oligoclonal immunoglobulin bands. The finding of oligoclonal bands by isoelectric focusing is not specific, however, for multiple sclerosis, and a parallel serum specimen is required. The same amounts of IgG in parallel CSF and serum samples are used, and oligoclonal bands are revealed with IgG specific antibody staining. Laboratories performing isoelectric focusing are advised to check their technique at least once a year, using "blind" standards for the 5 different CSF and serum patterns. Less sensitive are quantitative measurements of IgG production in the CNS. The albumin quotient was the preferred method for detection of blood-CSF barrier dysfunction; both total protein concentrations and CSF albumin were less satisfactory. The age of the patient and the local method of determination must both be taken into account when results are interpreted. Cells should be counted and results compared to the normal value, which does not exceed 4 cells/µL. Other tests offering potentially useful correlations with clinical indices include those for IgM, IgA, oligoclonal free light chains, or myelin basic protein concentrations.

Conclusions.—The essential test of CSF in the diagnosis of multiple sclerosis is that of oligoclonal IgG in CSF, determined by isoelectric focusing; this yields abnormal findings in more than 95% of cases of clinically definite multiple sclerosis. Among complementary tests, an increased IgG quotient and an increased cell count of more than 4/µL yield abnormal findings in 70% to 80% and 50% of cases, respectively.

▶ The consensus reports reemphasize the importance of oligoclonal bands in the laboratory-supported diagnosis of multiple sclerosis. Because the presence of oligoclonal bands is not a quantitative measurement, it is important that laboratories establish adequate quality standards to ensure proper interpretation. Uniformity with regard to the handling and processing of CSF immunoglobulins between laboratories is currently lacking, and it is hoped that the guidelines established in this study will be incorporated in all laboratories.—S. Sriram, M.D.

Increased Frequency of Interleukin 2–Responsive T Cells Specific for Myelin Basic Protein and Proteolipid Protein in Peripheral Blood and Cerebrospinal Fluid of Patients With Multiple Sclerosis
Zhang J, Markovic-Plese S, Lacet B, Raus J, Weiner HL, Hafler DA (Brigham and Women's Hosp, Boston; Harvard Med School, Boston; Dr L Willems-Instituut, Diepenbeek, Belgium)
J Exp Med 179:973–984, 1994   122-96-5–5

Background.—There is mounting evidence that multiple sclerosis (MS) is an autoimmune disease of the white matter of the CNS, mediated by T cells. The T-cell responses to both myelin basic protein (MBP) and proteolipid protein (PLP)—the most abundant myelin proteins—have been implicated in the development of MS. The number of CD4+ T cells recognizing these proteins is comparable in normal individuals and patients with MS. Therefore, if myelin-reactive T cells are pathogenetically important in MS, they might exist in a more active state in affected individuals.

Objective and Methods.—The frequency of MBP- and PLP-reactive T cells both at baseline and after stimulation was examined in 62 patients with a definitive diagnosis of MS, characterized by a relapsing-remitting course. Seven patients with other neurologic disorders and 17 normal subjects served as a control group. Limiting dilution analysis was carried out to determine the number of activated T cells recognizing myelin antigens after primary stimulation of T cells with recombinant interleukin-2 (rIL-2) and after stimulation with MBP, PLP, or tetanus toxoid (TT).

Findings.—Patients with definite MS and control subjects had similar numbers of MBP- and PLP-reactive T cells after primary antigenic stimulation. These cells—but not TT-reactive T cells—were significantly more frequent in patients with MS after primary stimulation with rIL-2. The reactive T cells were CD4+ and recognized the same MBP epitopes as did the MBP-reactive T-cell lines generated by primary stimulation with MPB. The number of MBP-reactive T cells in the CSF was more than 10 times greater than in paired blood samples. Patients with other neurologic diseases did not have MBP-reactive T cells in their CSF.

Implication.—A role for autoreactive T cells in the development of MS is supported.

▶ Proof of causality between the presence of autoreactive T cells and autoimmune disease is difficult in human T-cell–mediated autoimmune diseases, because autoreactive T cells are present in normal individuals. The presence of an increased precursor frequency of cells reactive to neural antigens in an activated T-cell population lends further credence to the role of both MBP and PLP in the development of MS. The ultimate test for the role of MBP and PLP in MS must come from therapeutic studies that show the reversal of MS after depletion of autoreactive T cells.—S. Sriram, M.D.

Quantitative Brain MRI Lesion Load Predicts the Course of Clinically Isolated Syndromes Suggestive of Multiple Sclerosis
Filippi M, Horsfield MA, Morrissey SP, MacManus DG, Rudge P, McDonald WI, Miller DH (Inst of Neurology, London)
Neurology 44:635–641, 1994   122-96-5-6

Background.—In many patients who have multiple sclerosis (MS), the first manifestation of the disease is an acute, unremitting, clinically isolated syndrome (CIS) involving the optic nerves, brain stem, or spinal cord. Semiautomated computer-assisted techniques can now provide reliable and reproducible measures of MRI lesion loads. Therefore, the brain MRI lesion load at presentation in patients with a CIS suggestive of MS was studied to determine its predictability of subsequent development of MS and to ascertain whether lesion load influenced the time in which the disease develops. In addition, lesion load at presentation was studied for its ability to predict later development of disability and the increase of lesion load in the next 5 years. Finally, the correlations between brain lesion load at follow-up and disability at follow-up were examined.

Patients and Findings.—Semiautomated quantitative measurements of brain MRI abnormalities were performed at initial presentation and 5-year follow-up in 84 patterns with an acute CIS of the optic nerves, brain stem, or spinal cord that was suggestive of MS. Thirty-four patients had clinically definite MS and 4 had clinically probable MS at follow-up. A higher lesion load was seen at presentation in patients who had MS develop subsequently compared who those who did not. A strong correlation was noted between the MRI lesion load at presentation and an increase in lesion load over the subsequent 5 years and disability at follow-up. In addition, a correlation between increasing initial lesion load and a decreasing time to development of MS was seen. Disability and brain lesion load were strongly correlated in patients who had MS develop.

Conclusions.—Magnetic resonance imaging at presentation in patients with CIS suggestive of MS effectively predicts the ensuing clinical course and the development of new MRI lesions. Quantitative MRI will be useful in selecting patients with early clinical MS for treatment trials and for subsequent monitoring of their treatment responses.

▶ Although MRI scans initially were a tool for making the diagnosis of CNS demyelinating disease, their value in prognosticating the course of MS has proven to be most interesting. This study by Filippi et al., has shown that in clinically isolated syndromes of MS, the presence of MRI lesions was a predictor of the ultimate course of MS. Magnetic resonance imaging will be an important tool both in the selection of patients for future clinical trials and in the evaluation of the natural history of MS.—S. Sriram, M.D.

Use of Proton Magnetic Resonance Spectroscopy for Monitoring Disease Progression in Multiple Sclerosis

Arnold DL, Riess GT, Matthews PM, Francis GS, Collins DL, Wolfson C, Antel JP (Montreal Neurological Inst and Hosp; McGill Univ, Montreal)
Ann Neurol 36:76–82, 1994   122-96-5-7

Background.—Decreased brain N-acetylaspartate (NAA) is related to neuronal loss or dysfunction. Changes in the NAA-to-creatinine resonance intensity ratio were measured by brain proton MR spectroscopy in 7 patients with multiple sclerosis to evaluate the progression of brain pathology.

Patients and Methods.—A history of relapses was noted in 4 patients, whereas 3 had a secondary progressive disease course. Clinical and MRI evidence of persistent neurologic abnormalities was noted in each patient. Proton MR spectra were obtained at 6-month intervals, and the NAA-creatinine ratio was determined. Volumes of hyperintense signal from lesions on standard MRI and Kurtzke Expanded Disability Status Scale scores were evaluated simultaneously. All patients were followed for 18 months, and findings were compared with those obtained in 13 normal controls.

Results.—At study initiation, the patient group had a significantly lower NAA-creatine ratio in central brain volumes compared with controls. The ratio further decreased in all patients in 12- and 18-month follow-up in accordance with progressive accumulation of neuronal damage. Conversely, the changes in lesion volume on MRI or disability status did not reach significance during this period. A significant association between increased or decreased NAA-creatinine ratios and changes in lesion volumes on MRI was observed at consecutive 6-month examinations in patients with a history of relapse.

Conclusions.—In patients with multiple sclerosis, the progression of cerebral damage may be effectively determined using proton MR spectroscopy and a novel quantitative index based on neuronal damage or dysfunction.

▶ With the implementation of a number of therapeutic trials in MS, an understanding of the role of surrogate markers that determine disability is strongly needed. Magnetic resonance spectroscopy offers crucial information on axonal loss and functions of neurons and, perhaps, a better guide to long-term disability in MS. It also offers a better picture of the metabolic state of the neuropil and should become an additional tool in the longitudinal analysis of patients with MS, especially those participating in clinical trials.—S. Sriram, M.D.

A Comparison of the Pathology of Primary and Secondary Progressive Multiple Sclerosis
Revesz T, Kidd D, Thompson AJ, Barnard RO, McDonald WI (Inst of Neurology, London)
Brain 117:759–765, 1994   122-96-5-8

Background.—The characteristics of primary progressive multiple sclerosis (MS) differ from those of the more common secondary progressive type. On MR studies, the frequency of enhancement of Gd-DTPA, a marker for blood-brain barrier dysfunction, has been found to be significantly less in patients with primary progressive as opposed to secondary progressive MS. The hypothesis that inflammation is less intense in these patients was examined.

Methods and Findings.—Postmortem material from 9 patients was studied. Case notes were retrospectively analyzed to determine whether the patients had primary progressive or secondary progressive disease. A total of 578 lesions were found. Significantly more inflammation was documented in material from patients with secondary progressive MS than in those with primary progressive disease. Greater inflammation was judged by the frequency of perivascular cuffing and cellularity of the parenchyma.

Conclusions.—Postmortem material from patients with secondary progressive MS showed significantly more inflammation than that from patients with primary progressive MS. However, these findings show unequivocally that primary progressive MS is an inflammatory disease. Thus, the effects of interferon-β in patients with primary progressive disease should be studied.

▶ This important study compares the pathology between primary and secondary progressive MS for the first time. It establishes the inflammatory nature of both primary and secondary progressive disease. The marked decrease in the degree of inflammation in primary progressive MS when compared with secondary progressive disease suggests that the underlying immunologic mechanisms may be different.—S. Sriram, M.D.

Induction of Nitric Oxide Synthase in Demyelinating Regions of Multiple Sclerosis Brains
Bö L, Dawson TM, Wesselingh S, Mörk S, Choi S, Kong PA, Hanley D, Trapp BD (Johns Hopkins Univ, Baltimore Md; Univ of Bergen, Norway)
Ann Neurol 36:778–786, 1994   122-96-5–9

Background.—It has been suggested that the free radical nitric oxide (NO) has a role in the development of multiple sclerosis (MS). Increased levels of messenger RNA (mRNA) for NO synthase (NOS) are found in animal models of autoimmune demyelination in the CNS. The histochemical stain NADPH diaphorase (NADPH-d) is a marker for NOS catalytic activity in the brain.

Objective.—The amount of mRNA encoding human inducible NOS as well as the presence and distribution of NADPH-d were determined in tissue sections from the brains of 19 patients with MS. Control specimens were taken from patients having viral or idiopathic encephalitis, adrenoleukodystrophy, or dementia, and from 3 neurologically normal subjects.

Findings.—The number of neurons stained by NADPH-d and the intensity of staining were similar in MS and control brains, but NADPH-d–positive cells were much increased in MS lesions. The cells were found in reactive astrocytes of actively demyelinating lesions and at the edges of chronic active demyelinating lesions. No positively staining astrocytes

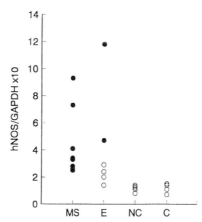

Fig 5–3.—Comparison of levels of human inducible nitric oxide synthase (*hNOS*) messenger RNA (mRNA) (corrected to levels of glyceraldehyde-3-phosphate dehydrogenase [GAPDH] mRNA) to the presence (*filled circles*) or absence (*open circles*) of NADPH diaphorase (NADPH-d)–positive astrocytes in *MS*, encephalitis (*E*), neurologic control (*NC*), and normal control (*C*) groups. Specimens that contained reactive astrocytes with NADPH-d activity contained significantly higher levels of hNOS mRNA than did specimens in which NADPH-d–positive astrocytes were not present ($P < 0.0001$). (Courtesy of Bö L, Dawson TM, Wesselingh S, et al: *Ann Neurol* 36:778–786, 1994.)

were found in control specimens. Levels of human NOS mRNA were markedly increased in MS brain specimens, compared with normal samples (Fig 5–3).

Conclusions.—Activation of NOS may be a key part of the pathogenesis of MS. If this is confirmed, it may prove feasible to direct treatment toward blocking NOS activity in MS lesions.

▶ The final pathway that leads to loss of myelinated axons in MS is most likely mediated by inflammatory cytokines. The role of free radicals such as NO in inflammatory regions substantiates a role for inflammatory mediators in the acute process. The presence of NO in other nondemyelinating CNS disorders would argue that other cytokines, perhaps acting in concert with NO, may be responsible for demyelination.—S. Sriram, M.D.

MRI in Acute Disseminated Encephalomyelitis

Caldemeyer KS, Smith RR, Harris TM, Edwards MK (Indiana Univ, Indianapolis)
Neuroradiology 36:216–220, 1994   122-96-5-10

Background.—Acute disseminated encephalomyelitis (ADEM) occurs acutely or subacutely usually after a viral infection or immunization. Pathologically, ADEM lesions are areas of demyelination. The MR and CT findings in one series of ADEM were reported.

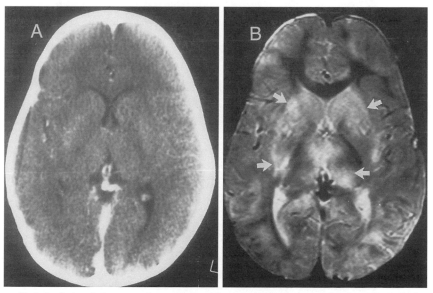

Fig 5–4.—Patient 3. **A,** computed tomography with contrast medium as normal. **B,** long-TR (2,500/80) MR image reveals abnormally increased signal in the basal ganglia, thalamus, and subcortical and periventricular white matter (*arrows*). (Courtesy of Caldemeyer KS, Smith RR, Harris TM, et al: *Neuroradiology* 36:216–220, 1994.)

Methods.—Twelve patients with a clinical diagnosis of ADEM were included in a retrospective study. Eleven initially had an acute onset of focal neurologic deficits, and 1 had generalized seizures. Findings on CT and MRI studies were analyzed.

Findings.—The lesions were most commonly found in the brain stem, periventricular white matter, subcortical white matter, and middle cerebellar peduncle. In 4 patients, high signal lesions were noted in the gray matter of the basal ganglia, thalamus, and/or temporal cortex (Fig 5–4). Gadolinium-diethylenetriamine pentaacetic acid enhanced images were performed at initial presentation in 5 patients. In 3, only some lesions were enhanced, demonstrated on long repetition time (TR) images (Fig 5–5). Of 2 patients undergoing spinal cord MRI, 1 had a white matter lesion at the C3-4 level, and the other had a lesion in the lumbar enlargement (Fig 5–6). Of 4 patients undergoing follow-up MRI after steroid treatment, 3 had a substantial reduction in the size and number of lesions, with complete resolution of many and no new lesions identified.

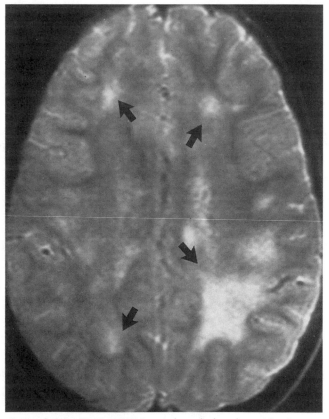

Fig 5–5.—Patient 8. Long TR (2,500/80) image above the lateral ventricles shows numerous symmetrical high signal areas of varying size in the white matter (*arrows*). (Courtesy of Caldemeyer KS, Smith RR, Harris TM, et al: *Neuroradiology* 36:216–220, 1994.)

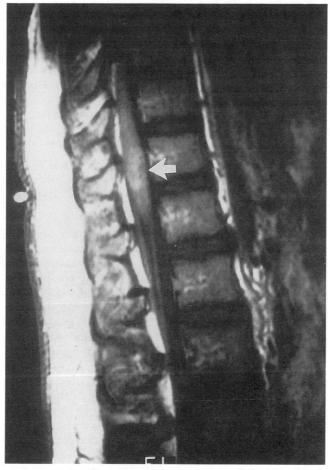

Fig 5–6.—Patient 11. Short-TR (483/20) sagittal image of the spine with lumbar enlargement (*arrow*). (Courtesy of Caldemeyer KS, Smith RR, Harris TM, et al: *Neuroradiology* 36:216–220, 1994.)

Conclusions.—In this series, MRI was the definitive modality for assessing the lesions of ADEM. All patients showed abnormalities consistent with their clinical diagnosis. Ten had abnormalities in the brain, and 3 had them in the spinal cord. Another 3 had evidence of optic neuritis. Computed tomography scans were normal in 6 of the 7 patients who underwent the procedure.

▶ The increased sensitivity of MRI compared with CT in demonstrating the intraparenchymal abnormalities of the brain and spinal cord is dramatically shown (Fig 5–4). Furthermore, the presence of the white matter lesions in the context of acute neurologic symptoms suggests the possibility that what some may occasionally incorrectly diagnose as acute MS may in fact be ADEM. The authors of this article make note of the periventricular matter, middle cerebellar peduncle, and MLF lesions, all of which are seen in MS. This article also again reminds us that an enlarged, enhanced spinal cord should not make one think exclusively of spinal cord tumor (Figure 5–6).—R.M. Quencer, M.D.

Antemortem Diagnosis of Baló Concentric Sclerosis: Correlative MR Imaging and Pathologic Features
Gharagozloo AM, Poe LB, Collins GH (State Univ of New York, Syracuse)
Radiology 191:817–819, 1994   122-96-5–11

Background.—Antemortem diagnoses of Baló sclerosis, a rare demyelinating disease, are uncommon. A patient whose antemortem MR images accurately paralleled the gross and microscopic pathologic findings on postmortem examination was described.

Case Report.—Woman, 32, was evaluated for initial left hemiparesis, which progressed to left hemihypesthesia and hemianopsia. A large lesion involving the right parietal lobe with mild mass effect and marginal enhancement was seen on initial brain MRI. Pathologic evaluation of a subsequent lesion biopsy specimen showed only demyelination of varying ages and perivascular collection of lymphocytes. Treatment with high-dose IV steroids led to some symptom improvement, although the left hemiparesis persisted. On subsequent spin-echo MR images, numerous areas of concentric demyelination, alternating with "spared" white matter, were noted. The rings were abruptly terminated at gray matter junctions. A diagnosis of Baló concentric sclerosis was made on the basis of MR findings. The remainder of the patient's clinical course was monophasic and relentless, resulting in death approximately 12 months after symptom onset. Pathologic examination of the brain showed multifocal lamellation of soft spongy yellow matter streaked in the white matter. Definite cortical and deep gray matter sparing was observed at all levels. A series of cavitary defects, arranged in concentric circles and usually measuring 5 mm to 6 mm × 2 mm to 3 mm, were noted. The white matter disease varied from simple myelin depletion to complete cystic necrosis, and it grossly involved the posterior body and splenium of the corpus callosum.

Conclusions.—The MR images of alternating ringlike lesions involving the deep and superficial white matter accurately corresponded to pathologic findings; therefore, MRI may play a principal role in the antemortem diagnosis of Baló concentric sclerosis. Accordingly, invasive diagnostic procedures can be reserved for ambiguous cases.

▶ Baló concentric sclerosis is a rare demyelinating disease of the CNS. Unlike multiple sclerosis, the disease is monophasic and invariably fatal. The ability to diagnose Baló disease by MRI may obviate the need for tissue biopsy. At present, there is no known treatment of the disease, and the use of corticosteroids has not been shown to alter the course of the disease.—S. Sriram, M.D.

6 Seizure Disorders

Lamotrigine Therapy for Partial Seizures: A Multicenter, Placebo-Controlled, Double-Blind, Cross-Over Trial
Messenheimer J, Ramsay RE, Willmore LJ, Leroy RF, Zielinski JJ, Mattson R, Pellock JM, Valakas AM, Womble G, Risner M (Univ of North Carolina, Chapel Hill; Univ of Miami, Fla; Univ of Texas, Dallas; et al)
Epilepsia 35:113–121, 1994   122-96-6-1

Background.—Lamotrigine (LTG), a new antiepileptic drug (AED) currently being developed, has been found to be effective against refractory partial seizures in several clinical trials. In a recent study, the efficacy of add-on LTG was evaluated in patients following a stable regimen of AEDs that was inadequate in controlling their partial seizures.

Methods.—Ninety-eight patients with refractory partial seizures were enrolled in the multicenter, randomized, double-blind, placebo-controlled, crossover study. Each treatment was given for 14 weeks. In most cases, LTG was titrated to a maintenance dose of 400 mg/day.

Findings.—Compared with placebo, the frequency of seizures decreased by at least 50% with LTG in one fifth of the patients. Overall median frequency of seizures was reduced by 25% among patients given LTG. These patients also had an 18% decrease in the number of seizure days (table). Investigator global assessment of overall patient clinical status favored LTG by 2:1. Plasma levels of LTG apparently were linearly related to dosage. Plasma levels of concomitant AEDs were not significantly

Changes in Seizure Frequency and Seizure Days as Compared With
Placebo by Category During Lamotrigine Maintenance Treatment

Variable	n	Decrease (%) ≥50	Decrease (%) 26–49	No change (25%)	Increase (%) 26–49	Increase (%) ≥50
Seizure frequency	88					
All patients (%)		20	24	38	7	11
Percent range*		(13–27)	(13–42)	(17–60)	(0–14)	(0–29)
Seizure days	88					
All patients		16	18	49	6	11
Percent range*		(0–29)	(0–40)	(14–60)	(0–14)	(0–29)

* Range for the percentage of patients in each category of change for the 7 study centers.
(Courtesy of Messenheimer J, Ramsay RE, Willmore LJ, et al: *Epilepsia* 35:113–121, 1994.)

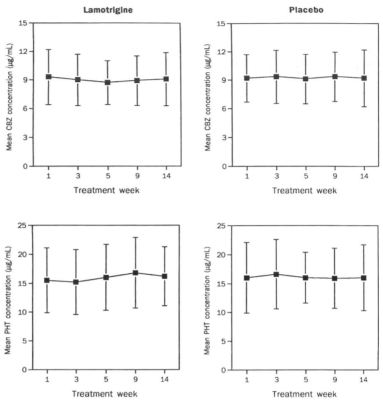

Fig 6–1.—Mean plasma concentrations (± SD) of phenytoin (*PHT*) and carbamazepine (*CBZ*) during placebo and lamotrigine treatment periods. (Courtesy of Messenheimer J, Ramsay RE, Willmore LJ, et al: *Epilepsia* 35:113–121, 1994.)

affected clinically by LTG (Fig 6–1). Adverse effects were generally minor. Central nervous system–related symptoms were most common; most of these symptoms were transient and resolved without the need to stop therapy.

Conclusions.—Twice-daily administration of LTG is effective and safe when added to the treatment of patients with previously uncontrolled partial seizures. The addition of LTG to existing AED regimens resulted in clinically and statistically significant decreases in the frequency of seizures and total number of seizure days.

▶ Lamotrigine is expected to be approved by the Food and Drug Administration for marketing this year. This paper presents the results of the controlled study upon which approval is based. Seizure frequency was significantly reduced during treatment with LTG and demonstrated the effectiveness in partial seizure. No interaction between LTG and either carbamazepine or phenytoin was found. Lamotrigine promises to be an important addition to the available anticonvulsants, which should be easy to use.—E.R. Ramsay, M.D.

Evaluation of the Mechanisms of Antiepileptic Drug-Related Chronic Leukopenia

O'Connor CR, Schraeder PL, Kurland AH, O'Connor WH (Univ of Medicine and Dentistry of New Jersey–Robert Wood Johnson Med School, Camden, NJ; Cooper Hosp–Univ Med Ctr, Camden, NJ)
Epilepsia 35:149–154, 1994   122-96-6-2

Background.—Leukopenia often occurs in patients receiving antiepileptic drugs (AEDs). It is especially a dilemma when the AED effectively controls seizures. One small series was studied to determine the possible mechanisms of leukopenia.

Methods and Findings.—The seven patients had a mean white blood cell (WBC) count of 3,000/µL and a mean of 42% polymorphonuclear leukocytes (PMNs). One patient was receiving carbamazepine alone; five patients, carbamazepine combined with phenytoin, primidone, phenobarbital, and/or valproate; and one patient, phenytoin alone. The results of bone marrow (BM) aspirate and PMN antibody studies with chemiluminescence were normal. Mild relative splenomegaly was found on 2 liver-spleen scans. After exercise, the WBC count in 7 cases increased by 54% as compared with 52% in control subjects. Antinuclear antibodies were positive in 1 case and absent in 6. Adhesion of PMNs to nylon wool was reduced (table).

Conclusions.—It is probably safe to continue AED treatment when leukopenia is stable and the percentage of PMN is normal. If the absolute PMN count is consistently less than 1,000/µL, caution is advised. Routine assessment of BM is not necessary for every patient with neutropenia caused by AEDs, especially if the leukopenia fluctuates between 2,000 and 4,000 cells/µL.

▶ Drug-induced reduction of the WBC count continues to be a concern for many physicians. The authors of this paper did not find antibodies against WBCs. Their results suggest that although counts may be low, WBC function and response to stress are normal. Therefore, in most cases, a low WBC count does not pose a clinically significant problem to the patient.—E.R. Ramsay, M.D.

| | White Blood Cells Per Microliter of Preexercise | | | |
| | Patients (*n* = 7) | | Controls (*n* = 5) | |
Parameter	Mean	Range	Mean	Range
Total WBC	3,000	2,000–3,800	4,800	3,900–6,500
PMN	1,260 (42%)	700–2,300	2,590 (54%)	1,600–3,730
Lymphocytes	1,530 (51%)	910–2,200	1,970 (41%)	1,480–2,230
Monocytes	150 (5%)	70–240	240 (5%)	80–480

Numbers in parentheses are percentages of the total WBC.
Abbreviations: WBC, white blood cell count; PMN, polymorphonuclear leukocytes.
(Courtesy of O'Connor CR, Schraeder PL, Kurland AH, et al: *Epilepsia* 35:149–154, 1994.)

Predictive Value of Induction of Psychogenic Seizures by Suggestion

Lancman ME, Asconapé J, Craven WJ, Howard G, Penry JK (Wake Forest Univ, Winston-Salem, NC)
Ann Neurol 35:359–361, 1994   122-96-6-3

Background.—Previous studies have indicated that induction by suggestion is effective in diagnosing psychogenic seizures. However, no one has reported the sensitivity and specificity of this procedure.

Methods.—The results of induction of psychogenic seizures by suggestion were analyzed in 93 patients with purely psychogenic seizures. Induction was also attempted in another 20 patients with epilepsy. Psychogenic seizure was diagnosed on the basis of a clinical event recorded on video-electroencephalography, the absence of clinical or electroencephalographic evidence of epilepsy, and the subsequent follow-up and withdrawal of anticonvulsants.

Findings.—Induction was positive in 72 patients with psychogenic seizures and in none of the patients with epilepsy. Therefore, the sensitivity of induction for diagnosing psychogenic seizure was 77.4% and the specificity, 100%. Its positive predictive value was 100%, and its negative predictive value was 48.7% (Tables 1 and 2).

Conclusions.—Induction technique by suggestion is a sensitive, specific technique for diagnosing PS. When the diagnosis of psychogenic seizure is suspected, this technique should be used to save hours of unnecessary monitoring. Although this technique is 100% specific for psychogenic seizures, however, it does not exclude the possibility that both psychogenic seizures and epileptic seizures are present.

▶ Differentiation of epilepsy from psychogenic seizures is often difficult. In this study, the authors found that placebo induction is very effective and specific for inducing nonepileptic seizures of psychogenic origin. No seizures were produced in patients with epilepsy. This procedure may be of value in the early evaluation of patients, thereby reducing the number of costly admissions in some instances.—E.R. Ramsay, M.D.

TABLE 1.—Sensitivity, Specificity, and Positive and Negative Predictive Values of Induction of Psychogenic Seizures by Suggestion in Our Population

	Psychogenic Seizures	Epilepsy	Total
Positive test	72	0	72
Negative test	21	20	41
Total	93	20	113

Sensitivity = 72/93 = 77.4%. Specificity = 20/20 = 100%. Positive predictive value = 72/72 = 100%. Negative predictive value = 20/41 = 48.7%.
(Courtesy of Lancman ME, Asconapé J, Craven WJ, et al: *Ann Neurol* 35:359–361, 1994.)

TABLE 2.—Clinical Findings in Our Population

Clinical Characteristics	*n*
Nonresponsiveness and generalized violent, thrashing, and uncoordinated movements	37
Nonresponsiveness and generalized trembling	21
Nonresponsiveness	13
Unilateral jerks, responsive	7
Generalized stiffness and nonresponsiveness	6
Staring	5
Incoherence	3
Generalized stiffness, responsive	1

(Courtesy of Lancman ME, Asconapé J, Craven WJ, et al: *Ann Neurol* 35:359–361, 1994.)

7 Pediatric Neurology

Neurodevelopment of Children Exposed In Utero to Phenytoin and Carbamazepine Monotherapy
Scolnik D, Nulman I, Rovet J, Gladstone D, Czuchta D, Gardner HA, Gladstone R, Ashby P, Weksberg R, Einarson T, Koren G (The Hosp for Sick Children, Toronto; Oshawa General Hosp, Ont, Canada; North York General Hosp, Ont, Canada; et al)
JAMA 271:767–770, 1994   122-96-7–1

Objective.—The lack of authoritative data on the relative risk and safety of antiepileptic drugs during pregnancy is causing confusion. Previous investigations have been difficult to interpret because of potential problems, such as confounding factors that may affect pregnancy outcome and polytherapy. Pregnancy outcome after phenytoin or carbamazepine monotherapy was compared with that in the general population, with emphasis on the cognitive function of offspring.

Study Design.—In a prospective, controlled, and blinded observational study, 36 mother-child pairs exposed to carbamazepine monotherapy and 34 pairs exposed to phenytoin monotherapy were compared with mother-child pairs exposed to nonteratogens, matched for maternal age, time of consultation, gravidity, parity, and socioeconomic status. The primary end point of the study was the children's global intelligence quotient (IQ), which was measured by the Bayley Mental Development Index or McCarthy Global Cognitive Index, according to the children's ages. Stepwise multiple regression analysis was used to verify whether the children's global IQ was affected by maternal age, IQ, and socioeconomic status.

Outcome.—All women were treated with phenytoin or carbamazepine during the first trimester; 29 women took phenytoin throughout pregnancy, and 30 continued taking carbamazepine. Children exposed to phenytoin in utero had a significantly lower mean global IQ score than their controls: the mean global IQ for children exposed to phenytoin was 103.1 compared with 113.4 in matched controls. Similarly, children exposed to phenytoin scored significantly lower on the Reynell developmental language scales. Seven children in the phenytoin group had a global IQ of 84 or less compared with only 1 among their matched controls, yielding a relative risk of 7 (95% confidence interval, 2.5–12.2). Maternal IQ, age, and socioeconomic status did not contribute to lowering children's global

IQ in the phenytoin group. In contrast, children exposed in utero to carbamazepine and their matched controls had similar results on the neurobehavioral tests.

Conclusions.—In utero exposure to phenytoin monotherapy has a clinically important adverse effect on neurobehavioral development, independent of maternal or environmental factors. Children exposed in utero to phenytoin have lower cognitive abilities than expected. In utero exposure to carbamazepine is not associated with similar effects. Carbamazepine therapy should be considered when clinically possible.

▶ This is a well-designed, prospective study. The results should be taken seriously and will influence my choice of anticonvulsants in pregnant women.—G.M. Fenichel, M.D.

Low-Dose Indomethacin and Prevention of Intraventricular Hemorrhage: A Multicenter Randomized Trial
Ment LR, Oh W, Ehrenkranz RA, Philip AGS, Vohr B, Allan W, Duncan CC, Scott DT, Taylor KJW, Katz KH, Schneider KC, Makuch RW (Yale Univ, New Haven, Conn; Brown Univ, Providence, RI; Maine Med Ctr, Portland)
Pediatrics 93:543–550, 1994   122-96-7–2

Background.—Risk for neurodevelopmental impairment is heightened in preterm infants with parenchymal intraventricular hemorrhage (IVH). Indomethacin may reduce the incidence of IVH in very-low-birth-weight infants because it modulates cerebral blood flow, serum prostaglandin levels, and germinal matrix microvascular maturation. The benefit of early administration of low-dose indomethacin on the incidence and severity of IVH in preterm neonates was evaluated.

Methods.—Two hundred nine neonates weighing 600–1,250 g with no evidence of IVH 6–11 hours after birth received IV indomethacin, 0.1 mg/kg, at 6–12 hours, with 2 additional doses given at 24-hour intervals; 222 neonates received an equal volume of saline placebo. Serial cranial ultrasound examinations and echocardiography were performed 24 and 48 hours after the first echocardiogram, on postnatal days 4, 5, 7, 14, and 21, and at 48 weeks.

Results.—Within the first 5 days, IVH developed in 25 neonates treated with indomethacin; only 1 had grade 4 IVH. Among placebo-treated neonates, 40 had IVH, of which 10 were grade 4. The death rates were comparable: 16 for indomethacin and 29 for placebo. However, the difference in survival time favored indomethacin treatment. Patent ductus arteriosus was noted in 86% of all neonates on the first postnatal day; with indomethacin, significant ductal closure occurred by the fifth day. Except for diminished urine output and confirmed or suspected necrotizing enterocolitis, the incidence of adverse events was comparable between treatments. None of the neonates with confirmed or suspected necrotizing enterocolitis died.

Conclusion.—Intravenous low-dose indomethacin administered at 6–12 hours of age is a beneficial addition to the medical management to neonates weighing less than 1,250 g, particularly those requiring assisted ventilation. This treatment significantly decreases the incidence and severity of IVH and causes few adverse drug events.

▶ The incidence of cerebral palsy in premature newborns has been increasing with the improved survival of very low-birth-weight newborns. Intraventricular-periventricular hemorrhage (PIVH) is one of the leading causes of chronic neurologic disability. Early treatment with low-dose indomethacin has been shown to prevent PIVH in animal models by reducing and modulating cerebral blood flow. This is the first study to show convincingly that indomethacin has a place in reducing the frequency and severity of PIVH in human infants. It is an important measure in the overall management of very low-birth-weight newborns.—G.M. Fenichel, M.D.

Rectal Diazepam for Prehospital Pediatric Status Epilepticus
Dieckmann RA (Univ of Calif, San Francisco)
Ann Emerg Med 23:216–224, 1994   122-96-7–3

Objective.—Parenteral diazepam is widely used for the prehospital management of pediatric status epilepticus. Because IV diazepam administration can cause apnea and respiratory depression, and because vascular access in young children is often difficult, the efficacy and safety of rectal diazepam in the prehospital management of pediatric status epilepticus were evaluated.

Methods.—During a 30-month study, 324 children with seizures were treated by paramedics in the field. Status epilepticus was defined as a generalized tonic-clonic, clonic, or tonic seizure that lasted for more than 15 minutes, or serial seizures lasting more than 20 minutes without intervening return of consciousness. Children with status epilepticus were treated with rectal diazepam, 0.2–0.5 mg/kg, or IV diazepam, 0.1–0.3 mg/kg, according to a prehospital protocol for pediatric seizures.

Results.—Thirty-six children (11%) met the criteria of status epilepticus. Sixteen children with a mean age of 3.0 years received rectal diazepam, and 13 (81%) of them stopped seizing within 10 minutes after receiving a single dose ranging from 0.16 to 0.57 mg/kg, but 4 of them had a recurrence before arriving at the emergency department (ED). The 3 children who did not stop seizing after rectal diazepam had serious underlying comorbidity. Fifteen children with a mean age of 9.1 years received IV diazepam, and all (100%) stopped having seizures after a single dose ranging from 0.03 to 0.33 mg/kg, but 9 of them had a recurrence before arriving at the ED. One child received both rectal and IV diazepam, and 6 received no drug therapy. None of the rectally treated children required prehospital endotracheal intubation for respiratory depression, but 2 were intubated in the emergency department. Two children who were treated with IV diazepam required prehospital intubation.

Conclusion.—Rectal diazepam is as effective as IV diazepam for the prehospital management of status epilepticus, and it is easier to administer.

▶ Diazepam suppositories are not commercially available in the United States, but they can be fabricated by a pharmacist. I regularly prescribe them for children with intractable epilepsy who have frequent episodes of status epilepticus. Parents administer a suppository at home when the child starts having repeated seizures. This approach has markedly reduced the number of emergency room visits and hospital admissions for this group of children. I recommend the use of diazepam suppositories as being safe and cost-effective.—G.M. Fenichel, M.D.

Autoantibodies to Glutamate Receptor GluR3 in Rasmussen's Encephalitis
Rogers SW, Andrews I, Gahring LC, Whisenand T, Cauley K, Crain B, Hughes TE, Heinemann SF, McNamara JO (VA Med Ctr, Salt Lake City, Utah; Duke Univ, Durham, NC; Salk Inst, La Jolla, Calif; et al)
Science 265:648–651, 1994   122-96-7–4

Introduction.—Rasmussen's encephalitis, a rare disease appearing in previously normal children, affects the cortex of a single cerebral hemisphere. The clinical features are intractable seizures, hemiparesis, and dementia. Standard therapy is surgical removal of the affected hemisphere. Behaviors typical of seizures and histopathologic features of Rasmussen's encephalitis were found in 2 rabbits immunized with the GluR3 protein during efforts to raise antibodies to recombinant glutamate receptors (GluRs).

Animal Model.—The rabbits had high titers of GluR3 antibodies and clinical features of the disease develop after 4 immunizations with GluR3 fusion protein. Microscopic examination of the brain revealed inflammatory changes consisting of microglial nodules and perivascular lymphocytic infiltration mainly in the cerebral cortex, together with lymphocytic infiltration of the meninges. These abnormalities were not observed in an asymptomatic rabbit immunized with GluR3 fusion protein.

Human Model.—Based on these findings, it was proposed that Rasmussen's encephalitis results from an autoimmune process directed at GluR3 protein. This idea was tested by measuring immunoreactivity toward GluR3 and other neural receptors in sera from 4 patients with Rasmussen's encephalitis, 4 age- and sex-matched children with epilepsy, 4 age- and sex-matched children without CNS disease, 5 children with active CNS inflammation, 4 other epileptic children, and 4 other normal children. Multiple sera samples from 2 patients with Rasmussen's encephalitis showed immunoreactivity to GluR3 fusion protein. A third patient exhibited weak reactivity to GluR2 fusion protein, and a fourth did not exhibit serum immunoreactivity to any tested antigen. No immunoreactivity was found in sera from 20 of 21 controls. One control showed immunoreactivity to GluR3 that was different from the serum GluR immunoreactivity observed in the patients with Rasmussen's encephalitis. Independent validation of GluR immunoreactivity in sera were obtained using transfected human embryonic kidney cells.

Conclusion.—When findings suggested that GluR3 antibodies could be pathogenic in Rasmussen's encephalitis, it was hypothesized that removal of GluR3 antibodies by recurrent plasma exchange might be beneficial. Repeated plasma exchanges in a severely ill child transiently reduced serum titers of GluR3 antibodies, decreased the frequency of her seizures, and improved neurologic function. An autoimmune process may thus underlie Rasmussen's encephalitis.

▶ Rasmussen's encephalitis is a poorly understood but well recognized clinical syndrome of childhood that is not established to be infectious or even inflammatory. *"Encephalitis"* is a misnomer. Like many things in neurology, case reports indicate a transitory beneficial response to the use of corticosteroids or intravenous immunoglobulin in affected children, although almost all affected children eventually require hemispherectomy to stop the seizures and progression of disease. The clinical and pathologic syndrome induced in rabbits is not a model of Rasmussen's encephalitis, but the presence of autoantibodies to GluR3 in affected children increases the interest in an immune-mediated basis for the disorder. Further work is needed to correlate the antibodies with the disease state and to explain the unilateral brain injury in response to a systemic abnormal immune response.—G.M. Fenichel, M.D.

Medical Treatment of Rasmussen's Syndrome (Chronic Encephalitis and Epilepsy): Effect of High-Dose Steroids or Immunoglobulins in 19 Patients

Hart YM, Cortez M, Andermann F, Hwang P, Fish DR, Dulac O, Silver K, Fejerman N, Cross H, Sherwin A, Caraballo R (Montreal Neurological Inst and Hosp, Canada; Hosp for Sick Children, Toronto, Canada; National Hosp for Neurology and Neurosurgery, London, England; et al)

Neurology 44:1030–1036, 1994   122-96-7–5

Introduction.—Rasmussen's syndrome (chronic encephalitis and epilepsy) is a rare progressive condition of unknown cause resulting in focal epilepsy, hemiparesis, and intellectual deterioration. Previous studies have suggested that intravenous immunoglobulins (IVIg), high-dose steroids, or both can control seizures and improve the end point of the disease. However, assessment of the efficacy of such treatments is difficult because of the rarity and variable progression of the condition.

Treatment.—Nineteen patients with Rasmussen's syndrome were treated with IVIg, high-dose steroids, or both, but the treatment protocols varied. The mean patient age at disease onset was 6 years, except for 2 patients with adult-onset disease. Fourteen patients had mild hemiparesis, 4 had evidence of intellectual deterioration, and 11 had epilepsia partialis continua. Biopsy specimens showed chronic encephalitis in all but 3 patients. The mean follow-up was 2 years.

Outcome.—Nine patients received IVIg, including 2 who concomitantly received high-dose steroids: 7 showed definite reduction in seizure frequency, although this was maintained in only 4 patients; 1 patient exhibited brief improvement in seizures and stabilization of the progress of the disease; and 1 showed no change. Seventeen patients were treated with steroids: 8 had greater than 50% reduction in seizure frequency and 2 showed a 25% reduction in seizure frequency. There was a slight improvement in hemiparesis, although this appeared to be related to improvement in seizure control. When steroids were withdrawn, seizure frequency increased in all but 2 patients whose improvement was maintained for at least 6 months after stopping steroids. Neither patient with adult-onset disease had significant improvement. There were no clear predictive factors for improvement, although patients receiving the highest doses of steroids tended to achieve greater improvement. The effect of treatment was not related to the duration of disease and age at onset. The side effects of the steroids were common, including steroid psychosis.

Summary.—The precise effect of IVIg and high-dose steroids in ameliorating the disease process in Rasmussen's syndrome is unknown. In view of the rarity of the condition, a central register should be developed using standardized treatment protocols. Treatment should be extended to children who have epilepsia partialis continua and who meet at least 1 of the following criteria to suggest the diagnosis of chronic encephalitis, including progressive neurologic deficit, progressive hemispheric atrophy on CT and/or MR imaging, presence of oligoclonal or monoclonal banding on CSF, and biopsy evidence of chronic encephalitis; and to children who do not have epilepsia partialis continua but have focal epilepsy and biopsy evidence of chronic encephalitis. Until more experience is gained, patients should be initially treated with IVIg. When there is no improvement, high-dose steroids should be tried.

▶ An immune-mediated basis for Rasmussen's syndrome is suspected because autoantibodies to GluR3 are detected in some affected children, and because corticosteroid and IVIg therapy sometimes are beneficial in reducing seizure frequency. Controlled clinical trials in Rasmussen's syndrome are almost impossible because the syndrome is relatively rare. Dr. Andermann and colleagues are proposing uniform diagnostic criteria and treatment protocols to use pooled multicenter data to evaluate currently suggested treatment regimens.—G.M. Fenichel, M.D.

Course and Outcome of Acute Cerebellar Ataxia
Connolly AM, Dodson WE, Prensky AL, Rust RS (Washington Univ, St Louis;

Univ of Wisconsin, Madison)
Ann Neurol 35:673–679, 1994   122-96-7–6

Background.—Acute cerebellar ataxia (ACA), a sudden disturbance in gait and balance, may develop in children after a variety of illnesses, usually varicella. Children with ACA in a major urban teaching hospital were studied to determine the long-term morbidity of ACA and to ascertain whether there are any clinical or laboratory predictors of outcome.

Methods and Findings.—All 73 children with a diagnosis of ACA who were seen at one center during a 23-year period were studied. Twenty-six percent had chickenpox; 52%, other viral illness; and 3%, immunization-related ataxia. No definite prodrome was identified in 19%. Sixty children were followed up for 4 months or more after the onset of ataxia. Ninety-one percent, including all those with chickenpox, completely recovered from ataxia. Eighty-nine percent of the children with non–varicella-related ACA had a complete recovery. Transient behavioral or intellectual problems occurred in 20% of the children followed up for more than 4 months. However, only 5 of 60 had sustained learning problems.

Conclusions.—This series is the largest reported, with the longest duration of follow up. Most patients recovered normal gait and fine motor control after 1–2 months. However, persistence of gait ataxia for 6 months did not predict outcome; most of these patients also fully recovered.

▶ The diagnosis of acute postviral cerebellar ataxia of childhood is made by its clinical features alone. The outcome is favorable. The disorder always has an explosive onset; symptoms are maximal at onset. Other disorders, such as neuroblastoma, need only be considered when the onset of symptoms progresses over several days or attacks are recurrent. Before the advent of CT and MRI, such children were never studied by arteriography or pneumoencephalography. Now they all have neuroimaging, and most have lumbar puncture. In obvious cases, it is more cost-effective to send the child home and consider only diagnostic testing if improvement is not seen after 2 weeks.—G.M. Fenichel, M.D.

High Prevalence of Antiphospholipid Antibodies in Children With Idiopathic Cerebral Ischemia

Angelini L, Ravelli A, Caporali R, Rumi V, Nardocci N, Martini A (Istituto Nazionale Neurologico "Carlo Besta," Milano, Italy; Universitá di Pavia, Italy)
Pediatrics 94:500–503, 1994   122-96-7–7

Background.—Numerous clinical studies have suggested that antiphospholipid antibodies (aPLs), identified as lupus anticoagulant (LA) or anticardiolipin antibody (aCL) on solid-phase assays, are frequently associated with thromboembolic phenomena. Several recent studies have also reported an association between stroke or transient ischemic attacks and aPLs in adults. Reported instances of aPL-positive primary stroke are limited in children, and no information on the prevalence of aPLs in unselected children with idiopathic cerebral ischemia is currently available. The frequency of LA and aCL in an unselected pediatric population with idiopathic cerebral ischemia was evaluated.

Patients and Methods.—Thirteen consecutive patients aged 5–16 years with idiopathic cerebral ischemia were prospectively evaluated. Of these, 8 had stroke, 3 had transient ischemic attack, and 2 had ocular ischemia. Twenty evidently healthy children within the same age range served as controls. Assessment of LA and aCL was performed within 3 days after the ischemic event and repeated at 3–6 months. Patients with either a positive LA test or positive IgG or IgM aCL at moderate-to-high levels in both determinations were considered aPL-positive. Various other laboratory and clinical evaluations were performed.

Results.—Positive determinations for either LA or aCL were noted in 10 of 13 patients. Cerebral CT scanning showed single or multiple hypodense areas in 6 of 8 patients with stroke and in 1 of 3 patients with transient ischemic attack. Isolated or multiple signal hyperintensities were noted in all patients with stroke or transient ischemic attack on MRI. No significant brain anomalies were detected via CT or MRI in patients with ocular ischemia. Clinical and radiologic features were similar between aPL-positive and aPL-negative patients, and laboratory findings were normal in all patients. In addition, no relationship between aPL status and results of evoked potentials, electroencephalography, and neuropsychometric assessment were observed. Five (50%) of those positive and 1 (33%) of the aPL-negative patients had a history of multiple ischemic events.

Conclusions.—Children with idiopathic cerebral ischemia have a very high prevalence of aPLs. Such patients should undergo evaluation for aPLs, because they have relevant treatment implications. Further studies using large samples are needed to determine the efficacy of various prophylactic regimens in children with persistent aPL positivity.

▶ This paper reinforces the many single case reports suggesting an association of aPLs with idiopathic thrombotic stroke in children. Most such children do not have lupus or other obvious immune-mediated disorders. Tests to measure aPLs are necessary in every child with thrombotic stroke, as positive results suggest the need for anticoagulation therapy.—G.M. Fenichel, M.D.

Cerebrovascular Disease in Children
Nagaraja D, Verma A, Taly AB, Veerendray Kumar M, Jayakumar PN (Natl Inst of Mental Health and Neurosciences, Bangalore, India)
Acta Neurol Scand 90:251–255, 1994   122-96-7–8

Introduction.—Stroke in children is rare because atherosclerosis generally is not a disorder of childhood. The causes of childhood stroke are difficult to diagnose and require extensive investigation. The clinical, radiologic, and biochemical characteristics of pediatric stroke patients were studied.

Methods.—Forty-three patients, aged 1–16 years, were given a diagnosis of nonhemorrhagic stroke over an 8-year period. Twenty-one were examined with cranial CT, 23 with angiography, and 11 with echocardiography. When indicated, hemorrhage and infection were excluded with a CSF examination. Blood and urine collections were analyzed.

Results.—The initial feature in most children was hemiplegia (86%), followed by convulsions (27%), fever (23%), speaking difficulty (23%), headache (11%), and altered consciousness (11%). Although 10 children had a history of fever before stroke, none had a preceding throat or ear infection, systemic or intracranial infection, enteric fever, or cardiac or pulmonary disease. Laboratory tests showed significantly reduced hemoglobin in 12 patients and an erythrocyte sedimentation rate above 20 mm/1st hour in 15. The CT showed infarction in 17 of 21 patients, it being bilateral in 5. Diffuse cortical atrophy was seen in 2 children, holo-hemispheric atrophy in 5, and focal atrophy in 5. The cortical, subcortical, and basal ganglia areas were involved in the infarctions. Cerebral angiography was abnormal in 18 children. Fifteen had bilateral abnormalities, including arteritis in 5, moyamoya disease in 6, fibromuscular dysplasia in 2, small vessel occlusion in 1, and superior sagittal sinus thrombosis in 1 patient. Three children had mitral valve prolapse proven by echocardiography.

Discussion.—Cranial CT and angiography are important and complimentary diagnostic modalities in the investigation of pediatric stroke. Angiographic evidence of arteritis in 6 patients without a history of systemic or intracranial infection suggests an immunologic etiology for the arteritis. The high incidence of basal ganglia involvement, detected by cranial CT, was a distinctive characteristic of pediatric stroke patients.

▶ Heart disease is no longer a major cause of stroke in children because the incidence of rheumatic fever has decreased and operative techniques for congenital heart disease have improved. Although the initial feature of stroke in children is hemiplegia, the underlying abnormalities are often bilateral vascular disease or an underlying coagulopathy. An intensive search for the cause is warranted in every child.—G.M. Fenichel, M.D.

The Brain in Infantile Autism: Posterior Fossa Structures Are Abnormal
Courchesne E, Townsend J, Saitoh O (Univ of California, San Diego, La Jolla)
Neurology 44:214–223, 1994   122-96-7-9

Background.—Early MRI studies found hypoplasia of posterior vermal lobules VI and VII and cerebellar hemispheres in most autistic patients. Recent autopsy analyses have found severe Purkinje neuron loss in the posterior vermis and hemispheres. Another type of cerebellar abnormality recently found in infantile autism is hyperplasia of posterior vermal lobules VI and VII. If the autistic samples in some MRI studies not detecting cerebellar hypoplasia were composed of both subtypes, then the autistic mean size reported in these studies would have appeared to be near the normal mean size only because it was the sum of the opposite subtypes.

Methods and Findings.—This possibility was tested by reassessing previously published vermal area measures of 78 autistic patients from 4 different studies. The autistic patient samples from these studies were composed of both the hypoplasia and hyperplasia subtypes. Cerebellar abnormalities were detected in 15 autopsy and quantitative MRI reports from 9 laboratories involving 226 autistic cases (Figs 7–1 and 7–2).

Conclusions.—Autism may be one of the first developmental neuropsychiatric disorders for which the location and type of neuroanatomical maldevelopment is in substantial accordance among several independent microscopic and macroscopic studies. Onset may occur as early as the second trimester. Discovering the etiologies underlying cerebellar maldevelopment may be key to understanding some of the causes of infantile autism.

▶ Hyperplasia and hypoplasia of the posterior vermal lobules VI and VII of the cerebellum are documented features of infantile autism. Autism is characterized primarily by cognitive and social disturbances and not by motor dysfunction. The importance of the cerebellar finding is that it dates the timing of the cerebral insult responsible for autism to the second trimester.—G.M. Fenichel, M.D.

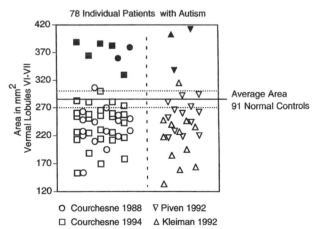

Fig 7–1.—Individual data from 4 studies showing the size of vermal lobules VI and VII in 78 autistic patients. Patients classed in the hypoplasia subtype are represented by *open symbols,* and those classed in the hyperplasia subtype are represented by *filled symbols.* The 2 studies of Courchesne et al. (*N Engl J Med* 318:1349–1354; *AJR* 162:123–130) are shown in the **left** column for comparison with data from Piven et al. (*Biol Psychiatry* 31:491–504, 1992) and Kleiman et al. (*Neurology* 42:753–760), which are shown in the **right** column. Autistic subjects represented in the **left** column had ranges of age and IQ very similar to those of autistic subjects represented in the right column. The mean size of vermal lobules VI and VII for 91 normal control subjects from 4 studies is marked by a *solid line,* with the 95% confidence interval (± 3 SE) marked by *dotted lines* above and below. (Courtesy of Courchesne E, Townsend J, Saitoh O: *Neurology* 44:214–223, 1994.)

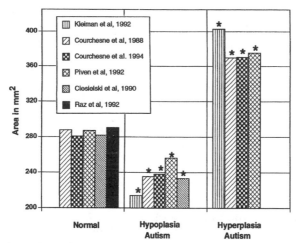

Fig 7–2.—Midsagittal area of vermal lobules VI and VII in autistic and normal subjects from 6 recent studies (see reference section of original article). Raz et al. conducted a normative study without autistic subjects. *Asterisks* denote areas significantly different from those of normal control subjects (*P* < .05). (Courtesy of Courchesne E, Townsend J, Saitoh O: *Neurology* 44:214–223, 1994.)

Rett Syndrome: Controlled Study of an Oral Opiate Antagonist, Naltrexone

Percy AK, Glaze DG, Schultz RJ, Zoghbi HY, Williamson D, Frost JD Jr, Jankovic JJ, del Junco D, Skender M, Waring S, Myer EC (Univ of Alabama, Birmingham; Baylor College of Medicine, Houston; Mayo Clinic and Found, Rochester, Minn; Med College of Virginia, Richmond)
Ann Neurol 35:464–470, 1994   122-96-7–10

Background.—Rett syndrome (RS) is characterized by mental retardation, movement, and communication dysfunction, breathing irregularities, growth failure, and seizures. The opiate antagonist, naltrexone, may be beneficial in individuals affected by this syndrome.

Methods.—Twenty-five patients with RS were enrolled in a randomized, double-blind, placebo-controlled crossover trial. The trial included 2 treatment periods lasting 4 months each, with an intervening 1-month washout.

Findings.—Because of significant sequence effects in the crossover design of the study, only data from the first part of the study were analyzed. Treatment had positive effects on certain respiratory characteristics, including reduced disorganized breathing during wakefulness. Forty percent of those receiving naltrexone progressed one or more clinical stages compared with none in the placebo group. The placebo group had a significantly higher adjusted end-of-treatment psychomotor test age. The other parameters measured did not change significantly.

Conclusions.—Naltrexone may modify some of the respiratory distur-bance in patients with RS. Reductions in motor function and more rapid disease progression suggest that it may have a deleterious effect.

▶ Rett syndrome is a devastating disorder of unknown etiology that occurs in infant girls. Several reports showing an increased concentration of β-en-dorphins in the CSF of affected girls led to several small trials of naltrexone which appeared to improve the abnormal breathing pattern. This controlled study shows that naltrexone may do more harm than good, and it should settle the question of its usefulness in Rett syndrome.—G.M. Fenichel, M.D.

Dystonia and Dyskinesia in Glutaric Aciduria Type I: Clinical Heteroge-neity and Therapeutic Considerations
Kyllerman M, Skjeldal OH, Lundberg M, Holme I, Jellum E, von Döbeln U, Fossen A, Carlsson G (Univ of Gothenburg, Göteborg, Sweden; Oslo Univ, Oslo, Norway; Huddinge Univ Hosp, Huddinge, Sweden; et al)
Mov Disord 9:22–30, 1994   122-96-7–11

Purpose.—Glutaric aciduria type I (GA-I) is a rare inherited neurometa-bolic disorder resulting from a glutaryl-CoA dehydrogenase deficiency, which causes defective degradation of tryptophan, lysine, and hydroxy-lysine. The onset of encephalopathy can be acute or insidious, and it usually occurs during the second part of the first year of life. Twelve new cases of GA-I were seen.

Patients.—Seven girls and 5 boys with GA-I, comprising all known cases in Norway and Sweden, received a diagnosis of GA-I at ages 9 months to 16 years. Ten children had a severe dystonic-dyskinetic disorder, 1 had a mild hyperkinetic disorder, and 1 was asymptomatic. Ten children under-went CT scanning of the brain and 3 were also examined with MRI.

Findings.—Two children died in a state of hyperthermia and shock. In 8 of 9 patients with an acute onset of encephalopathy, a severe dystonic syndrome developed and the patients became wheelchair bound. Dystonia and choreoathetosis had developed insidiously in 2 patients by age 4. One patient did not have any neurologic damage or functional impairment. Three children had macrocephaly. Radiographic examination revealed deep bitemporal spaces in 7 children. Neuropsychologic evaluation was performed in 8 children. All had extensive problems with verbal speech and motor performance. Three children had normal verbal comprehension and logical reasoning ability, 4 were mildly retarded, and 1 was in the severe mental retardation range. Treatment consisted of protein restric-tion, low lysine intake, and riboflavin supplementation. Supplementation with L-carnitine in patients with subnormal serum or muscle carnitine levels did not produce any clinical improvement. Drug therapy with L-dopa, baclofen, or sodium valproate was ineffective. Five long-term survivors gradually became emaciated. Percutaneous gastrostomy provided dramatic nutritional improvement within months accompanied by a marked reduction of the dystonia.

Conclusions.—Glutaric aciduria type-I has a much larger clinical variation than just severe dystonia. The diagnosis of GA-I is confirmed by enzyme assays of glutaryl Co-A dehydrogenase.

▶ The diagnosis of GA-I should be suspected in all infants who have dystonia develop during the first year of life. Dystonia usually occurs after an acute encephalopathy, but it may also develop insidiously. The abnormal urinary excretion of organic acids, which helps establish the diagnosis, is not constant. The optimal time to collect the specimen is during the encephalopathy or an intercurrent illness.—G.M. Fenichel, M.D.

Medium-Chain Acyl–Coenzyme A Dehydrogenase Deficiency: Clinical Course in 120 Affected Children
Iafolla AK, Thompson RJ, Roe CR (Duke Univ, Durham, NC)
J Pediatr 124:409–415, 1994   122-96-7–12

Objective.—Children with medium-chain acyl-coenzyme A dehydrogenase deficiency (MCAD), an autosomal recessively inherited disorder of β-oxidation, have episodic hypoglycemia, encephalopathy, apnea, and sudden death. Morbidity and mortality data were compiled in a retrospective study of 120 patients with MCAD.

Methods.—Physicians returned questionnaires on 120 patients with MCAD, aged 2–20 years. The parents of 48 patients also returned questionnaires. Twenty-two living patients were evaluated.

Results.—Nineteen percent of the children died before their disease was diagnosed. No children died of an illness related to MCAD after the disease was diagnosed. The average age at onset of symptoms was 12 months. At onset, 95% of patients required hospitalization or emergency care. In all patients, urine ketones were absent or lower than expected. In 85% of patients at onset, symptoms of infection were present. All 97 surviving patients were advised not to fast. The patients for whom medical and psychodevelopmental data were available were followed for an average of 2.6 years. Significant medical complaints included hypoglycemia, muscle weakness, seizures, failure to thrive, and "cerebral palsy." On routine developmental screening, 40% of children had abnormal results, including global developmental, behavioral, and speech disabilities, and attention deficit disorder (ADD). There was a significant association between ADD and female sex. Patients with ADD were older at diagnosis and were also significantly more likely to have seizures, encephalopathy, hyperammonemia, and more episodes of clinical illness.

Conclusion.—Newborns should be screened for MCAD deficiency, because children with this disease are at significant risk of death or developmental disabilities. Specific diagnostic tests for MCAD exist, and simple, effective, and inexpensive treatments are available.

▶ Four mitochondrial acyl-Coenzyme A dehydrogenases are described by the chain-length of their preferred substrates: short, medium, long, and very long. The first 3 types are located in the mitochondrial matrix, and deficiency causes recurrent coma or myopathy. Medium-chain acyl-coenzyme A dehydrogenase deficiency is the main cause of myopathy in "carnitine deficiency," which actually is a failure of carnitine to be transported across the mitochondrial membrane. Very long chain acyl-coenzyme A dehydrogenase is bound to the inner mitochondrial membrane, and deficiency causes exercise-induced myoglobinuria.—G.M. Fenichel, M.D.

8 Metabolic Disorders of the Nervous System

Clinical Diversity of Pyruvate Dehydrogenase Deficiency
Cross JH, Connelly A, Gadian DG, Kendall BE, Brown GK, Brown RM,
Leonard JV (Inst of Child Health, London; Hosp for Sick Children, London;
Univ of Oxford, England)
Pediatr Neurol 10:276–283, 1994   122-96-8-1

Background.—One of the most common causes of congenital lactic acidosis is pyruvate dehydrogenase deficiency (PDH). The majority of patients with PDH deficiency have a defect in the α-subunit of the E1 enzyme on the X chromosome. They are acutely ill and have a diverse range of clinical features in the neonatal period. The use of proton MR spectroscopy for the noninvasive examination of brain metabolites in children with suspected PDH was presented.

Methods.—Seven children (6 girls) with suspected metabolic disorder underwent proton MR spectroscopy. Plasma biochemistry, genetic testing, and spinal fluid analysis were also performed as part of the complete evaluation.

Results.—The early clinical problems of these patients were nonspecific and included failure to thrive, hypotonia, and developmental delay. Three children were seen with lactic acidosis in the neonatal period, and 2 had acute acidosis later in infancy. Those seen later had neurologic problems as well: 1 had Leigh encephalopathy and 1 had developmental regression after normal early development. No subsequent developmental progress was made by these infants, 3 had secondary microcephaly develop, and 3 had seizures develop. All had grossly increased lactate in their CSF as well as increased plasma levels of lactate. In 3 of the 4 children, PDH E1α immunoreactive protein was reduced. All of the children had MRI performed, and 6 demonstrated varying degrees of cerebral atrophy. The 6 children who also had proton MR spectroscopy performed demonstrated lactate in the brain in all cases. In those patients in whom 2 regions were examined regional variation in the lactate signal was observed.

Conclusions.—The diverse clinical presentation of children with PDH deficiency was confirmed. The biochemical basis of this diversity will be better understood with further genetic analysis and cranial MRI and MR spectroscopy.

▶ This report adds complexity to PDH deficiency, which is generally caused by mutations of the PDH E1α gene on the X chromosome. First, the phenotype is variable and, in some cases, is nothing more than arrest in development. Magnetic resonance spectroscopy or CSF measurement is required to demonstrate increased levels of lactate. Second, females with PDH deficiency are not uncommon. Inactivation of the X chromosome explains this in most patients, but the tissue variability of X chromosome inactivation may also render fibroblasts unsuitable for diagnostic studies. Biopsy of another tissue may be required!—D.A. Stumpf, M.D., Ph.D.

Carbohydrate-Deficient Glycoprotein Syndrome: Clinical Expression in Adults With a New Metabolic Disease
Stibler H, Blennow G, Kristiansson B, Lindehammer H, Hagberg B (Karolinska Hosp, Stockholm, Sweden; Univ Hosp, Lund, Sweden; East Hosp, Gothenburg, Sweden; et al)
J Neurol Neurosurg Psychiatry 57:552–556, 1994   122-96-8-2

Background.—The carbohydrate-deficient glycoprotein (CDG) syndromes are a newly identified group of recessively inherited disorders of glycoprotein metabolism. The symptoms of CDG syndrome type I in infancy and childhood are well described; the neurologic findings include psychomotor retardation, cerebellar and oculomotor dysfunction, peripheral neuropathy, comatose and strokelike episodes, epilepsy, and retinal pigmentary degeneration. The clinical findings of CDG syndrome type I in adults are less well known. The course and manifestations of CDG syndrome type I in 13 patients older than 15 years of age were described.

Patients.—The 13 patients (median age, 23 years) were drawn from 9 unrelated Swedish families. All patients had early-onset psychomotor retardation. Other features that were seen included slight facial dysmorphic features, some degree of hepatic dysfunction and, in 1 patient, pericardial effusion. Subcutaneous lipodystrophy and comatose or strokelike episodes occurred during childhood in about half the patients. After the age of 15 years, neurologic symptoms predominated, including nonprogressive ataxia associated with cerebellar hypoplasia, stable mental retardation, variable peripheral neuropathy, and strabismus. One third of the patients had generalized, usually sporadic, seizures. Retinal pigmentary degeneration and some degree of thoracic deformity were noted in all cases. None of the women had secondary sex characteristics develop, and the oldest woman had signs of premature aging. In contrast to pediatric patients, the adults had no severe internal organ symptoms. Serum concentrations of the biochemical marker carbohydrate-deficient transferrin were highly increased in all patients.

Conclusion.—The clinical expression of CDG syndrome type I in adults is described. The diagnosis is strongly suggested by the combination of early, nonprogressive mental retardation and cerebellar hypoplasia, variable peripheral neuropathy, strabismus, retinal pigmentary degeneration, thoracic deformity, and female hypogonadism. Analysis of serum transferrin isoforms confirms the diagnosis. Because the disease is nonprogressive, the patient can lead a socially functional, if dependent, lifestyle.

▶ About 80% of patients with CDG syndrome live into adulthood, and their neurologic disease stabilizes. Since its description in 1991, these authors have found the disorder in 60 patients on 3 continents, which suggests that the disorder may not be uncommon. The combination of mental retardation, ataxia, and strabismus is suggestive of the diagnosis. The history from childhood is more stormy, including seizures, strokelike episodes, and bouts of coma. Hypogonadism is prominent in females. A biochemical defect, not yet identified, likely affects catabolism or transport of glycoproteins. A variety of proteins are carbohydrate deficient, most notably transferrin, which is assayed by isoelectric focusing in several centers in the United States.—D.A. Stumpf, M.D., Ph.D.

Mitochondrial Encephalomyopathy: Correlation of P-31 Exercise MR Spectroscopy With Clinical Findings
Kuhl CK, Layer G, Träber F, Zierz S, Block W, Reiser M (Univ of Bonn, Germany; Ludwig-Maximilians-Universität, Munich, Germany)
Radiology 192:223–230, 1994   122-96-8-3

Objective.—Phosphorus-31 exercise MR spectroscopic studies of energy metabolism in muscle have been used to investigate mitochondrial encephalomyopathies. Routine clinical use of the technique has not been adopted because of problems with interpretation and evaluation of the spectra. The diagnostic capability and sensitivity of exercise MR spectroscopy were evaluated in 14 patients with mitochondrial encephalomyopathy.

Methods.—Phosphorus 31 spectra of calf muscles were obtained in 14 patients with mitochondrial encephalomyopathy and in 18 healthy, sedentary volunteers before, during, and after standard exercises. Lactate levels, pH time courses, and the phosphocreatine index (PCr) were determined.

Results.—All patients had external ophthalmoplegia and ragged red muscle fibers, 9 had paresis, and 11 were exercise intolerant. Myopathic changes were observed in 8 patients. Serum levels of creatine phosphate were elevated in 6 patients, and those of lactic dehydrogenase were increased in 5 patients. There was a significant correlation between the conventional test score and the PCr index. Conventional scores and PCr indices were significantly correlated with skeletal muscle involvement in 11 patients, with 1 patient having maximum skeletal muscle affects, 3 severe muscle affects, 2 mild disease, and 5 minor muscle affects. The pH parameters were not significantly correlated with clinical test scores.

Conclusion.—Phosphorus-31 exercise MR spectroscopy PCr indices represent a valuable diagnostic tool for determining the extent of muscle disease in patients with mitochondrial encephalomyopathy.

▶ Patients with mitochondrial myopathies frequently have exertional muscle weakness and sometimes pain, in combination with a progressive myopathy in many cases. Use of phosphorus-31 MR spectroscopy has previously been reported in a small number of cases to show a number of abnormalities of high-energy phosphate metabolism. This is one of the largest series of cases, and it shows examples of low PCr at rest, excessive depletion of PCr on exercise, and lack of exercise-induced acidosis. These findings suggest that phosphorus-31 exercise MR spectroscopy may be of value in noninvasive evaluation of such patients for diagnostic purposes.— W.G. Bradley, D.M., F.R.C.P.

Ophthalmoplegia Demylelinating Neuropathy, Leukoencephalopathy, Myopathy, and Gastrointestinal Dysfunction With Multiple Deletions of Mitochondrial DNA: A Mitochrondrial Multisystem Disorder in Search of a Name

Unicini A, Servidei S, Silvestri G, Manfredi G, Sabatelli M, Di Muzio A, Ricci E, Mirabella M, Di Mauro S, Tonali P (Univ of Chieti, Italy; Univ of Rome; UILDM Research Ctr for Neuromuscular Diseases of Rome, et al)
Muscle Nerve 17:667–674, 1994   122-96-8–4

Objective.—Mitochondrial multisystem disorders are characterized by a combination of cortical dysfunctions. Gastrointestinal dysfunction is a rare functional disorder. An occurrence of myopathy and neuropathy, external ophthalmoplegia, and gastrointestinal encephalopathy (MNGIE syndrome) was reported in a patient with multiple mitochondrial DNA (mtDNA) deletions.

Methods.—Motor and sensory nerve conductions were recorded, and muscle and sural nerve biopsies were performed. The DNA was extracted from muscle and blood and was mapped.

Results.—Woman, 37, had peripheral neuropathy, external ophthalmoplegia, and diarrhea. Motor conduction velocities were slow, there was extensive temporal dispersion, and cranial MRI was abnormal with focal hyperintensities. There were no signs of CNS involvement. Lactic acidosis was present. There was demyelination of the sural nerve. Muscle biopsy specimens showed ragged red fibers, and multiple deletions of mtDNA were detected in the muscle.

Conclusion.—Three previously reported cases appeared to be autosomal recessive for MNGIE, and the severity and duration of disease correlated with the number of deletions. In this patient, although a large number of deletions were found, there was only mild muscle weakness and a few ragged red fibers. This patient is the first to have this syndrome and multiple mtDNA deletions. It remains to be seen whether the multiple deletions are the cause of the syndrome or are a concurrent consequence.

▶ Mitochondrial disorders affect energy-consuming tissues: brain, muscle, heart, liver, and the renal tubule. Recently—but not surprisingly—the gastrointestinal mucosa was added to the list. Other tissues are sometimes affected, including the peripheral nerve or erythrocytes (sideroblastic anemia). Recognized, distinctive syndromes are Kearns-Sayre, MELAS, and MERFF. The new and emerging syndrome, which is further elucidated in this study and is referred to as MNGIE, POLIP, or MEPOP, produces encephalopathy, sensorimotor polyneuropathy, ophthalmoplegia, and pseudo-obstruction of the bowel (diarrhea, distension and cramping). Muscle biopsy and mtDNA analysis facilitate the diagnosis.—D.A. Stumpf, M.D., Ph.D.

Cerebral Hyperemia in MELAS
Gropen TI, Prohovnik I, Tatemichi TK, Hirano M (State Univ of New York, Brooklyn; Columbia-Presbyterian Med Ctr, New York)
Stroke 25:1873–1876, 1994   122-96-8-5

Background.—The pathophysiology of strokelike episodes in mitochondrial encephalomyopathy, lactic acidosis, and strokelike episodes (MELAS) remains unclear. A case report demonstrated findings to support the possibility that local production of lactic acid may be the basis of strokelike events.

Case Report.—Man, 24, was admitted to a hospital after a generalized seizure. Magnetic resonance imaging and CT revealed infarction in the left parietal, temporal, and occipital lobes. Quantitative planar ^{133}Xe regional cerebral blood flow examinations were done at 15 and 26 days and at 4 and 8 months after the strokelike episode. At 15 and 26 days, there was generalized hyperperfusion, which was highest in infarcted areas. Four and 8 months after the strokelike episode, the brain was still hyperemic, with highest flow occurring in the noninfarcted tissue. Reactivity to carbon dioxide was below normal within the infarct region when first tested at 26 days, but it was normal thereafter, improving on each subsequent examination. In the noninfarcted region, vasomotor reactivity was restricted at 4 months, when resting flows were at their peak.

Conclusion.—It is unclear whether the hyperemia persisting in this case report represents an attempt to compensate for metabolic imbalance or a passive response to tissue acidosis. The observations support the possibility that local production of lactic acid may be the basis for strokelike events and other cerebral signs of MELAS, and they emphasize the limitations of nonquantitative functional imaging in the investigation of diseases with diffuse alterations of cerebral flow.

▶ The pathophysiologic basis of the brain changes described as stroke in patients with MELAS remains uncertain. This study demonstrated increased cerebral blood flow throughout the normal brain of a patient with MELAS. The vasomotor reactivity to carbon dioxide was less than normal in the noninfarcted regions. It was suggested that the hyperemia was caused by local production of lactic acid resulting from the MELAS defect. The mechanism and pathology of the strokelike syndrome are still unknown.—W.G. Bradley, D.M., F.R.C.P.

9 Neurogenetics

Autosomal Dominant Cerebellar Ataxia With Pigmentary Macular Dystrophy
Enevoldson TP, Sanders MD, Harding AE (Natl Hosp for Neurology and Neurosurgery; London; Inst of Neurology, London)
Brain 117:445–460, 1994   122-96-9-1

Introduction.—Although the autosomal dominant cerebellar ataxias (ADCAs) were first described more than 100 years ago, their classification continues to pose problems. However, regardless of whether a clinical or pathologic classification is used, ADCA occurring with a pigmentary macular dystrophy is distinct from all other types. Previous reports of ADCA with pigmentary macular dystrophy have included no more than 4 small pedigrees. The clinical and genetic characteristics of 8 affected families were reviewed.

Patients.—The subjects of the review were 54 members of 8 families with a distinct ADCA associated with visual failure caused by pigmentary macular dystrophy. Thirty-four were male and 20 female; the age at onset ranged from 6 months to 60 years. The ratio of affected to unaffected offspring of patients or obligate carriers was 31:34. In two thirds of the cases, the symptom seen was ataxia only; the rest were seen with visual failure with or without ataxia. Patients with early disease manifestations often had subtle macular abnormalities, even those with moderately reduced visual acuity. Pyramidal tract signs and a supranuclear ophthalmoplegia were sometimes present as well. The clinical course was highly variable, even within families. Some patients had a rapidly progressive, infantile-onset phenotype; in these cases, transmission was always from an affected father.

Conclusion.—The genetic features of patients with ADCA with pigmentary macular dystrophy are similar to those reported in patients with myotonic dystrophy and Huntington's disease. Thus, gene mutation in ADCA with pigmentary macular dystrophy is also likely to consist of an unstable trinucleotide repeat expansion.

▶ Autosomal dominant cerebellar ataxias were once a classification nightmare, primarily because of the large phenotypic variation within single families. Modern genetics and good clinicians have brought clarity to the situation. The rather typical form (ADCA I) has now been mapped to 3 different chromosomes (6, 12 and 14). Molecular diagnosis is available for mutations of the one gene that has been cloned (SCA-I, chromosome 6). The variable age of onset, generally anticipation, correlates with amplification of trinucleotide repeats. Autosomal dominant cerebellar ataxia with retinal degeneration appear to be a distinct disease and, observing anticipation, the authors hypothesize another trinucleotide repeat mutation.—D.A. Stumpf, M.D., Ph.D.

Machado-Joseph Disease in Pedigrees of Azorean Descent is Linked to Chromosome 14

St George-Hyslop P, Rogaeva E, Huterer J, Tsuda T, Santos J, Haines JL, Schlumpf K, Rogaev EI, Liang Y, McLachlan DRC, Kennedy J, Weissenbach J, Billingsley GD, Cox DW, Lang AE, Wherrett JR (Univ of Toronto; The Hosp for Sick Children, Toronto; Hosp de Ponta Delgada, Ponta Delgada, Azores; et al)
Am J Hum Genet 55:120–125, 1994   122-96-9-2

Objective.—Machado-Joseph disease (MJD) is a pleomorphic neurodegenerative disease inherited as an autosomal dominant trait. It was originally found in patients of Azorean descent, but was recently detected in people of Japanese origin in whom a genetic defect was found on chromosome 14. It was determined whether MJD diagnosed in patients of Azorean descent also had a defect on chromosome 14, and the cause of the variability found with this disease was investigated.

Methods.—Five people with MJD pedigrees were classified as affected or asymptomatic. Their genomic DNA was isolated, and the genotype was established.

Results.—Testing of markers furnished significant proof of genetic linkage at chromosome 14q, with placement of MJD occurring between D14S67 and AACT. One homozygous patient had early onset of symptoms (age 16 years), whereas the disease usually manifests itself in the third, fourth, and fifth decades.

Conclusion.—It appears that the Azorean and Japanese patients have the same disease, but not necessarily the same mutation. There is much variability in the age at onset and severity of the disease. Additional phenotypic and molecular studies need to be done to refine the location of the MJD defect.

▶ The pace of genetic progress accelerates as more basic data accumulates. The research on ataxia is illustrative of this. Shortly after this article appeared, the MJD gene was cloned—at the time, the 7th trinucleotide repeat mutation and the 3rd cloned ataxia gene (1). Since then, the ataxia telangiectasia and vitamine E–deficient ataxia (2) genes were cloned, and the Wilson's, SCA1, and MJD genes were further characterized (3–5). The Freidreich's and SCA2 gene map regions are narrowing. We should not contain the excitement this brings, because it is uplifting to our patients, who now have tangible reasons for optimism.—D.A. Stumpf, M.D., Ph.D.

References

1. Kawaguchi Y, Okamoto T, Taniwaki M, et al: CAG expansions in a novel gene for Machado-Joseph disease at chromosome 14q32.1 *Nat Genet* 8:221–227, 1994.
2. Ouahchi K, Arita M, Kayden H, et al: Ataxia with isolated vitamin E deficiency is caused by mutations in the alpha-tocopherol transfer protein. *Nat Genet* 9:141–145, 1995.
3. Thomas GR, Forbes JR, Roberts EA, et al: The Wilson disease gene: Spectrum of mutations and their consequences. *Nat Genet* 9:210–217, 1995.
4. Kawakami H, Maruyama H, Nakamura S, et al: Unique features of the CAG repeats in Machado-Joseph disease. *Nat Genet* 9:344–345, 1995.
5. Ching SS, McCall AE, Cota J, et al: Gametic and somatic tissue-specific heterogeneity of the expanded SCA1 CAG repeat in spinocerebellar ataxia type 1. *Nat Genet* 10:344–350, 1995.

10 Behavioral Neurology

Performance-Based Driving Evaluation of the Elderly Driver: Safety, Reliability, and Validity
Odenheimer GL, Beaudet M, Jette AM, Albert MS, Grande L, Minaker KL
(Brockton/West Roxbury VA Med Ctr, Mass; New England Research Inst, Watertown, Mass; Harvard Med School, Boston)
J Gerontol 49:153M–159M, 1994   122-96-10–1

Objective.—An attempt was made to develop a road test encompassing a wide range of difficulty to evaluate elderly drivers possessing varying cognitive skills.

The Test.—A 10-mile test was designed to take about 45 minutes to complete. A closed-course component was intended to measure performance in difficult vehicular maneuvers, and also it served as a safety screen before the in-traffic phase. The driver was required to drive straight, turn to either side, back up, park at an angle and parallel, and drive between cones in both directions. The in-traffic part of the test progressed from driving on residential streets to congested areas and the freeway. It focuses on situations that tend to cause older drivers trouble, such as merging into rapid traffic and turning left at a busy intersection.

Validation.—Thirty licensed drivers older than 60 years of age were evaluated. Nine were referred from medical and dementia clinics, 4 from the community, and 17 from studies of normal aging. Each subject was accompanied by an instructor and 2 independent research raters who rode in the rear of the car. A masked design was used in which cognitive test scores were correlated with the raters' scores of driving performance.

Results.—Significant correlations were obtained between the "criterion standard" and both closed-course and in-traffic performance scores. In-traffic scores correlated with cognitive test scores (table). Inter-rater reliability was .84 for the closed-course part of the test and .74 for the in-traffic component. The values for internal consistency were .78 for closed-course and .89 for in-traffic. Age correlated negatively with both the instructor's global score and the in-traffic research score, but not with the closed-course ratings.

Conclusion.—This road test appears to be a safe and reliable means of assessing the driving ability of older individuals possessing varying cognitive skills.

Correlations Between Cognitive Tests and In-Traffic Scores

Measures	n	In-traffic Score	Age-adjusted In-traffic Score
Mini-Mental State Exam (20)	30	.72**	.72**
Traffic sign recognition	30	.65**	.69**
Visual memory (21)	30	.54**	.50**
Verbal memory (21)	29	.51**	.37*
Trials A (22)	29	.52**	.33*
Simple reaction time (23)	26	−.25	−.12
Complex reaction time (23)	16	−.70**	−.58**

A high score on all tests except the reaction time tasks indicates good performance. Therefore, reaction time scores are negatively correlated with the other tests.
* $P < 0.05$.
** $P < 0.01$.
Pearson r correlation coefficients (2-tailed).
Abbreviation: n, number of subjects completing the task.
(Courtesy of Odenheimer GL, Beaudet M, Jette M, et al: *J Gerontol* 49:153M–159M, 1994.)

▶ One of the most troubling problems in caring for elderly patients who have neurodegenerative disorders can be deciding when the patient must stop driving a car. On the one hand, giving up driving is a burdensome restriction on personal freedom, except perhaps in communities where stores and other amenities are geographically concentrated or public transport is readily available for those patients who can still manage to use it. On the other hand, an automobile is potentially a lethal weapon, both for those in it and for others on the street. This article describes a structured test of driving ability, using a real car. Other investigators have used simulators to test driving performance. What are needed are relatively clear, statistically validated guidelines relating performance in structured driving tests to the risk of driving in real life, to enable clinicians to provide more precise and, therefore, more confident information on when a patient must give up the privilege of driving a car.—J.P. Blass, M.D., Ph.D.

Are Semantic Systems Separately Represented in the Brain: The Case of Living Category Impairment
De Renzi E, Lucchelli F (Univ of Modena, Italy; S. Carlo Hosp, Milan, Italy)
Cortex 30:3–25, 1994   122-96-10-2

Introduction.—An occasional patient exhibits disproportionate impairment in his or her knowledge of certain types of objects, specifically animate objects such as animals, fruits and vegetables, and flowers. The deficit is apparent whether stimuli are presented in word or in picture form.

Case Report.—Woman, 49, was febrile and drowsy for a few days and became progressively confused. Encephalitis was diagnosed. The patient was comatose for 3 days despite acyclovir treatment but then regained consciousness. A CT study showed hypodense areas in the frontobasal region of the left hemisphere and the temporoinsular regions of both hemispheres. A month later, the patient was totally anosmic and exhibited severe anomia on confrontation testing. Visual naming of fruits, vegetables, and animals was impaired. The patient was markedly amnesic for past and recent memories of personal and public events. Periodic testing revealed a stable pattern characterized by a dissociation between the patient's semantic knowledge of living and nonliving things. Magnetic resonance imaging revealed damage to the anteromedial regions of both temporal lobes, more marked on the left side. Neuropsychological testing of the patient along with 10 normal age- and education-matched women confirmed that the patient's performance was most impaired for animals and flowers and moderately impaired for fruits and vegetables, but almost perfect for inanimate objects.

Interpretation.—This form of specific semantic impairment now is thought to be a possible result of herpes simplex encephalitis. The fundamental error involves a failure to retrieve those perceptual features that define categories of living objects. A block of access, rather than degradation in storage, probably is responsible. The deficit potentially can disrupt all types of category but, in the case of man-made objects, the close correspondence between shape and function provides an alternative means of access to their structured representations.

▶ This type of deficit has been reported mainly with *H. simplex* encephalitis but, also, in Alzheimer's disease, head trauma, and vascular disease. The fascination with this deficit lies in the fact that distinct semantic categories are affected while others are spared (in this case, animate vs. inanimate objects). In other category-specific anomias, syntactic rather than semantic categories, nouns may be spared while verbs are affected (e.g., foot/kick). The left temporal lobe is uniformly involved, although in one case of anomia for facial expressions, the right temporal lobe was injured. The recognition of animacy may be present in other animals, suggesting perhaps an innately special category for animate objects. Some have argued that studies do not adequately control for familiarity and frequency of occurrence, thereby leading to artifactual discrepancies between groups of words; however, by now these arguments have been adequately addressed, and the notion of category-specific aphasic disorders has been well established in the literature.—A.M. Galaburda, M.D.

A Potential Noninvasive Neurobiological Test for Alzheimer's Disease
Scinto LFM, Daffner KR, Dressler D, Ransil BI, Rentz D, Weintraub S, Mesulam M, Potter H (Brigham and Women's Hosp, Boston; Harvard Med School, Boston; Beth Israel Hosp, Boston)
Science 266:1051–1054, 1994   122-96-10–3

Background.—At present, Alzheimer's disease can only be definitively diagnosed by histologic examination of brain tissue taken at autopsy or biopsy. Accordingly, early, noninvasive, sensitive, and easily administered diagnostic tests are needed. In patients with clinically diagnosed Alzheimer's disease, a hypersensitivity to the pupil dilating effect of tropicamide, an acetylcholine receptor antagonist, has been observed. The tropicamide pupil dilation test was investigated for its ability to detect patients with Alzheimer's disease.

Patients and Methods.—The 58 participants were divided into 5 groups. Fourteen patients with probable Alzheimer's disease previously diagnosed according to standard clinical criteria comprised group 1. Group 2 included 4 patients with a diagnosis of non-Alzheimer's type dementia. The remaining 40 elderly individuals were assigned to 1 of 3 control groups, including 32 normal participants, 5 participants with suspected Alzheimer's, and 3 cognitively abnormal participants. After recording baseline measurements of pupil diameter, 1 drop of a very dilute tropicamide solution was placed in 1 eye, and 1 drop of sterile water was placed in the other eye. The individual applying the drops was blinded to solutions. Data on pupil diameter were obtained for each eye at scheduled times during a 1-hour period.

Results.—In comparison with normal controls, all of whom had a minimal increase in pupil diameter in 60 minutes, patients with a diagnosis of probable Alzheimer's disease showed a pronounced pupillary response. Those in the suspect Alzheimer's and cognitively abnormal control groups

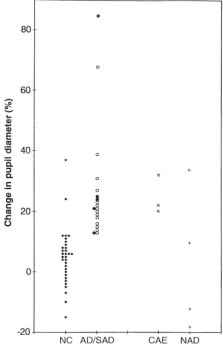

Fig 10–1.—Individual pupil dilation scores (percent change over baseline) at minute 29 for patients with probable Alzheimer's disease and all controls. *Abbreviations: NC,* normal elderly controls; *AD/SAD,* patients with Alzheimer's disease and those with suspected Alzheimer's dementia; *CAE,* cognitively abnormal elderly patients; *NAD,* patients with non-Alzheimer's type dementia. (Courtesy of Scinto LFM, Daffner KR, Dressler D, et al: *Science* 266:1051–1054, 1994.)

had a pattern of pupillary response similar to that seen in patients with clinically diagnosed probable Alzheimer's disease, whereas normal controls and those in the non-Alzheimer's dementia group had a comparable response. The complete set of data for the minute 29 sampling point (the point of maximal separation of patients with clinically diagnosed Alzheimer's disease and normal controls) showed a clear between-group distinction based on hypersensitivity to tropicamide (Fig 10–1). It was possible to distinguish 18 of the 19 individuals who were either diagnosed with or suspected of having Alzheimer's disease from 30 of the 32 normal elderly controls.

Conclusions.—The tropicamide pupil dilation test might be able to detect patients with Alzheimer's disease early in the disease process, when they could most benefit from therapies designed to slow disease progression. This test is safe, relatively noninvasive, sensitive, and easy to quantitate with available automated instrumentation, unlike other biochemical and physiologic tests currently in development.

▶ Alzheimer's disease is characterized by, among other things, failure of cholinergic systems, which in turn is considered an important factor in the memory loss seen in this disorder. This study indicates that the cholinergic innervation of the pupil also fails early in patients with Alzheimer's disease. This knowledge can be used to diagnose Alzheimer's disease early, at a time when any available therapy is more likely to be successful. Since the publication of this study, no other studies have been published to either support or refute these findings, but it is expected that other groups are attempting to confirm the findings before they can be accepted as clinically useful.— A.M. Galaburda, M.D.

ApoE ε4 Allelic Association With Alzheimer's Disease: Independent Confirmation Using Denaturing Gradient Gel Electrophoresis
Peacock ML, Fink JK (Univ of Michigan, Ann Arbor)
Neurology 44:339–341, 1994   122-96-10–4

Background.—Evidence suggests that apolipoprotein E (ApoE) is associated with Alzheimer's disease (AD). ApoE, deposited with β-amyloid in senile plaques, binds to β-amyloid in vitro. Generally, determining ApoE genotypes involves isoelectric focusing or techniques that rely on oligonucleotide hybridizations. Denaturing gradient gel electrophoresis (DGGE) was used to detect currently known and novel polymorphisms in the ApoE coding sequence.

Methods and Findings.—With denaturing gradient gel electrophoresis, ApoE ε2, ε3, and ε4 alleles were identified in 135 control subjects and 57 patients with AD. When compared with control subjects, patients with AD had a marked increase in ApoE ε4 allele frequency. The distribution of ApoE genotypes was almost identical to that predicted by the Hardy-Weinberg equation (table).

Apolipoprotein E Allele and Genotype Frequencies in Patients With Alzheimer's Disease and Control Subjects

	ApoE allele frequencies (%)			ApoE genotypes*					
	ϵ2	ϵ3	ϵ4	ϵ2, ϵ2	ϵ2, ϵ3	ϵ2, ϵ4	ϵ3, ϵ3	ϵ3, ϵ4	ϵ4, ϵ4
Clinically evaluated control subjects (n = 109)	10.5	75.7	13.8	1 (1)	17 (17)	4 (3)	65 (62)	18 (23)	4 (2)
Autopsy-evaluated control subjects (n = 26)	3.8	78.8	17.3	0 (0)	2 (2)	0 (0)	15 (16)	9 (7)	0 (1)
Autopsy-verified AD (n = 57)	4.4	55.3	40.3	0 (0)	3 (3)	2 (2)	17 (17)	26 (25)	9 (9)

* Values predicted by the Hardy-Weinberg equation are given in parentheses.
(Courtesy of Peacock ML, Fink JK: *Neurology* 44:339–341, 1994.)

Conclusions.—The independent finding of a marked association between ApoE ϵ4 allele and AD further suggests that ApoE plays a role in the pathogenesis of AD. In a population at genetic equilibrium, allele frequencies generally have a homogeneous distribution.

▶ A question regarding the association between ApoE ϵ4 and AD has been whether this simply represents a case of linkage disequilibrium. However, no relationship was detected with apolipoprotein C-II, which makes this interpretation unlikely. Instead, the inhomogeneity of allele representation in AD is likely to represent a true biological association with a possible causal role. However, AD appears to be a heterogeneous group of disorders with several possible loci of association, including loci on chromosome 21, chromosome 14 and, now, concerning ApoE ϵ4, on chromosome 19.—A.M. Galaburda, M.D.

Confirmation of the ϵ4 Allele of the Apolipoprotein E Gene as a Risk Factor for Late-Onset Alzheimer's Disease

Brousseau T, Legrain S, Berr C, Gourlet V, Vidal O, Amouyel P (Serlia INSERM U325, Lille, France; Hôpital P Brousse, Villejuif, France; INSERM U360, Villejuif, France)
Neurology 44:342–344, 1994   122-96-10–5

Background.—Family studies have suggested a link between the q13.2 region of chromosome 19 and Alzheimer's disease (AD). An apolipoprotein E isoform, whose gene maps in this region, is found more often in AD. The possible relationship between a genetic polymorphism of the apolipoprotein E gene and late-onset AD was investigated.

Methods and Findings.—The apolipoprotein E polymorphism distribution in 36 patients with sporadic late-onset AD and 38 control subjects of the same age was compared. All subjects were older than 65 years of age.

Forty-two percent of the patients and only 10.5% of the control subjects carried at least one ε4 allele.

Conclusions.—The distribution of apolipoprotein E genotypes differs between patients with late-onset AD and controls. Late-onset AD appears to be associated with the 19q13.2 region containing the apolipoprotein E gene locus.

▶ This is among the latest articles reporting a relationship between apolipoprotein E ε4 and late-onset Alzheimer's disease (AD). Moreover, the chromosome 19 locus for this protein is also linked to the clinical phenotype. Apolipoprotein E binds to the β-amyloid peptide and is present in senile neuritic plaques in AD, which indicates that the relationship between apolipoprotein E and AD is not likely to be fortuitous. In other disorders where amyloid is deposited, a relationship to apolipoprotein E ε4 has not been demonstrated.—A.M. Galaburda, M.D.

Nonsteroidal Anti-Inflammatory Drugs in Alzheimer's Disease

Rich JB, Rasmusson DX, Folstein MF, Carson KA, Kawas C, Brandt J (Johns Hopkins Univ, Baltimore, Md)
Neurology 45:51–55, 1995   122-96-10–6

Background.—Postmortem studies of the brains of patients with Alzheimer's disease (AD) have found evidence of immune-mediated autodestructive processes, suggesting that anti-inflammatory medications might play a therapeutic role in AD. Many lines of evidence support an inverse relationship between anti-inflammatory medications and AD, including the low prevalence of AD among patients with rheumatoid arthritis. A large sample of AD patients were reviewed to further examine the role of nonsteroidal anti-inflammatory drugs (NSAIDs) on the clinical features and progression of the disease.

Methods.—Of 210 consecutive patients with probable or possible AD, 32 were taking aspirin or NSAIDS on a daily basis and 177 were not. The 2 groups were compared by various clinical, cognitive, and psychiatric measures. Changes in neuropsychologic scores one year later were calculated to see if NSAID use affected the rate of progression of AD.

Findings.—At baseline, the NSAID group had a significantly shorter duration of illness than the non-NSAID group, 3.1 vs. 4.2 years. After adjustment for this difference, the NSAID group still showed significantly better performance on the Mini-Mental State Examination, the Boston Naming Test, and the delayed condition of the Benton Visual Retention Test. One year later, the NSAID patients demonstrated less decline on measures of verbal fluency, spatial recognition, and orientation than the non-NSAID group.

Conclusions.—Nonsteroidal anti-inflammatory drugs play a protective role in the risk, severity, and progression of AD. The protective function of NSAIDs may involve their primary anti-inflammatory properties, free-radical quenching, or a combination of these factors. Further studies are needed to address the issue of specificity by comparing the effects of NSAIDs with those of other medications.

▶ This is one of several articles suggesting an important role of inflammation in the pathogenesis of AD. Acute-phase proteins are elevated in the serum and are deposited in amyloid plaques. There are activated migroglia and stainable inflammatory cytokines, as well as complement components and C-reactive protein. On the other hand, these findings are not present in scrapie-induced amyloid in mice, suggesting that amyloid and inflammation are separate events and may be amenable to separate treatments.—A.M. Galaburda, M.D.

Pathologic Findings in a Case of Primary Progressive Aphasia
Scheltens P, Ravid R, Kamphorst W (Free Univ Hosp, Amsterdam; Netherlands Inst for Brain Research, Amsterdam)
Neurology 44:279–282, 1994   122-96-10–7

Objective.—The incidence of primary progressive aphasia (PPA) is rare and histopathologically heterogeneous, being associated with Alzheimer's disease, Pick's disease, or nonspecific cortical degeneration. The histopathologic and immunohistochemical changes in the brain of a patient with PPA who had Pick's disease diagnosed were presented.

Case Report.—Man, 59, with PPA for 9 years, had Pick's disease diagnosed on the basis of CT and MRI scans that showed widening of the sylvian fissures and severe atrophy of both temporal lobes. He was admitted to a nursing home because of unsociable behavior. His speech became monosyllabic; he ate and walked compulsively, had problems with dressing and urinating, and was restless at night. He died of bronchopneumonia 13 years after onset of the condition.

Results.—At autopsy, the patient's brain showed severe neuronal loss and intense gliosis throughout the cortex and the hippocampus. Many Alz-50–positive neurons were found, but no ubiquitin or spongiform changes were detected. No Pick bodies were found. There were no neuropathologic changes characteristic of either Alzheimer's disease or Pick's disease. The condition was considered to be nonspecific cortical degeneration.

Conclusion.—Primary progressive aphasia appears to be a clinical syndrome which needs to be verified histopathologically.

▶ Primary progressive aphasia is characterized by progressive language deficits with sparing of other functions, notably memory. The nature of the progressive aphasia primarily relates to the location of the pathologic changes. It appears that the clinical entity can be separated from other degenerative states by virtue of its behavioral findings rather than by its pathologic findings. Histologic findings of Pick's disease, neuronal achromasia and corticonigral degeneration, and Alzheimer's disease have been reported; when focal in the frontal and temporal lobes and sparing the hippocampal formation, they may result in this clinical picture.—A.M. Galaburda, M.D.

Cognitive Impairment After Stroke: Frequency, Patterns, and Relationship to Functional Abilities
Tatemichi TK, Desmond DW, Stern Y, Paik M, Sano M, Bagiella E
(Neurological Inst of New York, NY; Columbia Univ, New York)
J Neurol Neurosurg Psychiatry 57:202–207, 1994   122-96-10–8

Introduction.—Stroke in elderly patients often results in cognitive impairment as well as physical disability. To better characterize the nature and extent of the cognitive consequences of stroke, elderly patients who had no history of functional decline before stroke were compared with age-matched individuals living in the community who had no history of stroke.

Patients and Methods.—Cognitive function was examined in 227 patients, age 60 years of age or older, who had been given a diagnosis of acute ischemic stroke occurring within the previous 30 days. None had evidence of dementia or functional impairment before the stroke. Controls were 240 individuals older than 60 years of age; 17.3% were spouses of the patients with stroke. Patients and controls both underwent a battery of neuropsychological tests containing 17 scored items that assessed memory, orientation, language ability, visuospatial ability, abstract reasoning, and attention. Patients were classified by clinical syndrome and vascular territory.

Results.—The patients' raw neuropsychological scores indicated impairment on all 17 items. After adjusting for demographic factors, from 10.2% to 38.5% of patients with stroke performed below the fifth percentile. There was a significant difference between patients and controls in the mean number of failed tests. Forty percent of controls vs. 78% of patients failed 1 or more test items (Fig 10–2). When 4 or more failed tests were used as the cutoff for cognitive impairment, 35.2% of patients vs. 3.8% of controls fell

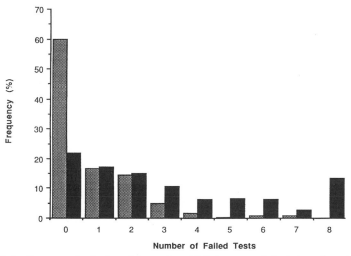

Fig 10–2.—Frequency distribution of the number of failed neuropsychological test items in patients with stroke (*filled bars*) and controls (*hatched bars*). (Courtesy of Tatemichi TK, Desmond DW, Stern Y, et al: *J Neurol Neurosurg Psychiatry* 57:202–207, 1994.)

into this category. None of the patients or controls classified as cognitively impaired failed only tests in a single cognitive domain. The most significant areas of impairment associated with stroke were memory, orientation, language, and attention. Cognitive impairment in the patient group varied by stroke syndrome and, to a lesser degree, by specific vascular territory and laterality (table). Women were more likely than men to experience cognitive impairment after stroke.

Conclusion.—Cognitive impairment is a common finding in elderly patients who have had an ischemic stroke. Memory, orientation, language, and attention are areas of function that are frequently affected. Cognitive impairment is a significant predictor of risk for dependent living after discharge, persisting after adjustment for age and degree of physical impairment.

▶ It is remarkable that it needs to be spelled out that the cognitive effects of stroke are real and separate from its physical effects. Clinicians are well aware that infarcts in "clinically silent" areas usually involve neurologic functions that are more subtle than silent. It is not surprising that even this study finds more problems relative to the left hemisphere, which indicates that the selection of tests does not address the kinds of disability usually associated with dysfunction in the right hemisphere. Nonetheless, clinicians should realize that deficits of the right hemisphere may be more subtle, but long-term survival and morbidity of right hemisphere infarcts may be more severely affected with right than with left hemisphere injury.—A.M. Galaburda, M.D.

Clinical Stroke Features and Frequency of Cognitive Impairment.
Percentages Indicate Proportions Within Subject Groups.

| | Cognitive impairment n(%) | |
| | Present | Absent |
Stroke feature	(n = 80)	(n = 147)
Stroke syndrome		
Major dominant	15 (18.8)	10 (6.8)
Major non-dominant	12 (15.0)	5 (3.4)
Minor dominant	10 (12.5)	25 (17.0)
Minor non-dominant	10 (12.5)	30 (20.4)
Lacunar	21 (26.3)	38 (25.9)
Brainstem-cerebellar	12 (15.0)	39 (26.5)
Stroke territory		
Left ICA*	2 (2.5)	3 (2.0)
Right ICA*	1 (1.3)	1 (1.4)
Left ACA	5 (6.3)	3 (2.0)
Right ACA	1 (1.3)	2 (1.4)
Left MCA	24 (30.0)	33 (22.4)
Right MCA	25 (31.3)	40 (27.2)
Left PCA	6 (7.5)	6 (4.1)
Right PCA	4 (5.0)	10 (6.8)
Vertebrobasilar	12 (15.0)	48 (32.7)

* Borderzone infarction.
Abbreviations: ICA, internal cerebral artery; *ACA,* anterior cerebral artery; *MCA,* middle cerebral artery; *PCA,* posterior cerebral artery.
(Courtesy of Tatemichi TK, Desmond DW, Stern Y, et al: *J Neurol Neurosurg Psychiatry* 57:202–207, 1994.)

11 Neurotrauma

β-Amyloid Protein Deposition in the Brain After Severe Head Injury: Implications for the Pathogenesis of Alzheimer's Disease
Roberts GW, Gentleman SM, Lynch A, Murray L, Landon M, Graham DI
(Smith Kline Beecham Pharmaceuticals, Harlow, England; Westminster Med School, London; Southern Gen Hosp, Glasgow, Scotland; et al)
J Neurol Neurosurg Psychiatry 57:419–425, 1994   122-96-11-1

Background.—A preliminary study recently reported that severe head injuries led to the deposition of β-amyloid protein (βAP) in the cortical ribbon of 30% of patients who survived for less than 2 weeks. To further investigate whether head injury triggers βAP deposition in the cortex, multiple cortical areas from patients with severe head injuries who survived between 4 hours and 2.5 years were examined and compared with findings from neurologically normal controls.

Patients and Findings.—A total of 152 patients (age, 8 weeks to 85 years) were investigated and compared with 44 controls (age, 51–80 years). Immunostaining with an antibody to βAP verified that head injury is associated with βAP deposits in 1 or more cortical areas in 30% of patients. Advancing age appeared to accentuate the degree of βAP deposition. No clear differences between βAP-positive and -negative patients were noted for sex, extent of coma on admission, operated hematoma, increased intracranial pressure, brain swelling, low blood pressure, or survival time. A statistically significant increase in the degree of clinically rated hypoxia was noted in the βAP-negative group, although this finding did not remain significant after applying the Bonferroni correction for multiple testing. β-Amyloid precursor protein (βAPP) immunoreactivity was elevated in the perikarya of neurons in the area of βAP deposits.

Conclusions.—Increased expression of βAPP is part of an acute stage response to neuronal injury in the human brain. Extensive overexpression of βAPP can result in deposition of βAP and the initiation of an Alzheimer's disease–type process within days. Consequently, head injury may be an important causal characteristic in Alzheimer's disease.

▶ A number of studies have shown a relationship between late-onset Alzheimer's disease and severe head injury. Diffuse axonal injury is associated with βAP deposition within hours after trauma. This study confirms and extends these findings. Although head injury may contribute to the cause of

Alzheimer's disease, genetic factors still remain the single most important causal characteristic of Alzheimer's disease.—A.M. Galaburda, M.D.

Fever of Central Origin in Traumatic Brain Injury Controlled With Propranolol

Meythaler JM, Stinson AM III (Univ of Alabama, Birmingham; Spain Rehabilitation Ctr, Birmingham, Ala)
Arch Phys Med Rehabil 75:816–818, 1994   122-96-11–2

Introduction.—Patients with traumatic brain injury (TBI) sometimes have central fevers develop, which are thought to result from injuries involving the hypothalamus. Beta-blockers are of known effectiveness in the treatment of hypertension produced by autonomic dysfunction, and one report has suggested the use of propranolol to control centrally mediated fevers in patients with TBI. The successful use of propranolol for this purpose was reported in 3 patients.

Patients.—All 3 patients sustained very severe TBI in motor vehicle accidents; their initial Glasgow Coma Score ratings were 3 or 4. On CT scans of the head, intraventricular hemorrhage was seen in 2 patients, although the third patient had no focal injury or bleeding. Decorticate posturing and autonomic dysfunction, manifested by tachycardia and profuse sweating, developed in all 3 patients. During hospitalization, the patients had high fevers of 38.9°C to 40.6°C. No infectious or inflammatory cause could be found, so the fevers were thought to be centrally mediated.

Treatment and Outcomes.—All patients were treated with propranolol, 20–30 mg every 6 hours. Within 48 hours, the temperature decreased by at least 1.5°C. Whenever weaning from propranolol was attempted, the patients' temperature increased to more than 38.0°C within 3 days. Again, no infectious or inflammatory causes of the fevers could be found, and they were reduced again when propranolol was restarted. Propranolol treatment was therefore continued until all signs of autonomic dysfunction cleared at 1–2 months after discharge.

Discussion.—Although further studies are needed, propranolol appears to have a role in the treatment of central fevers in patients with TBI. Administration of the β-blocker is followed by a dramatic reduction in such fevers, which return when use of the drug is discontinued. Propranolol has also been reported to reduce central fevers in children with decerebrate posturing, and there is pharmacologic, neurophysiologic, and anatomical evidence to suggest that the CNS plays an important role in regulating blood pressure and temperature.

▶ There is increasing experimental and clinicial evidence that hyperthermia is markedly detrimental to the brain in patients with head injury and stroke. This study suggests that propranolol may be of benefit for central neurogenic hyperthermia. The 3 patients with severe head injury also had signs of autonomic dysfunction, including tachycardia and profuse sweating; therefore, they were given propranolol. This dramatically reduced central body temperature, and the fever returned when medication was withdrawn. The mechanism of central hyperthermia remains undetermined, but it presumably is hypothalamic in origin.—W.G. Bradley, D.M., F.R.C.P.

12 Neurologic Complications of General Medical Diseases

Assessment of Neurological Prognosis in Comatose Survivors of Cardiac Arrest
Edgren E, Hedstrand U, Kelsey S, Sutton-Tyrrell K, Safar P, and BRCT I Study Group (Univ Hosp, Uppsala, Sweden; Univ of Pittsburgh, Pa)
Lancet 343:1055–1059, 1994   122-96-12–1

Introduction.—Patients frequently remain unconscious for a time after being resuscitated from cardiac arrest. This may reflect either severe, permanent brain damage or merely a reversible metabolic disorder.

Objective.—A statistical modeling exercise was done using data from the Brain Resuscitation Clinical Trials I Study Group in an attempt to find a reliable means of predicting at an early stage the outcome from the clinical neurologic findings. It was hypothesized that it would be possible to reliably predict a permanent vegetative state within a few days after cardiac arrest.

Study Population.—Twelve hospitals in 9 countries contributed 262 patients seen in cardiac arrest who were initially comatose and had no purposeful motor response to painful stimulation 10 minutes after circulation was restored. Advanced life support was followed by a standard protocol of intensive care and, in some cases, thiopentone administration. The Glasgow coma score and its Pittsburgh modification were determined after 8, 16, and 24 hours and on days 2 through 7. The patients were followed for 1 year after the arrest.

Results.—At entry to the study, positive predictive values indicating a good outcome ranged from 42% for seizures and the pupillary light reflex to 73% for eye opening on painful stimulation. Absence of the pupillary light response correctly predicted a poor outcome (negative predictive value) in 82% of cases. All Glasgow and Glasgow-Pittsburgh coma scores were significantly correlated with a poor neurologic outcome. Both these

TABLE 1.—Negative Predictive Value (Percentage of Correct Predictions of Poor Outcome, Cerebral Performance Category 3 to 5) for Some Neurologic Signs in the Glasgow-Pittsburgh Coma Score

Neurologic sign	Negative predictive value (%) at:									
	Entry	8 h	16 h	24 h	Day 2	Day 3	Day 4	Day 5	Day 6	Day 7
No eye opening to pain	69	77	85	92	93	100	95	93	92	100
No motor response to pain	75	84	89	91	92	100	100	93	100	100
No response to verbal stimulus	67	70	71	75	89	94	96	97	97	100
Absence of pupil light response	83	96	100	93	94	100	100	100	100	100
Absence of selected cranial nerve reflexes	68	84	86	91	93	96	95	100	92	100
Seizures	69	90	92	88	88	100	100	100	100	100

This table concerns the 131 standard treatment patients. All listed signs had statistically significant correlation with poor outcome in univariate analysis. (Courtesy of Edgren E, Hedstrand U, Kelsey S, et al: *Lancet* 343:1055–1059, 1994.)

TABLE 2.—Ability of Neurologic Signs to Predict Bad Outcome on Day 3 in 109 Unconscious Survivors

	Best outcome (CPC)			
	1	2	3	4
Scores	6	7	15	81
Glasgow score ≤5	0	0	0	45
Glasgow score >5	6	7	15	36
Glasgow-Pittsburgh ≤22	0	0	1	47
Glasgow-Pittsburgh >22	6	7	14	34
Neurological sign				
Response to pain:				
No eye opening	0	1	4	45
Some eye opening	6	6	11	36
No motor response	0	0	0	43
Some motor response	6	7	15	38
Extensor posturing	0	0	2	11
No extensor posturing	6	7	13	70
Pupil light response				
None	0	0	0	18
Some	6	7	15	63
Selected cranial nerve reflexes				
Absent	2	0	4	42
Present	4	7	11	39
Seizures				
Yes	0	1	3	13
No	6	6	12	68

Numbers refer to best outcome achieved at any time during follow-up.
Abbreviation: CPC, cerebral performance category.
(Courtesy of Edgren E, Hedstrand U, Kelsey S, et al: *Lancet* 343;1055–1059, 1994.)

scores had a negative predictive value of 69%. The predictive accuracy of the various measures improved over time (Table 1). On day 3, the best predictor of a severely disabled or permanently comatose outcome was the absence of a motor response to pain (Table 2). The status of 131 patients who received standard treatment with thiopental is illustrated in (Fig 12–1).

Conclusion.—Pending confirmation of these findings in large multi-center studies, it would appear that 3 days of observation under intensive care makes it possible to predict the neurologic outcome well enough to make informed decisions regarding life support in comatose patients who have survived cardiac arrest.

▶ The ability to restore cardiac function in patients who have cardiopulmonary arrest has improved progressively over the years. Unfortunately, this results in the initial survival of many patients who have had severe hypoxic-ischemic brain damage. Since the trail-blazing studies of Plum and Posner (1) first appeared, there have been many attempts to improve our prognostic abilities with regard to the degree of recovery of such patients. Completely reliable criteria would allow definitive advice to be given to grieving relatives; would assist in the establishment of medical, legal and social guidelines for withdrawal of life support systems; and would assist in limiting expenditure for the continuing care of patients for whom there is no hope.

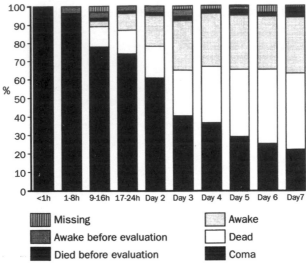

Missing

Awake before evaluation

Died before evaluation

Awake

Dead

Coma

Fig 12–1.—Status of 131 patients receiving standard treatment during the first week of care. Each *column* describes the status of patients at the beginning of the period indicated. The most common outcomes are the 3 in the right-hand part of the *key* (awake, dead, coma). (Courtesy of Edgren E, Hedstrand U, Kelsey S, et al: *Lancet* 343:1055–1059, 1994.)

This multicenter study quantifies the reliability of good and poor prognostic indicators that should be helpful in everyday clinical practice and in planning future larger studies. One of the crucial questions is the false negative rate for each of these criteria, because there continue to be rare patients who have some bad prognostic features and yet somehow "beat the odds" to make a moderate functional recovery.—W.G. Bradley, D.M., F.R.C.P.

Reference

1. Plum F, Posner J: *The Diagnosis of Stupor and Coma*, ed 3. Philadelphia, F.A. Davis, 1980.

Sensitivities of Noninvasive Tests for Central Nervous System Vasculitis: A Comparison of Lumbar Puncture, Computed Tomography, and Magnetic Resonance Imaging

Stone JH, Pomper MG, Roubenoff R, Miller TJ, Hellmann DB (Johns Hopkins Univ, Baltimore, Md; Tufts Univ, Boston)
J Rheumatol 21:1277–1282, 1994   122-96-12–2

Purpose.—Central nervous system vasculitis may occur as primary angiitis of the CNS (PACNS), as a complication of rheumatic or vasculitic disorders, or as a result of a number of diverse CNS insults. In patients with suspected CNS vasculitis, the decision to perform invasive diagnostic tests (i.e., angiography or biopsy) is based on the results of noninvasive

Sensitivities of LP, CT, and MRI in Patients With Angiograms Positive for CNS Vasculitis

Test	Proportion	Percent: CI
LP sensitivity	8/15	(53%; CI: 27–79)
CT sensitivity	11/17	(65%; CI: 38–86)
MR sensitivity	12/16	(75%; CI: 48–93)
Sensitivity of LP and CT	11/12	(92%; CI: 62–100)*
Sensitivity of LP and MR	12/12	(100%; CI: 74–100)†
Sensitivity of CT and MR	10/13	(77%; CI: 46–95)

*Result different from LP sensitivity ($P = 0.04$) by Fisher's exact test.
†Result different from LP sensitivity ($P = 0.007$).
(Courtesy of Stone JH, Pomper MG, Roubenoff R, et al: *J Rheumatol* 21:1277–1282, 1994.)

tests, such as lumbar puncture (LP), CT, and MRI. There is, however, little information on the sensitivities of these tests. These sensitivities were examined in a sample of patients with angiography-positive CNS vasculitis of diverse causes.

Methods.—The retrospective study included 12 females and 8 males (mean age, 44 years). Etiologic categories were PACNS in 7 patients; rheumatologic illnesses in 8, including 4 with systemic lupus erythematosus; and other causes in 5, including CNS infections in 2. The noninvasive tests reviewed included LP in 15 patients, CT in 17, and MRI in 16.

Results.—Calculated sensitivities were 53% for LP, 65% for CT, and 75% for MRI. Greater sensitivity was achieved when LP was added to either CT or MRI: 92% for LP and CT and 100% for LP and MRI. The sensitivity of CT plus MRI was no higher than that of either test alone (table). A blinded reviewer agreed with the original interpretation of the CT scans in 94% of cases and MRI scans in 92% of cases.

Conclusions.—The noninvasive tests of LP, CT, and MRI have only modest sensitivities for angiography-positive CNS vasculitis. The CT and MRI findings may be completely normal. The addition of CT or MRI to LP testing may aid in the diagnosis of CNS vasculitis; patients with a normal LP test and a normal CT or MRI scan are unlikely to have a positive CNS angiogram.

▶ The problem with CNS vasculitis is that it is relatively rare but enters into the differential diagnosis of many common diseases, such as dementia, stroke, and epilepsy. The gold standard undoubtedly should be pathologic confirmation, but autopsy series are undoubtedly biased toward a poorer prognosis, and few—if any—centers undertake "blind" brain biopsies without very strongly suggestive preliminary studies. Angiogram-positive vasculitis may not be the gold standard, for many pathologically proven cases have involvement of vessels that are too small to be detected by routine angiography. This paper adds to the discussion of this difficult topic. This is truly the area where the experienced neurologist needs to use "his own personal computer," i.e., his experience as an integrating mechanism of determining weighting factors related to the likelihood of the diagnosis on clinical grounds, the chance of producing worthwhile improvement if the diagnosis is proven, and the risks to the patient (relating to age, infirmity, etc.) resulting from a brain biopsy.—W.G. Bradley, D.M., F.R.C.P.

Leptomeningeal Metastases: Analysis of 31 Patients With Sustained Off-Therapy Response Following Combined-Modality Therapy
Siegal T, Lossos A, Pfeffer MR (Hadassah Hebrew Univ Hosp, Jerusalem)
Neurology 44:1463–1469, 1994   122-96-12–3

Background.—At 1 center, the treatment protocol for leptomeningeal metastases (LM) specifies the length of therapy and requires treatment withdrawal at the completion of the predetermined schedule. Experience with patients who were followed for at least 6 months after treatment withdrawal was summarized. This was the first study in which treatment withdrawal adhered to strict guidelines and represented the only report on long-term follow-up of such a policy.

Patients and Findings.—Of 137 patients undergoing treatment for LM, 31 were evaluated. All 31 had obtained a sustained off-therapy response of

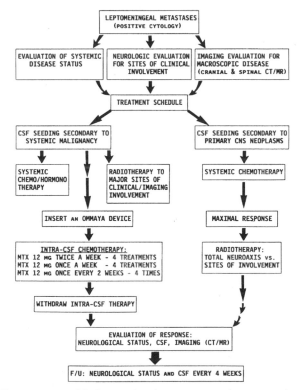

Fig 12–2.—Treatment protocol for leptomeningeal metastases secondary to systemic malignancy or to primary CNS neoplasms. *Abbreviation: F/U,* follow-up. (Courtesy of Siegal T, Lossos A, Pfeffer MR: *Neurology* 44:1463–1469, 1994.)

at least 6 months' duration after undergoing standard treatment, including radiation therapy and intra-CSF chemotherapy (Fig 12–2). Equal distribution was noted for various tumors: lymphoma (29%), breast carcinoma (20%), and other tumors (19%). After performing neuroimaging of the neuraxis, subarachnoid deposits were observed in 70%, with unexpected findings seen in 55%. A complete response was achieved in all 13 patients with lymphomas at therapy withdrawal. A partial response was noted for 61% of those with other tumors. Nine patients experienced an off-therapy relapse after a median of 12 months, but this was not associated with the type of attained response. A second prolonged response occurred in 5 patients, primarily by systemic therapy. Eight patients receiving only systemic therapy responded to treatment, 4 of whom achieved a complete response. All other patients underwent both systemic and intra-CSF treatment and maintained a systemic response. Late complications were noted in 58%. Leukoencephalopathy equally affected those exposed and not exposed to cranial irradiation. A median survival of 23 months was noted for the entire group.

Conclusions.—With the exception of lymphomas, a partial response is compatible with an extended off-therapy response in LM. Because LM may respond to systemic therapy, a prospective reevaluation of intra-CSF therapy, with its associated complications, is warranted.

▶ Two major points of interest are made in this review of treatment consisting of systemic and intrathecal chemotherapy for patients with LM. The first is that even a partial response to therapy may yield a prolonged period of freedom from symptoms. The second is that some patients may respond to systemic chemotherapy alone. This second finding suggests to the authors that a reevaluation of intrathecal chemotherapy is necessary. It is not surprising that systemic chemotherapy is sometimes effective. Animal experiments have shown that once LM are established, disruption of the blood-CSF barrier enables entry of parenteral chemotherapeutic agents that normally do not enter CSF. Nevertheless, intrathecal chemotherapy allows the delivery of high doses of the chemotherapeutic agent to the site of the tumor with minimal systemic toxicity.—J.D. Posner, M.D.

Superficial Hemosiderosis of the Central Nervous System

River Y, Honigman S, Gomori JM, Reches A (Hadassah Univ Hosp, Jerusalem; Haemek Hosp, Afula, Israel)
Mov Disord 9:559–562, 1994   122-96-12–4

Background.—Superficial hemosiderosis of the CNS is a rare condition caused by repeated subarachnoid hemorrhage, with progressive superficial siderosis of the CNS. A patient with superficial hemosiderosis who was seen with progressive movement disorder and the treatment he received were studied.

Case Report.—Man, 47, was seen with a 5-year history of progressive speech disturbances and unsteady gait with recurrent falls. He complained of occasional involuntary closure of the left eye, which was followed within 5–20 seconds by spasm of the left side of the mouth and cheek. In addition, the patient had hearing loss and memory deterioration. Examination revealed bilateral horizontal nystagmus, decreased hearing on both sides, dysarthria, hyperactive tendon reflexes, the Babinski sign elicited on the right side, and ataxic gait. The patient's CSF iron levels were 6.9 μmol/L, compared with an average of 1.6 μmol/L in a control group of 20 patients. Brain stem auditory evoked potentials were bilaterally abnormal. Computed tomography scan revealed symmetric atrophy of the cerebellum, and a MRI scan showed on T1- and T2-weighted images severe atrophy of the cerebellum. The patient was treated with an iron-chelating agent, trientine dihydrochloride, 2 g/day. Symptoms of hemifacial spasm completely resolved within 6 months of therapy, and a 2-year follow-up showed no further deterioration in neurologic condition. Examination of the CSF showed a marked improvement, with a reduction of iron levels to 3 μmol/L and a decrease in ferritin levels to 55 μmol/L.

Conclusion.—This case report provides evidence to suggest that CSF levels of iron and ferritin could be a useful additional diagnostic criterion for superficial hemosiderosis of the CNS. In addition, these levels may provide a possible means of evaluating the efficacy of different treatment approaches. A further trial to study chelation therapy is required in a selected group of patients.

▶ This paper describes an unusual patient who, at the age of 13 years, had a cerebellar tumor removed and then received irradiation of the posterior fossa. It is possible that the superficial hemosiderosis of the nervous system resulted from chronic bleeding from the operative site, because no other etiology was identified. This study offers the opportunity to review the uncommon condition of superficial hemosiderosis, its diagnosis by iron levels in the CSF, and the possible therapeutic benefit of iron chelation therapy.—W.G. Bradley, D.M., F.R.C.P.

Delayed Cerebellar Ataxia Complicating Falciparum Malaria: A Clinical Study of 74 Patients

Senanayake N, de Silva HJ (Univ of Peradeniya, Sri Lanka; Univ of Kelaniya, Sri Lanka)
J Neurol 241:456–459, 1994   122-96-12–5

Introduction.—Infrequently, falciparum malaria is complicated by a self-limited form of cerebellar dysfunction termed delayed cerebellar ataxia (DCA). It occurs as the only abnormality in a patient who is conscious and otherwise well after a malarial attack.

Series.—Data were reviewed on 74 patients seen over 2 years in Sri Lanka who had ataxia after a documented attack of *Plasmodium falciparum* malaria. The patients, all but 8 of whom were male, were aged 16–56 years and had a median age of 28 years.

Clinical Findings.—Most patients had received chloroquine, but 11 were not given any antimalaria treatment. Half the patients had had previous episodes of malaria. The median interval between the onset of the last febrile episode and the appearance of ataxia was 13 days. Mainly midline-trunkal signs were evident. All the patients were markedly ataxic. There was no evidence of cerebral dysfunction, and no features suggesting another cause of cerebellar pathology.

Investigations.—Serum antibody titers to *P. falciparum* were significantly elevated. The results of cranial CT with contrast enhancement were negative in the 11 patients examined. Nerve conduction studies and electromyographic study of the extremity muscles consistently gave normal results.

Outcome.—The 66 patients who were followed up recovered spontaneously and totally within 3 months of the onset of ataxia. The 8 remaining patients had improved when last seen. Two of 3 patients with a subsequent attack of malaria again became ataxic.

Conclusion.—Delayed cerebellar ataxia appears to be a postinfective neurologic disorder that may have an immunologic origin.

▶ The phenomena of delayed cerebellar ataxia occurring after infection with *P. falciparum* is a poorly understood phenomenon. This large study from Sri Lanka emanates from the same investigators who first described the disorder a little more than 10 years ago. The key features of the disorder are midline cerebellar findings, onset within two weeks of the onset of fever, and frequent spontaneous recovery within 3 months. The pathogenesis of the disorder remains uncertain. The authors propose that it may be the consequence of immune-mediated damage of the cerebellum. However, other possibilities include the effects of hyperthermia, injury resulting from small vessel occlusion, or a peculiar effect of the antimalarial agents used to treat the infection. More intensive investigations will be required to determine the precise cause.—J.R. Berger, M.D.

Hepatic Myelopathy: A Rare Complication of Portacaval Shunt
Mendoza G, Marti-Fàbregas J, Kulisevsky J, Escartin A (Autonomous Univ of Barcelona, Spain)
Eur Neurol 34:209–212, 1994   122-96-12–6

Background.—Hepatic myelopathy is associated with progressive paraparesis and extensive collateral portal circulation. In 3 cases, hepatic myelopathy followed surgical performance of a portacaval shunt.

Case Report.—Man, 66, who had portal cirrhosis and a previous episode of reversible encephalopathy, had difficulty walking. Examination revealed spastic paraparesis, brisk tendon jerks, bilateral ankle clonus, and extensor plantar responses. A hemogram was near normal; albumin, 28.1 g/L; gammaglobulin, 25.5 g/L; total bilirubin, 22 µmol/L; direct bilirubin, 9 µmol/L; aspartate transaminase, 50 units/L; and HBcAG, strongly positive. Magnetic resonance imaging done 7 weeks later during an episode of encephalopathy revealed high signal lesions in the periventricular white matter and cerebellar vermis atrophy. Paraparesis progressed;

after 2 months, the patient could not walk. Encephalopathic episodes followed dietary transgressions. After 5 years, sudden weakness and paresthesia developed in the left arm, and the patient was bedridden. Magnetic resonance imaging showed lacunar ischemic lesions in the right lenticular nucleus. The patient died of terminal liver failure one year later.

Discussion.—The clinical features of hepatic myelopathy include progressive spastic paraparesis, hyperreflexia, and extensor plantar responses; sensory symptoms and incontinence are rare. Surgical portacaval shunt precedes symptom development by 4 months to 10 years. Although the rate of progression and the final degree of impairment vary, most cases are severely affected. No therapeutic measure has been shown to forestall the progression of paraparesis, although protein restriction with oral antibiotic therapy and lactulose has been beneficial in some patients. Although portacaval shunt surgery is no longer performed to manage esophageal variceal hemorrhage, hepatic myelopathy may still occur as a result of spontaneous shunting.

▶ Encephalopathy is the usual neurologic complication of acute hepatocellular dysfunction, and this can be recurrent in patients with portacaval shunts. The original of this paper describes 3 new cases of a relatively uncommon syndrome of progressive myelopathy, the predominant feature of which is a progressive spastic paraparesis. I have also seen one case in whom posterior column features with lower limb sensory ataxia was the most striking finding.—W.G. Bradley, D.M., F.R.C.P.

Cutaneous Nerve Fibre Depletion in Vibration White Finger
Goldsmith PC, Molina FA, Bunker CB, Terenghi G, Leslie TA, Fowler CJ, Polak JM, Dowd PM (Univ College and Middlesex School of Medicine, London; Royal Postgraduate Med School, Hammersmith Hosp, London)
J R Soc Med 87:377–381, 1994   122-96-12–7

Introduction.—The disorder called vibration white finger, or hand-arm vibration syndrome, consists of episodic blanching of the fingers on cold exposure in an individual who works with hand-held vibrating tools. In contrast to Raynaud's phenomenon, paresthesias and pain often persist in the hand and arm between attacks of blanching. Nearly all those who are affected are male.

Objective and Methods.—The digital skin of 15 men with vibration white finger was biopsied to determine the distribution of immunoreactive nerves and vasoactive peptides. The study group included 5 coal miners, 4 riveters, and 6 road diggers. Six healthy road diggers and 26 men not exposed to vibrating tools served as a control group.

Findings.—In control biopsy specimens, immunoreactivity for calcitonin gene-related peptide (CRGP) appeared as beaded fibers in the epidermis and surrounding subepidermal and dermal vessels. The fibers that were immunoreactive for CGRP and protein gene product (PGP) 9.5 were significantly depleted in the epidermis and papillary dermis of biopsy specimens from patients with vibration white finger. There were no significant differences in immunoreactivity for neuropeptide Y, vasoactive intestinal peptide, endothelin-1, or von Willebrand factor. Nerve conduction studies in 6 affected road diggers showed that 5 of them had sensory action potentials in the low normal range. The most severely symptomatic of these patients had the most marked loss of immunoreactive nerve fibers.

Conclusions.—The concomitant loss of CGRP and PGP immunoreactivity may explain both the vascular and neurologic abnormalities of vibration white finger. The disorder may be diagnosable immunohistochemically.

▶ Thirty years ago, medical schools taught that chronic exposure to vibrating tools gave rise to precipitation of Raynaud's phenomenon. This paper clearly delineates that the episodic blanching of the fingers in response to cold is different from typical Raynaud's phenomenon in the presence of paresthesia and pain between attacks. It also demonstrates that there is a terminal nerve fiber degeneration in the skin biopsy specimens of such patients with loss of CGRP immunoreactive nerve fibers, but there is no loss of fiber staining with neuropeptide Y and other factors. The cause of nerve degeneration remains undetermined.—W.G. Bradley, D.M., F.R.C.P.

13 Neurotoxicology

Neurological Sequelae Following Carbon Monoxide Poisoning Clinical Course and Outcome According to the Clinical Types and Brain Computed Tomography Scan Findings
Lee MS, Marsden CD (Yongdong Severance Hosp, Seoul, Korea; Yonsei Univ, Seoul, Korea; Inst of Neurology, London)
Mov Disord 9:550–558, 1994   122-96-13-1

Background.—Carbon monoxide is a common but frequently misdiagnosed cause of poisoning. For patients who survive CO poisoning—especially those who have persistent neurologic complications develop after recovering from the initial coma—the prognosis is uncertain. In an attempt to identify factors predicting the final disability, 31 patients with sequelae of carbon monoxide poisoning were reviewed.

Methods.—The patients were 19 women and 12 men (mean age, 51 years) with the sequelae of carbon monoxide poisoning. The course was classified as progressive in 8 patients who did not show initial recovery but progressed to a vegetative state. The other 23 patients were classified as having a delayed relapsing course, with recovery from the initial encephalopathy but later deterioration in motor and mental function. The patients all underwent CT scanning of the brain within 1 week after acute poisoning or after the onset of delayed sequelae. All were followed up for more than 1 year.

Outcomes.—The patients with a progressive course had a persistent akinetic-mute state develop, and 50% died. In the delayed-relapsing group, 9 patients developed a parkinsonian state with behavioral and cognitive impairment, although they were able to walk. The other 14 patients had further progression to an akinetic-mute state and were bedbound. In both of these subgroups, deterioration occurred rapidly, over a few days to a week. Sixty-one percent of those in the delayed-relapsing group had subsequent improvement; 13% died.

Prognostic Factors.—Mean age was 37 years in patients who had a progressive course without initial recovery compared with 55 years in those with a delayed-relapsing course. The mean duration of the initial coma was 10 and 2 days, respectively. There was no difference in the initial carbon monoxide hemoglobin levels of the 2 groups. The CT scan was normal in 10 patients; white matter low-density lesions were seen in 13 patients, and globus pallidus low-density lesions were seen in 4. The outcomes were not accurately predicted by these findings, although the prognosis was bad for all patients who had both globus pallidus and white matter low-density lesions. Follow-up CT scanning was performed in 8 patients. Although all had progressive changes, new lesions, or both, 3 patients improved. The prognosis was poor for 4 of 5 patients who had globus pallidus and white matter low-density lesions at their follow-up scan.

Conclusions.—Most patients with carbon monoxide poisoning have a period of more or less complete recovery, followed by abrupt relapse. Patients with progressive-type sequelae are younger and have a longer coma duration than those with delayed-relapsing sequelae; they also have a worse prognosis. Although the brain CT findings are not good predictors of outcome, patients who have both globus pallidus and white matter low-density lesions appear to have a poor prognosis.

▶ Exposure to carbon monoxide remains one of the most common causes of acute fatal poisoning. Among early survivors, neurologic sequelae may include progressive coma leading to death or a delayed relapse with deficits ranging from mild bradykinesia to akinetic-mutism. In Lee and Marsden's patients, neither the initial CT scan nor the carbon monoxide hemoglobin level predicted the nature or severity of eventual neurologic dysfunction. Despite progressive neurologic deficits, some follow-up CT scans remained normal, whereas others demonstrated low-density lesions in the hemispheric white matter or globus pallidus. In some cases, clinical improvement occurred despite apparent progression of the CT lesions. Although neither lesion, when present alone, predicted poor outcome, patients with white matter ₐnd globus pallidus lesions were least likely to improve.

The reasons for ischemic vulnerability of the globus pallidus in carbon monoxide poisoning remain unclear; they probably relate more to it being an end-arterial zone of the anterior choroidal and lenticulostriate vessels than to the regional differences in intrinsic metabolic activity.—A.R. Berger, M.D.

Methylmercury Poisoning: Long-Term Clinical, Radiological, Toxicological, and Pathological Studies of an Affected Family
Davis LE, Kornfeld M, Mooney HS, Feidler KJ, Haaland KY, Orrison WW, Cernichiari E, Clarkson TW (Univ of New Mexico, Albuquerque; Univ of Rochester, NY)
Ann Neurol 35:680–688, 1994   122-96-13–2

Introduction.—The acute effects of methylmercury poisoning have been well described, but there is little information on the long-term sequelae. The findings of a 22-year follow-up of a family with severe methylmercury poisoning were reported.

Methods.—A family, including a pregnant mother and 3 children, aged 20, 13, and 8, consumed methylmercury-contaminated pork for 3 months and were severely intoxicated. The infant was born with CNS damage, and the other children showed signs of neurologic disorder. They were treated with chelation therapy. Twenty-two years later, the surviving members were examined and underwent MRI. Autopsy tissues were examined from the child who was poisoned at age 8 years and died at age 30, and from an unrelated control subject.

Results.—The 2 older children demonstrated improved neurologic function, although the MRI scans revealed persistent damage in the calcarine cortices, parietal cortices, and the cerebellum, accounting for the clinical dysfunction. The younger children remained in a vegetative state until death. The parents and 2 other family members were asymptomatic, although the mother had cerebellar atrophy on MRI. The brain weight of the autopsied child was profoundly reduced, and almost all of the lobes were atrophic. The corpus callosum was thin, and the lateral and third ventricles were enlarged. There was variable neuronal loss, mostly pseudolaminar, in most of the cerebral cortex, especially in the paracentral and parietooccipital areas, where there were no neurons, and in the thalamus. There was myelin loss and gliosis in the adjacent white matter. The brain stem and spinal cord had severe secondary degeneration. Inorganic mercury levels in the brain of this patient were 50 times greater than those found in the control patient.

Discussion.—The poisoned family members lived at least 21 years, suggesting that methylmercury is a potent neurotoxin but is not lethal. Although there was some improvement in the older children, chelation therapy failed to reverse the neurologic damage. Because methylmercury easily crosses the blood-brain barrier but inorganic mercury does not, the biotransformation must have occurred inside the brain of the 8-year-old child.

▶ This paper illustrates the pathologic changes that result from remote intoxication with methylmercury. The severity of the long-term sequelae appears to be highly dependent on the individual's age at the time of exposure. Children are at greatest risk for the development of persistently severe neurologic deficits. In adults exposed to methylmercury, improvement occurred over time. The pathologic findings included neuronal dropout, predominantly in the cerebrum and cerebellum. Methylmercury freely enters and leaves the CNS, and it may possibly be converted to inorganic mercury, which poorly penetrates the blood-brain barrier. Although clinical deficits may relate to the intensity of methylmercury intoxication, persistent exposure to inorganic mercury may be important in the genesis of long-term deficits.—A.R. Berger, M.D.

Solvent Vapor Abuse Leukoencephalopathy: Comparison to Adrenoleukodystrophy
Kornfeld M, Moser AB, Moser HW, Kleinschmidt-DeMasters B, Nolte K, Phelps A (Univ of New Mexico, Albuquerque; Johns Hopkins Univ, Baltimore, Md; Univ of Colorado, Denver)
J Neuropathol Exp Neurol 53:389–398, 1994   122-96-13-3

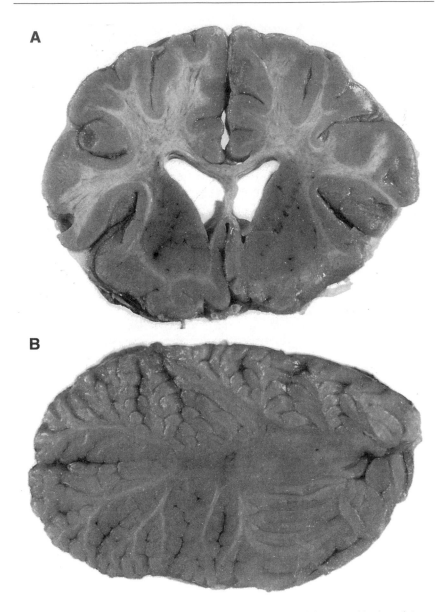

Fig 13–1.—A, white matter has a mottled appearance and is retracted along some blood vessels in case 1. **B,** uneven gray discoloration of the cerebellar white matter. (Courtesy of Kornfeld M, Moser AB, Moser HW, et al: *J Neuropathol Exp Neurol* 53:389–398, 1994.)

Introduction.—The chronic inhalation of the vapors of volatile organic solvents can cause severe, permanent CNS damage. Although there are many reports detailing the clinical findings in such patients, there is little information about the pathology. The pathologic findings in the CNS of 2

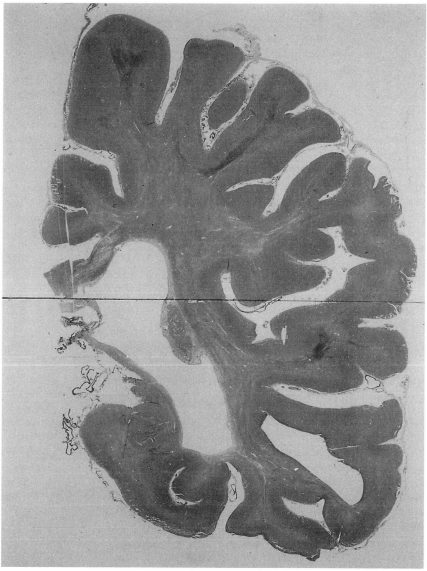

Fig 13–2.—Patchy loss of myelin in central, convolutional, and callosal white matter (LFB-PAS; magnification, ×2). (Courtesy of Kornfeld M, Moser AB, Moser HW, et al: *J Neuropathol Exp Neurol* 53:389–398, 1994.)

solvent vapor abusers, including gross, light, and electron microscopic evidence and chemical analyses, were described.

Methods.—The tissues, including whole brain slabs, were obtained from the 2 patients at autopsy and were examined after immunostaining. The cholesterol esters were extracted and measured from white matter.

Results.—Both patients had reduced brain weight. Both patients had patchy gray discolorations in the white matter of cerebral and cerebellar lobes (Fig 13–1), which corresponded to a patchy loss of myelin that is mostly, but not entirely, around the blood vessels (Fig 13–2). Myelin loss was accompanied by fewer oligodendrocytes and gliosis and was followed by a slower axonal loss. Irregularly round mononuclear cells with a granular, strongly periodic acid-schiff (PAS)–positive cytoplasm, marked with antibodies CD-68 and HAM-56, were found throughout the cerebral and cerebellar white matter, either singly in the parenchyma in areas with more myelin or grouped in the perivascular spaces in areas with more severe myelin loss. These cells contained lamellar aggregates almost exclusively. The brain stem appeared grossly normal but had a severe loss of myelin, and the PAS-positive macrophages were scattered throughout. The cholesterol esters of the brain had increased amounts of very long chain fatty acids.

Discussion.—The pathologic findings in these patients were consistent with a demyelinating process. The ultrastructural finding of trilamellar accumulation in the cytoplasm of the PAS-positive macrophages is a finding similar to that found in some forms of adrenoleukodystrophy. However, the myelination patterns in adrenoleukodystrophy are more uniformly profound and differentiated from normal areas than were seen in these patients.

▶ Chronic solvent abuse remains a prevalent problem in many parts of the world. The clinical syndrome includes cerebellar ataxia, cognitive impairment, spasticity and weakness, and blindness and deafness. This paper illustrates the pathologic findings that underlie both the clinical deficits and the MRI appearance of multifocal demyelination and cortical atrophy. Although widespread demyelination is the end result of both adrenoleukodystrophy and solvent vapor abuse leukoencephalopathy, the difference in pathologic findings, as reported in this paper, probably reflects different pathogenetic mechanisms.—A.R. Berger, M.D.

Aseptic Meningitis Associated With High-Dose Intravenous Immunoglobulin Therapy: Frequency and Risk Factors
Sekul EA, Cupler EJ, Dalakas MC (National Inst of Neurological Disorders and Stroke, Bethesda, Md)
Ann Intern Med 121:259–262, 1994   122-96-13–4

Background.—The initial use of IV immunoglobulin therapy was in the treatment of immune deficiency states, but it has also been shown to be effective in thrombocytopenic purpura, Kawasaki disease, Guillain-Barré syndrome, and dermatomyositis. It has also been used in the treatment of Graves' disease, systemic lupus erythematosus, and myasthenia gravis among others. Although immunoglobulin therapy is considered safe, there have been reports on the rare occurrence of acute renal failure, anaphylactic reactions, and aseptic meningitis. The frequency of aseptic meningitis in patients undergoing IV immunoglobulin therapy was determined.

Methods.—During a 4-year period, 54 consecutive patients, 7–79 years of age, with various immune-related neuromuscular disorders participated in a high-dose trial (2 g/kg) of IV immunoglobulin. Aseptic meningitis was based on symptoms. If the patient was symptomatic, CSF was cultured for bacteria, fungi, and other variables. The serum levels of IgG, glucose, and albumin were determined when the CSF was sampled. A second infusion was administered later to see if the meningitis was related to various infusion parameters.

Results.—Six of the 54 patients had aseptic meningitis within 24 hours after completing the infusion protocol. Treatment cleared symptoms in all patients in 3–5 days. The CSF showed evidence of pleocytosis (4 patients), eosinophilia (3 patients), and IgG elevation (all patients). Cultures of the fluid were negative. Fifty percent of the patients with a history of migraine had meningitis develop. Despite different immunoglobulins and rates of infusion, meningitis still occurred in patients with a history of migraine.

Conclusion.—High-dose IV immunoglobulin therapy can lead to aseptic meningitis. Patients with a history of migraine headaches seem to be particularly susceptible despite using different suppliers and infusion rates. The possible factors leading to meningitis include the IgG preparation, stabilizing compounds, cytokine release, or cerebrovascular sensitivity.

▶ With increased experience with the use of any drug, there comes recognition of side effects that have previously gone unnoticed. As IV immunoglobulin is more widely used, it is to be expected that we shall gain experience of its relatively rarer complications. This study is useful, because it reports on 54 patients who received IV immunoglobulin, 2 g/kg. Although it is unclear from the report, it seems likely that these patients received this dosage as a single infusion in one day, which is ultra-high-dose therapy. Eleven percent had the syndrome of aseptic meningitis develop, the clinical and laboratory features of which are well characterized in this study. There seemed to be no specific relationship to the batch of drug, different commercial preparations, or corticosteroid therapy. There may have been some relationship to a previous history of migraine, and this association is of interest. I have seen approximately the same frequency of severe headache with the more standard regimen of 0.4 g/kg/day given for 5 days.

The cause of the aseptic meningitis remains unclear. Many patients have such a reaction with one infusion and then do not have a recurrence with later infusions. Treatment with nonsteroidal anti-inflammatory medications appears to be relatively effective in suppressing the symptoms, and these can be used prophylactically. The condition frequently does not occur on rechallenge, although occasionally it does so and prevents further usage of this treatment. The aseptic meningitis is to be added to the other complications of IV immunoglobulin therapy, including those of hyperviscosity, such as stroke, myocardial infarction, and congestive failure, as well as rashes and phenomenon.—W.G. Bradley, D.M., F.R.C.P.

Early Diagnosis of *n*-Hexane–Caused Neuropathy

Pastore C, Marhuenda D, Marti J, Cardona A (Hosp Universitari Sant Joan D'Alacant, Spain; Univ of Alicante, Spain)
Muscle Nerve 17:981–986, 1994   122-96-13–5

Background.—The neurotoxin *n*-hexane produces peripheral and, probably, central axonal abnormalities, chiefly those involving distal sensory and motor nerves. The severity of the neuropathy depends on the duration of exposure. The neurotoxicity has been associated with 2,5-hexanedione (2,5-HD), a metabolite formed by the biotransformation of *n*-hexane and methyl *n*-butyl ketone. Those who are affected usually have progressive numbness develop in the distal parts of the extremities. Motor changes develop much later and only in those who are severely affected.

Objective.—An attempt was made to diagnose this disorder electrophysiologically and at an early stage in those whose neuropathy was subclinical. Twenty overtly healthy individuals occupationally exposed for prolonged periods to solvents containing *n*-hexane were studied. All had urinary 2,5-HD levels higher than 5 mg/L, which is the recommended biological exposure index. The mean level was 11 mg/L.

Findings.—Myotactic limb reflexes were preserved. Only 6 of the 20 subjects described sporadic numbness in the fingers and toes when directly questioned. Conduction velocities were consistently normal, but affected individuals had significantly reduced sensory nerve action potential (SNAP) amplitudes in the sural, median, and ulnar nerves compared with healthy adults matched for age. The SNAP amplitudes in the sural and median nerves correlated inversely with the time of exposure to a significant degree.

Conclusion.—Measuring SNAP amplitudes in the peripheral nerves may permit an early diagnosis of neuropathy caused by exposure to *n*-hexane.

▶ Nerve conduction abnormalities in neuropathy resulting from *n*-hexane show a combination of axonal and demyelinating features. This article reports that an early change in asymptomatic subjects exposed to *n*-hexane involved reductions in median, ulnar, and sural sensory potential amplitudes. These findings need to be interpreted with caution. The control group was not representative of the exposed subjects, and there was no controlling of variables such as sex, height, and finger circumference, all of which are known to affect conduction parameters.—A.R. Berger, M.D.

14 Infectious Diseases

Herpes Simplex Virus Infection as a Cause of Benign Recurrent Lymphocytic Meningitis
Tedder DG, Ashley R, Tyler KL, Levin MJ (Univ of Colorado, Denver; The Children's Hosp, Denver, Colo; Denver Veterans Affairs Med Ctr, Colo; et al)
Ann Intern Med 121:334–338, 1994   122-96-14-1

Objective.—Reactivation of latent herpes simplex virus (HSV) infection from sensory ganglia can cause encephalitis and meningitis. Except for 1 patient, it has not been possible to isolate HSV from the CSF of patients with recurrent meningitis. The role of HSV in benign recurrent lymphocytic meningitis was studied using new diagnostic techniques.

Methods.—In CSF specimens, HSV DNA was detected using the polymerase chain reaction (PCR), followed by hybridization with an HSV-specific DNA probe. Herpes simplex virus types 1 and 2 DNA products were distinguished by digestion with restriction enzymes and analysis by gel electrophoresis. Immunoblotting was used to detect anti-HSV antibodies.

Patients.—Between 1990 and 1993, 20 consecutive patients with a presumptive diagnosis of benign recurrent lymphocytic meningitis were seen. Thirteen patients met the criteria for recurrent benign lymphocytic meningitis. These patients had 3 to 9 attacks of meningitis (mean, 4.6 attacks) during periods ranging from 2 to 21 years (mean, 8.4 years). Analysis of CSF showed 48 to 1,600 cells/μL and normal levels of glucose (> 2.22 mmol/L) and protein (41–240 mg/dL).

Results.—In 11 patients (84.6%; confidence interval, 55% to 98%), HSV DNA was detected by PCR in CSF specimens. Of them, 10 patients had HSV type 2 DNA and HSV type 2 antibodies, and 1 had HSV type 1 DNA and HSV type 1 antibodies. The remaining 2 patients had no detectable HSV DNA, although both had anti-HSV type 2 antibodies. Only 3 patients with HSV DNA and antibody in their CSF had a history of recurrent genital herpes simplex, but none had mucocutaneous lesions at the time of their meningitis.

Conclusion.—Herpes simplex virus, predominantly HSV type 2, is a major causative agent in benign recurrent lymphocytic meningitis. Herpes simplex virus type 2 in sensory neurons of sacral dorsal root ganglia may seed the CSF subarachnoid space and produce meningitis. This raises the possibility that therapy may abort attacks of meningitis or prevent recurrent attacks, although treatment with acyclovir has not yet been shown to definitely alter the natural history of the disease.

▶ In as much as 25% of the population in the United States, HSV type 2 can be demonstrated in sacral ganglia. Seroepidemiologic data confirm this seemingly high rate of infection. Most, if not the majority, of these infections are subclinical. Tedder and colleagues have detected HSV type 2 infection by PCR as the cause of benign recurrent lymphocytic (Mollaret's) meningitis in 77% of patients, confirming prior observations that suggested HSV type 2 was responsible for the overwhelming preponderance of these cases. Of practical importance is the value of prophylactic acyclovir in the treatment of this disorder. In my own experience, acyclovir, given in daily doses as low as 400 mg, has been effective in preventing recurrences.—J.R. Berger, M.D.

Human Spongiform Encephalopathy: The National Institutes of Health Series of 300 Cases of Experimentally Transmitted Disease
Brown P, Gibbs CJ Jr, Rodgers-Johnson P, Asher DM, Sulima MP, Bacote A, Goldfarb LG, Gajdusek DC (Natl Insts of Health, Bethesda, Md)
Ann Neurol 35:513–529, 1994   122-96-14–2

Background.—There has been a recent trend to redefine the spongiform encephalopathies as "prion dementias" based on molecular biology and genetics. Therefore, it seems appropriate to summarize the clinical, pathologic, and biological features of experimentally transmitted cases occurring between 1963 and 1993.

Cases and Findings.—The review included 300 experimentally transmitted cases of spongiform encephalopathy from among more than 1,000 cases of various neurologic disorders inoculated into nonhuman primates in the past 30 years. There were 278 subjects with Creutzfeldt-Jakob disease (CJD), of whom 234 had sporadic disease; 36, familial; and 8, iatrogenic disease. Eighteen patients had kuru, and 4 had Gerstmann-Sträussler-Scheinker (GSS) syndrome. Sporadic CJD had an average age at onset of 60 years, with the frequent early appearance of cerebellar and visual/oculomotor signs and a broad spectrum of clinical features. The disease was usually fatal in less than 6 months. All but 2 patients had characteristic spongiform neuropathology. Microscopically visible kuru-type amyloid plaques were noted in 5% of patients with CJD, 75% of those with kuru, and all of those with GSS syndrome. A brain biopsy specimen was diagnostic in 95% of the cases confirmed subsequently at autopsy. Proteinase-resistant amyloid protection was identified in Western blots of brain extracts from 88% of the subjects tested. Experimental rates of transmission were greatest for iatrogenic CJD at 100%, kuru at 95%, and sporadic CJD at 90%. They were considerably lower, at 68%, for most familial forms of disease (table).

Conclusions.—The National Institutes of Health series of 300 experimentally transmitted cases of spongiform encephalopathy were reviewed.

Summary of Experimental Primate Transmission Attempts From Patients With Spongiform Encephalopathy Referred to the NIH Laboratory of CNS Studies, 1963–1993

Disease	Transmitted	No. of Cases* Untransmitted	Inconclusive	No. of Animals
Creutzfeldt-Jakob (CJD)				
Sporadic	225	24[†]	78[‡]	1,167
Familial	36	11	14	197
Iatrogenic	8	0	0	45
Gerstmann-Sträussler-Scheinker	4	5	4	42
Fatal familial insomnia	0	3§	2[||]	18
Kuru	18	1	7	445
Totals	291¶	44	105	1,914

* Criteria used to classify cases as transmitted, untransmitted, or inconclusive are described in the Methods section of the original article.
† One of these cases transmitted to guinea pigs in another laboratory.
‡ Two of these cases transmitted to marmosets or mice in other laboratories.
§ All members of the same family; a total of 6 animals inoculated with cerebral cortical homogenates survived well beyond the maximum limit for inconclusive cases in chimpanzees (2) and squirrel monkeys (4).
|| Unrelated recent cases (1993), each inoculated into 6 animals (pairs of animals were inoculated with homogenates prepared from 3 different brain regions; cerebral cortex, basal ganglia/cerebellum, and thalamus).
¶ Nine additional cases of sporadic Creutzfeldt-Jakob disease (CJD) transmitted exclusively to nonprimates (6 were not inoculated into primates, and 3 did not transmit to primates), bringing the total transmitted cases to 300.
(Courtesy of Brown P, Gibbs CJ Jr, Rodgers-Johnson P, et al: Ann Neurol 35:513–529, 1994.)

Infectivity reached average levels of almost 10^5 median lethal doses per gram of brain tissue but was present irregularly in tissues outside the brain.

▶ This large review of human spongiform encephalopathies confirms a number of earlier observations, including the almost equal male to female ratio, a median age of onset of 60 years (range, 16–82 years), and a gradual onset of the illness occurring over a period of weeks to months in the overwhelming majority (87%) of patients. The illness was heralded by pro-dromal symptoms in 26%, and pyramidal, extrapyramidal, cerebellar, and visual/oculomotor findings were common. Myoclonus was ultimately observed in 78%, and periodic EEGs were done in 60%. The median duration of illness was 4.5 months, and the mean duration was 8.0 months. Although high levels of infectivity were found in brain tissues, it was inconsistently present and only in much lower titers in tissues outside of the brain. Furthermore, CSF was the only body fluid that was demonstrated to be infective. The latter observations should be reassuring to health care providers and the families of these patients.—J.R. Berger, M.D.

Iatrogenic Creutzfeldt-Jakob Disease: An Example of the Interplay Between Ancient Genes and Modern Medicine

Brown P, Cervanáková L, Goldfarb LG, McCombie WR, Rubenstein R, Will RG, Pocchiari M, Martinez-Lage JF, Scalici C, Masullo C, Graupera G, Ligan J, Gajdusek DC (National Inst of Neurological Disorders and Stroke, Bethesda, Md; Inst for Basic Research in Developmental Disabilities, Staten Island, NY; Western General Hosp, Edinburgh, Scotland; et al)
Neurology 44:291–293, 1994   122-96-14-3

Objective.—Mutations of amyloid protein are involved in the pathogenesis of familial spongiform encephalopathies. The same mutations are suspected in nonfamilial disease. The DNA from patients with iatrogenic Creutzfeldt-Jakob disease (CJD) was tested for the presence of mutations of the amyloid gene.

Methods.—The DNA samples extracted from the brains of 15 patients infected by contaminated electroencephalogram electrodes or corneal or dura mater homografts, 11 patients infected with contaminated human growth hormone, and 110 controls were compared. The DNA was analyzed for mutations at codons 102, 178, 200, and 129.

Results.—None of the specimens showed any relationship to familial forms of the disease. Homozygosity in the polymorphic codon 129 was detected in 92% of the patients and 50% of the controls.

Conclusion.—Patients who are homozygous at codon 129 appear to be more susceptible to iatrogenic infections. This is important for patients receiving homografts or growth hormone, who might thereby be exposed to the causative agent of CJD.

▶ This study is important because it confirms and expands the observations of Collinge and colleagues (1) regarding the importance of homozygosity for valine at codon 129 in the development of CJD after iatrogenic exposure. Why has CJD not occurred in each of the recipients of contaminated pooled human growth hormone? One possible explanation may be the varying susceptibility to the disease determined by the presence homozygosity for valine or methionine at codon 129. Perhaps these amino acids render the protein more likely to undergo conformational change to an insoluble form when exposed to the infectious prion. Codon 129 also appears to be important not only in the rapidity with which the disease will develop after exposure, but also in its phenotypic expression.—J.R. Berger, M.D.

Reference

1. Collinge J, Palmer MS, Dryden AJ: Genetic predisposition to iatrogenic Creutzfeldt-Jakob disease. *Lancet* 337:1441–1442, 1991.

Polymerase Chain Reaction for Rapid Diagnosis of Tuberculous Meningitis in AIDS Patients
Folgueira L, Delgado R, Palenque E, Noreiga AR (Hospital Doce de Octubre, Madrid, Spain)
Neurology 44:1336–1338, 1994   122-96-14–4

Objective.—Central nervous system involvement is especially significant in HIV-seropositive patients with tuberculosis. However, it is difficult to detect *Mycobacterium tuberculosis* microbiologically. The use of the polymerase chain reaction (PCR) technique to detect *M. tuberculosis* in 11 CSF samples from 10 HIV-seropositive patients was documented.

Methods.—Results from 11 CSF samples taken from HIV-seropositive patients were compared with those of control groups including 6 HIV-seropositive and 8 HIV-seronegative patients with neurological illnesses other than tuberculosis. The assay detected the 123-bp region in the mycobacterial DNA-complex.

Results.—Six of 10 patients had abnormal neurologic signs, and 8 of 10 had suspected tuberculosis. The cultures were positive in 5 of these patients. Polymerase chain reaction results were positive in 9 samples from the patients with suspected tuberculosis and negative in the control group samples.

Conclusion.—In this limited study, PCR was faster and more sensitive in diagnosing tuberculosis in patients with HIV than were conventional tests.

▶ Even in the present day, tuberculous meningitis has a poor prognosis, particularly when the diagnosis is delayed. In the old days, pathologists were extremely skilled at searching Ziehl-Neelsen–stained smears of CSF for the one single characteristic *M. tuberculosis* bacterium that was sufficient to diagnose the disease. Proof of the infection by culture is much slower. The PCR technique is the mechanism by which a suspected diagnosis of tuberculous meningitis should be confirmed.—W.G. Bradley, D.M., F.R.C.P.

Use of Thallium-201 Brain SPECT to Differentiate Cerebral Lymphoma From Toxoplasma Encephalitis in AIDS Patients
Ruiz A, Ganz WI, Post MJD, Camp A, Landy H, Mallin W, Sfakianakis GN
(Univ of Miami, Fla)
AJNR 15:1885–1894, 1994   122-96-14-5

Objective.—Because of the difficulty in distinguishing between cerebral lymphoma and toxoplasmic encephalitis in HIV-infected patients using CT or MRI, a prospective study of brain single-photon emission CT (SPECT) imaging was undertaken in these patients.

Methods.—Included were 37 patients with AIDS in whom CT or MRI, or both, had demonstrated mass lesions in the CNS. Planar SPECT imaging began 5 minutes after the injection of 5 mCi of radiothallium. All patients underwent high-resolution CT scanning followed by a double-dose contrast study of the brain. Six patients also had MRI before and after gadopentetate dimeglumine injection.

Results.—Twelve of the 37 patients with negative serum antitoxoplasmosis IgG antibody titers had increased thallium uptake that, in each case, matched the patient's findings on CT or MRI, or both. Five patients had more than 1 parenchymal lesion. The biopsy and autopsy findings confirmed primary brain lymphoma in each patient. The remaining 25 patients lacked cerebral uptake of radiothallium. Six of these patients had a single CNS lesion. All the patients except 1 with tubercular infection had positive antitoxoplasmosis IgG antibody titers and improved when receiving antitoxoplasmosis medication. Serial CT scanning showed that the lesions resolved within 2–6 weeks.

Conclusion.—Cerebral SPECT imaging with ^{201}Tl in patients with AIDS with mass lesions of the CNS may help confirm or rule out lymphoma and may also allow earlier radiation therapy when CNS lymphoma is diagnosed.

▶ The importance and extreme usefulness of the thallium SPECT imaging technique in patients who have AIDS and an intracerebral mass (or masses) are emphasized by this article. Ruiz and his colleagues have demonstrated the ability to differentiate between the 2 most common causes of intraparenchymal masses in AIDS: toxoplasmosis and lymphoma. Rather than adding cost to a patient's workup, this procedure can quicken the time to diagnosis, prompting early biopsy and radiation therapy if the ^{201}Tl SPECT results are positive and lymphoma is suggested. Integrating this imaging into a patient's evaluation is recommended.—R.M. Quencer, M.D.

Persistent Enhancement After Treatment for Cerebral Toxoplasmosis in Patients With AIDS: Predictive Value for Subsequent Recurrence
Laissy JP, Soyer P, Parlier C, Lariven S, Benmelha Z, Servois V, Casalino E, Bouvet E, Sibert A, Vachon F, Menu Y (Hôpital Bichat, Paris)
AJNR 15:1773–1778, 1994   122-96-14–6

Introduction.—Toxoplasmosis is the most common opportunistic brain infection among patients with AIDS in western Europe. At least one fourth of patients may be affected. The advent of retroviral drugs has increased the likelihood that cerebral toxoplasmosis will recur.

Objective and Methods.—In a retrospective study, it was determined whether CT or MR findings, or both, are able to predict recurrences of toxoplasmosis in the brain. Forty-three patients, 32 without and 11 with recurrences, were examined by CT scanning before and after intravenous contrast injection, and 22 also had MRI. Three radiologists independently interpreted the findings without knowledge of the patients' clinical status. The patients were initially treated with both sulfadiazine and pyrimethamine.

Findings.—The patients with recurrences did not differ clinically from those without recurrences to a significant extent, but in most patients with recurrences, toxoplasmosis was the initial feature of conversion to a positive HIV status. Patients with recurrences tended to have fewer lesions at the time of diagnosis and more ring-enhancing lesions. Almost three fourths of the patients had sequelae such as encephalomalacia, persistent focal subcortical enhancement, and hemorrhage. Persistent enhancement correlated with recurrences, but areas of encephalomalacia did not. Recurrences did not develop in patients lacking brain sequelae.

Implication.—The more aggressive treatment of patients exhibiting cerebral sequelae of toxoplasmosis, using combination antibiotherapy, might minimize the risk of serious neurologic impairment.

▶ In both western Europe and North America, toxoplasmosis is the most common opportunistic infection of the brain. As with most other infections in patients with AIDS, secondary prophylaxis is required to prevent recurrence of the disorder. Dr. Laissy and colleagues report on the predictive value of persistent contrast enhancement of these lesions for recurrence, and they suggest that this radiographic feature may be valuable in identifying those individuals who require more aggressive prophylactic antitoxoplasmosis therapy. The regimen that they used for secondary prophylaxis is somewhat different than that commonly used in the United States. Despite that, physicians should exercise a higher degree of vigilance in those patients with toxoplasmosis who have persistent enhancement. Whether an alteration in the standard secondary prophylactic regimen is necessary will require further study.—J.R. Berger, M.D.

Cytomegalovirus Encephalitis in Acquired Immunodeficiency Syndrome (AIDS)

Holland NR, Power C, Mathews VP, Glass JD, Forman M, McArthur JC
(Johns Hopkins Univ, Baltimore, Md)
Neurology 44:507–514, 1994   122-96-14-7

Background.—The specific clinical features of cytomegalovirus encephalitis (CMVE) have not yet been fully defined. As such, this condition is frequently diagnosed only post mortem. The clinical, radiologic, and laboratory features of CMVE were determined in a retrospective case-control study.

Patients and Findings.—Fourteen autopsy-verified patients with CMVE were compared with a control group of 17 demented patients with AIDS but not CMVE or any other pathologically identified CNS opportunistic processes. Cytomegalovirus encephalitis occurred more frequently in homosexual men. In addition, a subacute onset of CMVE was more typical, with a mean duration of presenting symptoms of 3.5 weeks compared with 18 weeks in demented controls. The median survival times were 4.6 and 28 weeks for patients with CMVE and control patients, respectively. At autopsy, CMVE was accompanied by prominent systemic cytomegalovirus (CMV) infection. This included CMV adrenalitis in 92%, CMV pneumonitis in 42%, systemic *Mycobacterium avium-intracellulare* (MAI) in 58%, and CMV retinitis in 58%. In addition, hyponatremia and MAI bacteremia were noted in 58% of the patients with CMVE. The CMV genome, identified via polymerase chain reaction (PCR) of CSF samples, was also found in 33% of the patients with CMVE. Periventricular enhancement on CT and periventricular lesions with meningeal enhancement on MRI scans were found to be associated with CMVE (Fig 14–1).

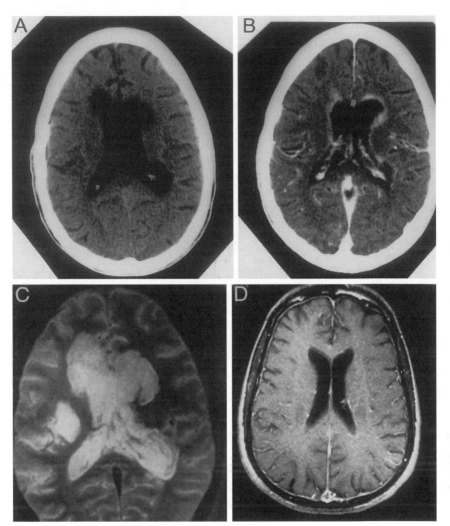

Fig 14–1.—Case 10. Imaging of a patient with severe cytomegavovirus encephalitis. **A,** CT scan showing atrophy with periventricular hypointensity. **B,** CT with contrast showing periventricular enhancement extending beyond the periventricular region. **C,** T2-weighted MRI scan showing periventricular hyperintensity with a right parenchymal lesion. **D,** MRI scan from case 2 showing meningeal enhancement. (Courtesy of Holland NR, Power C, Mathews VP, et al: *Neurology* 44:507–514, 1994.)

Conclusions.—Cytomegalovirus encephalitis should be strongly suspected in homosexual men with subacute encephalopathy who have had AIDS for more than 12 months and a prior history of systemic CMV infection. In addition, periventricular lesions, hyponatremia, and identification of the CMV genome in CSF via PCR may provide further support for a diagnosis of CMVE.

▶ One pathogen frequently seen in the brain in patients with AIDS with dementia is CMV. In some pathologic studies, evidence for CMVE has been detected in as many as 40% of demented patients with AIDS. Although the value of therapy directed at CMVE remains to be decisively established, ganciclovir and foscarnet have shown efficacy in other illnesses caused by CMV in patients with AIDS. They and the anti-CMV agents currently being developed are likely to have value in the treatment of CMVE as well. Identifying reliable markers for the presence of CMVE, as Holland and colleagues have done in this paper, is the first step toward developing rational therapy. Instituting therapy directed against CMV in patients with AIDS with dementia accompanied by adrenal insufficiency, periventricular lesions on MRI, or a history of systemic CMV infection should be considered irrespective of the results of CSF viral culture and PCR studies for CMV.— J.R. Berger, M.D.

Varicella-Zoster Virus Infection of the Central Nervous System in the Acquired Immune Deficiency Syndrome
Gray F, Bélec L, Lescs MC, Chrétien F, Ciardi A, Hassine D, Flament-Saillour M, de Truchis P, Clair B, Scaravilli F (Université Paris-Val de Marne, France; Université Paris V, France; Université Paris VI, France, et al)
Brain 117:987–999, 1994   122-96-14–8

Background.—Varicella-zoster virus (VZV) infection has been considered an uncommon opportunistic CNS infection in patients with AIDS. Using immunocytochemistry and in situ hybridization, 11 patients with AIDS with productive VZV infection of the CNS were identified. Just 4 of these patients had the characteristic skin eruption of zoster. These and 11 previously reported cases were analyzed to clarify the different clinicopathologic patterns of VZV infection of the CNS in patients with AIDS.

Findings.—Five different clinicopathologic patterns, which could occur simultaneously, were revealed. Four of the 11 patients had a multifocal encephalitis that predominantly involved the white matter, and this was most likely caused by a hematogenous spread of the VZV infection. Three patients had vasculitis, 2 of whom had complete acute or chronic necrosis of the ventricular wall with marked vasculitis. The third patient in this group had an irregular-appearing ependymal lining with foci of VZV-infected cells, some of which protruded into the ventricular lumen.

Two patients had acute hemorrhagic meningo-myeloradiculitis with necrotizing vasculitis; this was associated with ventriculitis in 1 patient, perhaps the result of the shedding of infected cells into the ventricular lumen and secondary seeding of the CSF. One patient had focal necrotizing myelitis after cutaneous herpes zoster; this was believed to result from neural spread from the diseased dorsal root ganglion, similar to previously reported cases of encephalitis limited to the visual system after VZV ophthalmicus, or bulbar encephalitis after trigeminal zoster. Four patients had vasculopathy involving the leptomeningeal arteries and causing cerebral infarcts. In most cases, this vasculopathy was associated with meningitis.

Conclusions.—In patients with AIDS, VZV infection of the CNS appears to be more frequent than previously thought. The diagnosis of VZV infection should be considered in patients with AIDS who have encephalitis, ventriculitis, focal myelitis, acute myeloradiculitis, or cerebral infarcts. The spread of VZV to the CNS may occur through various routes.

▶ This study highlights the myriad ways that herpes VZV may affect the nervous system in patients with AIDS. Furthermore, only 4 of the 11 patients in this study exhibited skin lesions suggestive of herpes VZV infection, rendering the diagnosis difficult. A high index of suspicion for herpes VZV is required when one is confronted with multifocal encephalitis, stroke, myelopathy, or myeloradiculitis in a patient with AIDS. The application of polymerase chain reaction to CSF samples may be of value in detecting the infection, but additional studies will be required to establish the sensitivity and specificity of this test. High doses of acyclovir are warranted in treating these disorders.—J.R. Berger, M.D.

Clinicopathologic Correlations of HIV-1–Associated Vacuolar Myelopathy: An Autopsy-Based Case-Control Study

Dal Pan GJ, Glass JD, McArthur JC (Johns Hopkins Univ, Baltimore, Md)
Neurology 44:2159–2164, 1994   122-96-14-9

Background.—Autopsies of patients dying of AIDS frequently show HIV-1–associated vacuolar myelopathy (VM), a spongiform degeneration of the spinal cord. There are few reports, however, on the clinical correlates of HIV-associated VM, the frequency of this condition in patients with AIDS, or its relationship to other AIDS-related illnesses. The clinical features of patients with AIDS who had pathologically proven VM (cases) were compared with those of patients with AIDS without VM (controls).

Methods.—The study group was drawn from 251 autopsies of patients with AIDS. In 215 autopsies, the brain and spinal cord were examined. These records and hospital charts were reviewed for the presence of AIDS-defining illnesses. Data on neurologic diagnoses were recorded for each patient seen by the study institution's AIDS neurology consultation service.

Results.—One hundred (46.5%) of the 215 autopsies were classified as cases and 115 (53.5%) as controls. The VM cases were slightly older than the controls, but the 2 groups were similar in HIV-1 risk behaviors. The frequency of VM showed no temporal trend during the study years (1983–1991). Median survival after the initial diagnosis of AIDS was 12.1 months for cases and 12.6 months for controls; only 5 patients, all without VM, survived more than 39 months after diagnosis. There was a strong association between an increasing number of AIDS-defining illnesses—particularly *Mycobacterium avium-intracellulare* infection and *Pneu-*

mocystis carinii pneumonia—and the likelihood of VM (Fig 14–2). Cases were also more likely to have multinucleated giant cells in the brain and to have sensory neuropathy. Only 26.8% of the cases with VM who had undergone detailed neurologic evaluations had signs and symptoms of myelopathy. There was a significant correlation between pathologic severity and the presence of symptomatic myelopathy.

Conclusions.—Although VM is a common neuropathologic finding at autopsy in patients who have died of AIDS, the condition is often unrecognized during life. The correlation between VM and the number of AIDS-defining illnesses suggests that VM is associated with severe immunosuppression and advanced HIV disease. A certain threshold level of structural damage appears to be necessary before myelopathy is clinically evident.

▶ In this study correlating autopsy and clinical data, the frequency of pathologically documented VM significantly exceeded its detection by examination. There was an apparent association between the degree of immunosuppression and the likelihood of detecting the disorder clinically, as evidenced by the increased numbers of opportunistic infections and other AIDS-defining illnesses. The specific mechanism by which this myelopathy arises remains unclear. Some studies have demonstrated a poor correlation between the presence of VM and the presence of HIV-1 in the affected areas of the spinal cords, suggesting that indirect effects of the virus may be responsible. When confronted with an HIV-infected individual with myelopa-

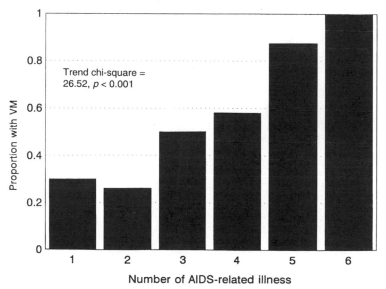

Fig 14–2.—Probability of vacuolar myelopathy (*VM*) as a function of the number of AIDS-defining illnesses. Cases and controls were grouped according to the number of AIDS-defining illnesses (range, 1–6). For each number, the proportion with VM was determined. Trend chi-square analysis indicates a significant increase in the proportion with VM as the number of illnesses increases. (Courtesy of Dal Pan GJ, Glass JD, McArthur JC: *Neurology* 44:2159–2164, 1994.)

thy, the physician must also consider other etiologies (in particular, those that are potentially treatable, such as the encroachment on the spinal cord by lymphoma or syphilitic meningomyelitis). Magnetic resonance imaging of the involved spinal cord and detailed examination of the spinal fluid for evidence of opportunistic infection, syphilis, and malignancy are mandatory.—J.R. Berger, M.D.

Acute Lumbosacral Polyradiculopathy in Acquired Immunodeficiency Syndrome: Experience in 23 Patients
So YT, Olney RK (Univ of California, San Francisco)
Ann Neurol 35:53–58, 1994   122-96-14–10

Background.—Acute lumbosacral polyradiculopathy is uncommon, occurring in less than 2% of seropositive patients referred for neurologic consultation. The distinctive clinical features, differential diagnosis, and temporal course of this syndrome were studied in 1 series.

Patients and Findings.—Twenty-three patients with AIDS and acute lumbosacral polyradiculopathy were included in the review. All had a distinctive syndrome of rapidly progressive flaccid paraparesis and areflexia often associated with sphincter disturbances. Fifteen patients had persuasive laboratory evidence of a cytomegalovirus polyradiculopathy. Ganciclovir treatment resulted in clinical stabilization, though worsening in the first 2 weeks was common. Severe residual deficits were noted in most patients with CMV polyradiculopathy. In two other cases, metastasis from systemic lymphoma was responsible for the polyradiculopathy. The

---

Symptoms and Physical Findings in 23 Patients With Acute
Lumbosacral Polyradiculopathy

	No. of Patients
Symptoms	
Leg weakness	23
Bladder and bowel dysfunction	19
Leg paresthesias	15
Low-back pain	9
Fever	8
Neurological findings	
Weakness	23
Depressed or absent tendon reflex in legs	23
Early areflexia	14
Depressed initially, later areflexic	4
Depressed but present in at least 1 site	5
Sensory loss	19
Lower limbs	19
S4 and S5 dermatomes	12
Weak contraction of anal sphincter	14
Pain with straight-leg raising	8
Lumbosacral spine tenderness	7

(Courtesy of So YT, Olney RK: *Ann Neurol* 35:53–58, 1994.)

remaining 6 patients had a more benign syndrome, characterized by a slower clinical progression and less severe neurologic deficits at the nadir than in patients with CMV polyradiculopathy. In addition, the CSF in the former group showed a predominantly mononuclear pleocytosis, unlike in patients with CMV infection. Spontaneous improvement without treatment was common in those with more benign disease (table).

Conclusion.—This and other experiences suggest that the acute lumbosacral polyradiculopathy in AIDS has different etiologies and variable clinical outcomes. Recognizing this heterogeneity is important in the management of individuals and in the interpretation of treatment results (Fig 14–3).

▶ In their attempt to define the clinical syndromes of lumbosacral polyradiculopathy occurring in patients with AIDS, So and Olney describe 3 entities: CMV polyradiculopathy, metastatic lymphoma, and a relatively benign syndrome without identified pathogen. With additional clinical experience, it

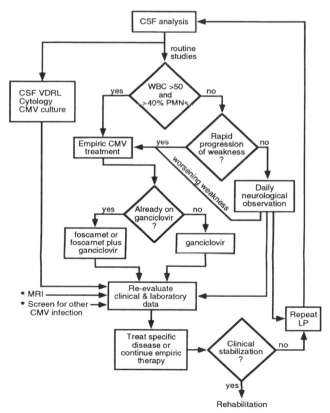

Fig 14–3.—Proposed algorithm in the empirical management of patients with AIDS and acute lumbosacral polyradiculopathy before an etiologic diagnosis is established. *Abbreviations: CMV,* cytomegalovirus; *LP,* lumbar puncture; *PMNs,* polymorphonuclear cells; *WBC,* white blood cell count. (Courtesy of So YT, Olney RK: *Ann Neurol* 35:53–58, 1994.)

is not unlikely that the latter disorder will be better characterized and, perhaps, other disorders with similar manifestations identified. The value of their observations is in distinguishing between these entities, establishing a prognosis, and instituting a sensible therapeutic option. As demonstrated in this study, an acute, progressive polyradiculopathy occurring in patients with AIDS is usually the consequence of CMV infection, and appropriate therapy often results in clinical improvement.—J.R. Berger, M.D.

Cytomegalovirus Multifocal Neuropathy in AIDS: Analysis of 15 Consecutive Cases

Roullet E, Assuerus V, Gozlan J, Ropert A, Saïd G, Baudrimont M, El Amrani M, Jacomet C, Duvivier C, Gonzales-Canali G, Kirstetter M, Meyohas M-C, Picard O, Rozenbaum W (Hôpital Saint-Antoine, Paris; Hôpital Rothschild, Paris; Hôpital Bicêtre, France)
Neurology 44:2174–2182, 1994   122-96-14–11

Background.—Cytomegalovirus (CMV), the most common opportunistic pathogen of late-stage HIV-1 infection, is responsible for a wide range of neurologic complications. Two peripheral nerve syndromes caused by CMV in patients with AIDS are polyradiculomyelopathy (PRAM) and multifocal neuropathy (CMV-MN). There are a number of studies on the clinical features and treatment of PRAM, whereas only 8 cases of CMV-MN have been reported. Therefore, 15 consecutive cases of CMV-MN were reviewed, and the clinical and electrophysiologic aspects of the syndrome were illustrated.

Patients and Methods.—The patients, all men with confirmed HIV-1 infection, were examined between May 1989 and August 1992. Diagnosis of CMV-MN was based on the findings of markedly asymmetric neuropathy, fewer than 100 CD4+ cells per mm^3, and exclusion of other causes of neuropathy. In addition, 2 patients had characteristic CMV cytopathic changes on neuromuscular biopsy, 2 had positive CSF cultures for CMV, and 11 showed clinical improvement on anti-CMV therapy given for either concurrent extraneurologic CMV disease or neuropathy.

Results.—Two patients did not receive specific anti-CMV therapy. One was soon lost to follow-up, and the other died 6 months after onset of neurologic symptoms, leaving 15 patients for analysis. Initial symptoms were paresthesias, pain, weakness, and numbness. Moderate or severe sensorimotor asymmetric neuropathy developed after a mean of 11 weeks. Deficits were purely motor in 1 patient, purely sensory in 1, and mixed in 13. Before treatment, 1 patient was bedridden, 2 used a wheelchair, and 2 needed bilateral walking aids. The polymerase chain reaction technique showed cytomegalovirus DNA in the CSF of 90% of patients tested. Extraneurologic involvement included retinitis in 7 patients and pneumonopathy in 2. Nerve biopsy, performed in 8 patients, showed endoneurial inflammation in 4, and typical CMV inclusions in 2. There was mild or moderate neurogenic atrophy in all muscle biopsy specimens. All patients were treated with specific anti-CMV drugs: ganciclovir (5 mg/kg IV every 12 hours) in 12 patients, and foscarnet (100 mg/kg IV every 12 hours) in 10 patients. Fourteen patients showed improvement, starting at a mean of 3 weeks after initiation of therapy. Of 13 patients who received maintenance therapy, 3 had a relapse of neuropathy, and 5 had probable or confirmed CMV encephalitis. Twelve patients died during follow-up, 9 of CMV infection. Death occurred at a mean of 6.6 months after the start of therapy and 9.5 months after the onset of symptoms.

Conclusions.—Most patients previously reported with CMV-MN died soon after diagnosis. The patients often showed a milder course and responded to treatment. The clinical pattern of CMV-MN is homogeneous, with painful sensory symptoms present at onset. Electrophysiologic abnormalities are suggestive of an axonal neuropathy. Both drugs that were used yielded a high rate of initial response. A useful diagnostic marker for the syndrome is the polymerase chain reaction detection of cytomegalovirus DNA in the CSF.

▶ Several neuropathic syndromes occur in HIV infection, including the Guillain-Barré syndrome, chronic inflammatory demyelinating polyneuropathy, vasculitic neuropathy, a chronic, painful, distal sensory polyneuropathy, and CMV-associated PRAM. This paper emphasizes the last condition and a rarer entity, CMV-associated multifocal neuropathy. Treatment of these patients with ganciclovir or foscarnet resulted in considerable improvement in most patients, although maintenance therapy was required in the majority.—W.G. Bradley, D.M., F.R.C.P.

Acute Rhabdomyolysis in Patients Infected by Human Immunodeficiency Virus
Chariot P, Ruet E, Authier FJ, Lévy Y, Gherardi R (Hôpital Henri Mondor, Créteil, France)
Neurology 44:1692–1696, 1994   122-96-14–12

Introduction.—Various muscle disorders can develop in patients with HIV infection. In rhabdomyolysis, creatine kinase and myoglobin escape from muscle cells because of direct injuries or an imbalance between energy production and use in muscle. There have been several case reports of HIV-related rhabdomyolysis, with varying causes and clinical courses. Toward defining the spectrum of HIV-related rhabdomyolysis, 9 new and 11 previously reported cases were studied.

Patients and Findings.—Rhabdomyolysis occurred at all stages of HIV infection. The patients were classified into 3 groups. Seven of the 20 patients were considered to have HIV-associated rhabdomyolysis, in which there was no concurrent illness or other condition to explain their findings. In 3 patients, acute rhabdomyolysis occurred coincidentally with primary HIV infection—these cases were considered acute myoglobinuric viral infection. Two patients had recurrent rhabdomyolysis in which HIV infection may have played a pathogenetic role. Two patients had isolated rhabdomyolysis; in one case, this was believed to result from HIV-associated polymyositis. All patients in this group recovered, most spontaneously.

Six patients had probable drug-induced rhabdomyolysis. One case appeared related to both psychotropic drug overdose and compression. A direct toxic effect may have been operative in 2 cases of didanosine-associated rhabdomyolysis. In the remaining 3 patients in this category, the mechanism of muscular toxicity—related to sulfamethoxazole in 2 cases and pentamidine in another—was unclear. Two patients in this group died; the rest recovered, 3 after withdrawal of the causative drug.

In 7 patients, rhabdomyolysis occurred at the end stage of AIDS. This category included 4 patients with diffuse opportunistic infections involving skeletal muscle: 2 had systemic toxoplasmosis, and 2 had *Staphylococcus aureus* septicemia. Three of these patients recovered after therapy against the infecting organism. In the other 3 patients in this category, rhabdomyolysis occurred as part of a multiorgan failure with no definite cause of muscle damage.

Conclusions.—Rhabdomyolysis may occur under widely varying circumstances in patients at all stages of HIV infection. The prognosis depends partly on the cause of rhabdomyolysis, so it is important to recognize drug-induced or opportunistic, infectious muscle disorders.

▶ The most common forms of muscle disease seen in association with HIV-1 infection are a mitochondrial myopathy occurring as a consequence of zidovudine use and an inflammatory myopathy, presumably caused by HIV-1 itself. Rhabdomyolysis occurring with HIV-1 infection is rare. In this study by Dr. Chariot and colleagues, 20 cases of rhabdomyolysis with HIV-1 infection are reviewed. The disorder did not appear to have a predilection for any particular stage of AIDS, and it was attributed. to a broad spectrum of etiologies, including opportunistic infections, drug exposure, compression, multiorgan failure, and no identifiable etiology other than HIV-1. Although rare, clinicians should be aware of acute rhabdomyolysis as a potential cause of rapidly evolving weakness in a patient with HIV-1 infection, and they should also be aware of the potentially treatable causes of this entity.—J.R. Berger, M.D.

Cytokine Expression in the Muscle of HIV-Infected Patients: Evidence for Interleukin-1α Accumulation in Mitochondria of AZT Fibers
Gherardi RK, Florea-Strat A, Fromont G, Poron F, Sabourin J-C, Authier J (Hôpital Henri Mondor, Créteil, France; Hôpital Necker, Paris)
Ann Neurol 36:752–758, 1994   122-96-14–13

Objective.—Biopsy specimens from muscles of patients with HIV infection were examined for the presence of interleukin-1α (IL-1α), IL-1β, IL-6, and tumor necrosis factor-α (TNF-α) to examine the potential role of those cytokines in HIV-associated muscular disorders. The most common muscular disorders in such patients are an HIV-associated myopathy that usually fulfills the criteria for polymyositis, zidovudine (AZT) myopathy, and the HIV-wasting syndrome.

Patients and Methods.—Biopsy specimens were from 20 patients, 10 with typical AZT-induced mitochondrial myopathy, 5 with HIV-associated myopathy not treated by AZT, and 5 with the HIV-wasting syndrome. In addition, specimens from 12 patients seronegative for HIV were examined: 2 had normal muscle and 10 had genetically induced mitochondrial cytopathy. Immunocytochemistry was performed to identify cytokine expression.

Results.—Patients with HIV infection showed positive reactions in vessels (IL-1) and in inflammatory cells (primarily IL-1 and TNF-α), including perivascular hemosiderin-laden macrophages in 5 patients. A majority of AZT fibers, atrophic ragged-red fibers with marked myofibrillar alterations, showed mild to marked expression of IL-1 in specimens from patients with AZT myopathy. The expression of IL-1 in the other mitochondrial myopathies proved to be much weaker. In situ hybridization demonstrated IL-1β messenger RNA in muscle fibers, suggesting the production of IL-1 in muscle cells. Specimens from a patient with AZT myopathy, when examined by immunoelectron microscopy, revealed that IL-1α was mainly bound to mitochondrial membranes in AZT fibers.

Conclusion.—Strong cytokine expression was observed in muscle biopsy specimens from HIV-infected patients with muscular symptoms. Vascular structures showed IL-1β reactivity, mononuclear inflammatory cells exhibited IL-1α , IL-1β, and TNF-α reactivities, and the AZT-induced ragged-red fibers had IL-1α and IL-1β reactivities. The proinflammatory and destructive effects of these cytokines may cause several of the myopathologic changes seen in HIV-infected patients.

▶ Paralleling the observation of cytokine expression in the HIV-infected brain, Gherardi and colleagues have demonstrated cytokine expression in muscle biopsy specimens from HIV-infected subjects with muscular symptoms. There appeared to be a difference in the nature of the cytokine expression, namely, the type of cytokine and the location of its expression (i.e., in the vessel wall, mononuclear cell, or muscle fiber) between the different muscle disorders (HIV polymyositis, HIV wasting syndrome, and zidovudine myopathy). However, there was no statistical confirmation of these differences, perhaps as a result of small numbers of patients assessed.

The authors suggest that the inflammatory and destructive effects of the cytokines may be responsible for the muscle disorders observed with HIV infection. In light of there being significant expression of IL-1β in the muscle fibers of AZT myopathy, they also propose that the myofibrillar changes within AZT fibers could be related to the proteolytic effect of IL-1. It is conceivable that therapies directed at these cytokines and their pernicious effects may be effective in alleviating some of the symptoms of these HIV-associated muscle disorders.—J.R. Berger, M.D.

15 Neuro-Ophthalmology

Bilateral Simultaneous Optic Neuropathy in Adults: Clinical, Imaging, Serological, and Genetic Studies
Morrissey SP, Borruat FX, Miller DH, Moseley IF, Sweeney MG, Govan GG, Kelly MA, Francis DA, Harding AE, McDonald WI (Inst of Neurology, London; Queen Elizabeth Hosp, Birmingham, England; Univ of Birmingham, England)
J Neurol Neurosurg Psychiatry 58:70–74, 1995   122-96-15–1

Objective.—Clinically isolated acute unilateral optic neuritis (AUON) is a relatively common condition in adults, and up to three fourths of affected patients show progression to clinically definite multiple sclerosis. In many patients with AUON, brain MRI reveals cerebral white matter lesions that are indistinguishable from the lesions of multiple sclerosis. Bilateral simultaneous optic neuropathy (BSON) is much less common in adults. Some proportion of these patients have Leber's hereditary optic neuropathy (LHON), and a few have progression to multiple sclerosis. The diagnosis of LHON can be made by detecting specific mutations in mitochondrial DNA. In patients with AUON, the findings of brain MRI, HLA typing, and CSF electrophoresis all influence the risk of progression to multiple sclerosis. An attempt was made to clarify the causes of acute or subacute BSON in adults.

Methods.—The follow-up study included 23 patients with clinically isolated BSON of unknown cause. Their mean age at the onset of BSON was 31 years, and the mean age at follow-up was 37 years. The patients underwent clinical assessment, brain MRI, HLA typing, and mitochondrial DNA analysis. Although CSF electrophoresis was not performed, results were available from 11 previously studied patients.

Findings.—Fourteen patients were still classified as having clinically isolated BSON of uncertain cause at a mean follow-up of 50 months. Five patients (mean follow-up, 121 months) had clinically definite multiple sclerosis. The diagnosis of LHON was made by mitochondrial DNA analysis in 4 men: 3 had the 11778 mutation, and 1 had the 14484 mutation.

On brain MRI, all 5 patients with clinically definite multiple sclerosis showed characteristic multiple periventricular and discrete cerebral hemisphere white matter lesions; 4 had additional infratentorial lesions. Three of the 4 patients with LHON had normal brain MRI findings. Eight of the 14 patients with clinically isolated BSON had normal brain MRI findings; 3 had a single small white matter lesion; and 3 had multiple cerebral white matter lesions compatible with multiple sclerosis. The visual outcome was good—defined as visual acuity of 6/9 or better in both eyes—in 9 of 14 patients with isolated BSON at follow-up. The visual outcome was also good in 4 of 5 patients with multiple sclerosis, but it was poor in all patients with LHON. The CSF studies showed oligoclonal IgG bands in 4 of 4 patients who had multiple sclerosis develop vs. 1 of 7 patients with isolated BSON.

Conclusions.—The identification of a firm diagnosis was reported in 39% of patients with BSON: multiple sclerosis in 22%, and LHON in 17%. Progression to multiple sclerosis appears to be less common in patients with BSON than in those with AUON. Most patients who still have isolated BSON at follow-up do not show oligoclonal IgG bands in CSF or multiple white matter lesions on brain MRI. Overall, patients with isolated BSON have a low frequency of paraclinical risk factors for multiple sclerosis, which suggests that they have a low probability of future progression to multiple sclerosis.

▶ The authors present convincing data that BSON may less frequently evolve to the clinical picture of multiple sclerosis. Their thorough study of MRI, CSF electrophoresis, and HLA typing suggests a low probability of future progression to multiple sclerosis in those with isolated BSON. They describe a 20% occurrence rate for multiple sclerosis and, with predictive factors being predominantly negative in the remaining group, it seems that BSON will remain well below the multiple sclerosis rate of 70% seen in patients with long-term follow-up of AUON.

Although this paper does not address the alternative diagnostic considerations in the 61% of patients with BSON who remain without a diagnosis, when encountering BSON, a thorough investigation to exclude known etiologies, such as pituitary apoplexy and infiltrative sarcoid optic neuropathy, should be undertaken, as should a careful screening for vasculitis.—N.J. Schatz, M.D.

Late Onset Dysthyroid Optic Neuropathy
Chou P-I, Feldon SE (Doheny Eye Inst, Los Angeles; Univ of Southern California, Los Angeles)
Thyroid 4:213–216, 1994   122-96-15–2

Background.—Optic neuropathy is a vision-threatening manifestation of thyroid-associated ophthalmopathy (TAO). Three patients who had the condition several years after stabilization of the ophthalmopathy were studied.

Case 1.—Man, 54, complained of progressive bilateral dimness of vision during a period of 6 weeks. He had been given a diagnosis of TAO 7 years previously and had been maintained with prednisone, 10 mg twice daily. On ocular examination, his best corrected visual acuity was right eye (R.E.):20/50+1 and left eye (L.E.):20/40. He had color vision loss, and Humphrey visual field examination showed diffuse depression, greater in the right eye than the left. The patient was treated with prednisone, 100 mg/day. One month later, visual acuity had improved to R.E.20/25 and L.E.20/20, color vision had also improved, and the Humphrey visual fields improved in both eyes. Reduction of prednisone dosage brought a return in vision loss, so the patient was maintained with 20 mg of prednisone daily.

Case 2.—Man, 71, complained of decreased vision in the right eye of 3 months' duration. Fifteen years previously, he had been treated for hyperthyroidism with ^{131}I, and had been maintained on levothyroxine sodium, .1 mg/day. Ocular examination revealed visual acuity of R.E.: 20/30 and L.E: 20/20. A 1+ right afferent pupillary defect was seen. The patient correctly identified 7 of 15 pseudoisochromatic plates for color vision testing. He was treated with 80 mg of prednisone daily, and his vision improved within 2 months. He remained symptom free while receiving a daily dose of 10 mg of prednisone.

Case 3.—Woman, 79, was seen with a 6-month history of declining eye vision in the right eye and decreased vision in the left, along with decreased color vision. She had had diplopia secondary to TAO 12 years previously. Her best corrected visual acuity was R.E.:20/400 and L.E.:20/40. There was a 2+ right afferent pupillary defect. The patient started receiving prednisone, 80 mg/day for 1 month. Her vision increased, and Humphrey visual fields showed marked improvement; however, corticosteroids were poorly tolerated. Bilateral transantral orbital decompression was, therefore, done. Six months later, her visual acuity was R.E.:20/30+2 and L.E.:20/30, and color vision had improved to identification of 7 of 15 pseudoisochromatic plates. Humphrey visual fields also improved.

Conclusion.—A rare, delayed optic neuropathy occurring years after the onset of TAO was studied. It is thought that apical compression of the optic nerve caused by progressive or late-onset fibrosis of the extraocular muscles is the likely cause. Standard methods of therapy (e.g., corticosteroid treatment, radiation, and orbital decompression) appear effective.

▶ Optic neuropathy secondary to enlarged eye muscles and compression of the optic nerve occurs at the orbital apex. External signs of thyroid orbitopathy may be minimal. The activity of orbitopathy does not correlate with thyroid dysfunction and may occur at any time. Measurements of eye muscle size may be most helpful in diagnosis. Enlargement secondary to fibrosis seems unlikely.—N.J. Schatz, M.D.

Spontaneous Palpebromandibular Synkinesia: A Localizing Clinical Sign

Pullicino PM, Jacobs L, McCall WD Jr, Garvey M, Ostrow PT, Miller LL (State Univ of New York, Buffalo)
Ann Neurol 35:222–228, 1994   122-96-15–3

Objective.—In corneomandibular reflex (CMR), corneal stimulation results in anterolateral jaw movements. In 14 patients, eyelid blinks produced the same type of jaw movement. The relationship of this spontaneous palpebromandibular synkinesia (SPMS) to CMR was investigated.

Methods.—In 11 of the 14 patients, CMR and SPMS were both present. Corneomandibular reflex, but not SPMS, was blocked by corneal anesthesia. Four patients had brain stem lesions, 5 had cerebral and upper brain stem lesions, and 5 had evidence of cerebral dysfunction.

Results.—Mandibular kinesiography; latency of synkinesia; the number of voluntary blinks with or without electromyographic discharge; and amplitude, velocity, direction, and duration of jaw movement of SPMS and CMR were similar.

Conclusion.—Spontaneous palpebromandibular synkinesia and CMR appear to be similar reflexes, although SPMS does not demand corneal stimulation to produce jaw movement. The synkinesias arise centrally, probably in the pons. Because patients with these synkinesias have upper brain stem or cerebral lesions, SPMS may be a clinically useful indicator.

▶ Spontaneous palpebromandibular synkinesia and CMR are demonstrated to be the same reflex mechanism (in 11 of 14 patients tested, the phenomena co-existed). The mechanism of release of this reflex remains unclear, but since present in normal neonates, cerebral activity appears to suppress this reflex. Bilateral cerebral lesions or upper brain stem lesions are required to release this phenomenon.—N.J. Schatz, M.D.

Role of Pontine Nuclei Damage in Smooth Pursuit Impairment of Progressive Supranuclear Palsy: A Clinical-Pathologic Study
Malessa S, Gaymard B, Rivaud S, Cervera P, Hirsch E, Verny M, Duyckaerts C, Agid Y, Pierrot-Deseilligny C (Hôpital de la Salpêtrière, Paris)
Neurology 44:716–721, 1994　　　　　　　　　　122-96-15–4

Background.—The degeneration of the pontine nuclei in the basis pontis may be associated with the development of progressive supranuclear palsy. A quantitative anatomical study of the pontine nuclei in the basis pontis and a semiquantitative examination of the extrapontine structures involved in smooth pursuit in progressive supranuclear palsy were done.

Methods.—Autopsy was performed on 4 patients with severe horizontal smooth pursuit impairment and histopathologically confirmed progressive supranuclear palsy. After autopsy, each brain was hemisected; half was used for neuropathologic study and half was used for quantitative analysis of the pontine nucleus.

Results.—Regular histopathology showed that the cytoarchitecture of the frontal eye field region, the parieto-temporo-occipital region, and the cerebellum was preserved. However, neocortical neurofibrillary tangles were found in the small cells of layers V and VI and in the vestibular nuclei of the patients with the most severe lesions. Samples from these patients also had a few starlike tufts of fibers without degenerative features or amyloid cores in the cerebral cortex. Torpedoes of degenerative Purkinje cells were found in the cerebellar flocculus and in the vermis. Neuronal density was significantly lower in the pontine nucleus and basis pontis of the patient group compared with that of the control group.

Conclusion.—It appears that degenerative lesions affecting the pontine nuclei may be responsible in large part for the horizontal smooth pursuit impairment in progressive supranuclear palsy.

▶ This clinicopathologic study demonstrates that in patients with progressive supranuclear palsy, horizontal smooth pursuits and saccadic velocity are reduced with time.

Postmortem studies demonstrate maximum loss of pontine nuclei with relative sparing of extrapontine structures. Neuronal loss in the pontine nuclei seemed mainly responsible for the marked horizontal smooth pursuit abnormalities in these patients.—N.J. Schatz, M.D.

Risk Factors for Ischemic Ocular Motor Nerve Palsies

Jacobson DM, McCanna TD, Layde PM (Wills Eye Hosp, Philadelphia; Med College of Wisconsin, Milwaukee)

Arch Ophthalmol 112:961–966, 1994   122-96-15–5

Background.—Diabetes-associated ophthalmoplegia is a well-described condition that appears to result from microvascular infarction of an ocular motor nerve in its subarachnoid or cavernous segment. However, similar ophthalmoplegias have also been reported in patients without diabetes who have other overt or unrecognized vascular risk factors. There have been no systematic studies to evaluate the risk factors associated with this condition. Therefore, the influence of diabetes and other risk factors on the occurrence of ischemic ocular motor nerve palsies were examined in a case-control study.

Methods.—Sixty-five patients, at least 50 years of age, who had ischemic ophthalmoplegia, were evaluated. Strict inclusion and exclusion criteria were used to increase the chances that the patients had no alternative cause of ophthalmoplegia. A sex- and age-matched control was randomly selected for each patient from a population of patients undergoing a comprehensive medical evaluation. The well-defined risk factors evaluated included diabetes, hypertension, hypercholesterolemia, coronary artery disease, left ventricular hypertrophy, adiposity, tobacco use, previous ocular motor nerve palsy, and hematocrit.

Results.—Including newly diagnosed patients, 71% of the cases had either diabetes or glucose intolerance, and 66% had hypertension. Three risk factors remained significant after adjustment for potential confounders: previously diagnosed diabetes (odds ratio [OR], 5.75); left ventricular hypertrophy (OR, 5.20); and hematocrit (OR, 1.35 per percentage increase).

Conclusions.—Important risk factors for ischemic ocular motor nerve palsy, in addition to diabetes, are left ventricular hypertrophy and elevated hematocrit. The findings, which should be confirmed in further studies, highlight the importance of testing for abnormal glucose metabolism in apparently nondiabetic patients who are evaluated for ischemic ocular motor nerve palsies. If any of the identified risk factors are noticed, the patient can be treated appropriately; if not, the patient should be followed up, as appropriate, for alternative causes of the ophthalmoplegia.

▶ The results of risk factors in these 65 patients with ischemic ocular motor palsies are unique. Previously diagnosed diabetes has been a recognized risk, but this article suggests that poor control may predispose patients to such palsies.

The association with left ventricular hypertrophy of a threefold increase in risk and the finding that an increase in hematocrit of a single percentage point was associated with an average increase of 35% in the risk for ocular motor palsy must be substantiated by others. The authors suggest a rational diagnostic approach: obtain a fasting and standard 2-hour postprandial glucose tolerance test, hemoglobin A_{1c} levels, blood pressure, EKG and hematocrit.—N.J. Schatz, M.D.

Saccadic Lateropulsion in Wallenberg's Syndrome May be Caused by a Functional Lesion of the Fastigial Nucleus
Helmchen C, Straube A, Büttner U (Ludwig-Maximilians-Universität München, Germany; Klinikum Großhadern, München, Germany)
J Neurol 241:421–426, 1994   122-96-15–6

Introduction.—One of the oculomotor symptoms in Wallenberg's syndrome is saccadic lateropulsion, consisting of hypermetric saccades to the ipsilateral and hypometric saccades to the contralateral side. The structure responsible for this condition remains unclear. Twelve patients with Wallenberg's syndrome were prospectively examined to determine the lesion site related to saccadic lateropulsion.

Patients and Methods.—The patients, 7 men and 5 women, ranged in age from 29 to 72 years. All came to the emergency room with acute neurologic symptoms and showed at least 3 typical clinical signs of Wallenberg's syndrome. None had multiple infarctions of different vascular territories in the brain stem, nor did they show a cerebellar lesion on CT or MRI. Eye movement recordings were performed between 1 day and 3 weeks after the stroke. The data recorded included the gain of the initial saccade and the number of corrective saccades. Saccades with a gain greater than 0.96 were classified as hypermetric and those with a gain of less than 0.91 as hypometric.

Results.—The lesion was left-sided in 7 patients and right-sided in 5. Eight patients had at least 1 predisposing factor for cerebrovascular disease. Six patients had MRI evidence of a medullary lesion, and 4 who

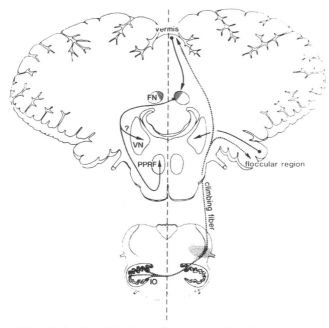

Fig 15–1.—Schematic drawing of the climbing fiber pathway (*dotted line*), which is damaged in the lateral medullary infarction (LMI). The lesion of the climbing fiber input to the Parkinje cells causes disinhibition of the Purkinje cell simple spike resting activity and, as a direct result, increased inhibition of the saccadic neurons in the caudal fastigial nucleus. *Abbreviations: IO,* inferior olive; *PPRF,* paramedian pontine reticular formation; *VN,* vestibular nuclei; *FN,* fastigial nucleus. *Hatched area* in FN indicates fastigial oculomotor region. *Dotted area* in brain stem shows region of LMI. (Courtesy of Helmchen C, Straube A, Büttner U: *J Neurol* 241:421–426, 1994.)

underwent vertebral angiography had occlusion of the ipsilateral vertebral artery or the posterior inferior cerebellar artery. All patients showed hypermetric saccades to the ipsilateral side and hypometric contralateral saccades. This finding was comparable with the effects of cerebellar lesions on saccadic accuracy in monkeys. Overall, the more hypermetric ipsiversive saccades were, the more hypometria occurred in contraversive saccades.

Conclusion.—These patients with Wallenberg's syndrome but no signs of a cerebellar lesion consistently exhibited hypometric contraversive saccades and hypermetric saccades to the lesion side. On the basis of recent animal studies, it is hypothesized that saccadic lateropulsion in lateral medullary infarction is essentially identical with cerebellar saccadic dysmetria. Its cause appears to be a disruption of afferent olivocerebellar climbing fibers that leads to functional disinhibition of the cerebellar cortex and increased inhibition of the deep cerebellar nuclei (Fig 15–1).

▶ Saccadic lateral pulsions in lesions limited to the lateral medullary plate are localizing and lateralizing. They do not require a concomitant cerebellar lesion but reflect disruption of afferent olivocerebellar climbing fibers, which leads to functional cerebellar disinhibition.

The saccadic lateral pulsion is ipsilateral to the lesion. The eyes tend to shift toward the ipsilateral side, and ipsilateral saccades are hypermetric.— N.J. Schatz, M.D.

Jerk-Waveform See-Saw Nystagmus Due to Unilateral Meso-Dien-cephalic Lesion
Halmagyi GM, Aw ST, Dehaene I, Curthoys IS, Todd MJ (Royal Prince Alfred Hosp, Sydney, Australia; Univ of Sydney, Australia; Algemeen Ziekenhuis, Bruges, Belgium)
Brain 117:789–803, 1994   122-96-15–7

Introduction.—In the eye movement disorder known as see-saw nystagmus, one eye intorts and elevates, whereas the other extorts and depresses. A pendular waveform is present in most patients, but certain unilateral mesodiencephalic lesions can also cause a see-saw nystagmus. In the latter case, a jerk-waveform is observed, with the torsional fast phases beating toward the side of the lesion. The clinical and MRI findings for 3 patients with the disorder were reported.

Patients.—The patients, all of whom were white and right-handed, were a 53-year-old man, a 36-year-old woman, and a 26-year-old woman. All had a unilateral mesodiencephalic lesion resulting in a jerk-waveform see-saw nystagmus. In each case, the torsional component of the nystagmus fast phases rotated the upper poles of the eyes toward the side of the lesion. The disorder typically came after a thalamic hemorrhage (Fig 15–2), and the nystagmus was unaffected by changes in eye or head position, or in vergence angle. Two of the patients have had no change in nystagmus or other neurologic signs in more than 2 years; nystagmus was absent in the 36-year-old woman at the time of her last examination.

Discussion.—Oculography is helpful in distinguishing a pendular-waveform nystagmus from a jerk-waveform nystagmus (Fig 15–3). Because the 2 eyes are making different movements, the distinction is particularly difficult in cases of see-saw nystagmus. The jerk see-saw nystagmus is proposed to be a result of unilateral inactivation of the torsional eye-velocity integrator, located in the interstitial nucleus of Cajal. There is sparing of the torsional fast-phase generator, thought to be in the adjacent rostral interstitial nucleus of the medial longitudinal fasciculus. Jerk see-saw nystagmus can be associated with a paroxysmal ocular tilt reaction, a tonic ocular tilt reaction, or with both.

▶ Pendular see-saw ocular movements localize to lesions in the midline, invading or compressing the brain stem. Oculographic recordings have demonstrated a type of see-saw nystagmus with a jerk-waveform that would appear to be anatomically specific for unilateral mesodiencephalic lesions.

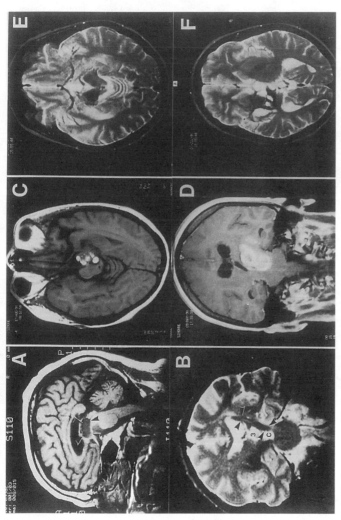

Fig 15-2.—A and B, MRIs from a man, 53, 4 years after a left thalamic hemorrhage. (A) T1-weighted parasagittal and (B) T2-weighted coronal images showing a hemosiderin-containing lesion (*arrowbeads*) extending from the internal capsule through the medial thalamus to the subthalamus and the region of the internodular cortex and rostral interstitial nucleus of the medial longitudinal fasciculus (3 = 3rd ventricle; C = interpeduncular cistern). C and D, MR images from a woman, 36. Coronal T1-weighted image with gadolinium, 2 weeks after her fourth left thalamic hemorrhage in 8 years (D). At the left mesodiencephalic junction there is a largely high-signal-intensity lesion (not enhanced with gadolinium) that involves the region of the INC and riMLF. No major blood vessel supplies the lesion. A nonenhanced axial T1-weighted image 3 months later (C) shows a multilobulated lesion of mixed signal intensity. This appearance is typical of a cavernous hemangioma containing hemosiderin and methemoglobin from extravasated blood of different ages. E and F, MRIs from the 26-year-old woman, 1 year after a right thalamic hemorrhage. T2-weighted axial images show a lesion extending from the subcortical white matter of the parietal lobe through the thalamus and the internal capsule, into the right cerebral peduncle and involving the region of the INC. The lesion contains CSF and hemosiderin, indicating that it is a resolving hematoma communicating with the ventricular system. (Courtesy of Halmagyi GM, Aw ST, Dehaene I, et al: *Brain* 117:789–803, 1994.)

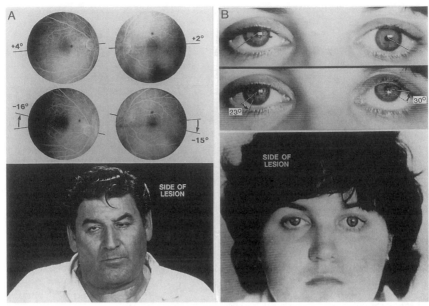

Fig 15-3.—A, man, 53 years. The first row shows fundus photographs of the position of the eyes during a null period of the jerk see-saw nystagmus. There is 4 degrees of clockwise extorsion of the right eye and 2 degrees of clockwise intorsion of the left eye. The second rows show the positions of the eyes during nystagmus, at the end of a fast phase. The total amplitude of the counter-clockwise torsional component of the fast phase was 20 degrees in the right eye and 17 degrees in the left with respect to the null-period torsional position. The bottom figure shows that, during nystagmus, the patient also has a 20-degree right/left skew deviation as well as ~6 degrees of left esotropia develop. The patient had a constant clockwise head tilt of ~20 degrees. The black spot on the fundus photographs was a heat-sink in the camera lens system and was not visible to the patient. B, woman, 26, with a right thalamic hemorrhage. The top and bottom figures show the position of the eyes at the start of a fast phase of the jerk see-saw nystagmus. The middle figure shows the position of the eyes at the end of the same fast phase of the nystagmus, showing the maximal clockwise torsional displacement of the eyes. A line has been drawn on each eye joining the position of an iris landmark—indicated by the single discontinuity in the line—and the pupil center. The interrupted line in the middle figure indicates the position of the iris landmark at the beginning of the fast phase and is the same as the position shown in the top figure. From the torsional displacement of this line (i.e., the angle between the 2 lines), the amplitude of the torsional component of the jerk see-saw nystagmus was estimated to be 30 degrees in the left eye and 23 degrees in the right. The amplitude of the vertical component of the jerk see-saw nystagmus was ~30 degrees in the left eye and < 2 degrees in the right so that each fast phase produced a left/right skewing of the eyes. There is ~4 degrees of right/left skew deviation at the start of the fast phase (*top figure*). Each figure is a photograph of one frame of videotape recording. (Courtesy of Halmagyi GM, Aw ST, Dehaene I, et al: *Brain* 117:789–803, 1994.)

The authors' conclusion that jerk see-saw nystagmus is secondary to a unilateral mesodiencephalic lesion is well illustrated by the reports of 3 patients with the disorder.

Distinguishing pendular see-saw nystagmus from jerk-waveform see-saw on clinical grounds would not appear to be a difficult task. Mesodiencephalic jerk see-saw nystagmus, however, is indistinguishable from the torsional-vertical nystagmus induced by lesions of the medulla oblongata. This differentiation requires careful oculography and evaluation of the accompanying neurologic signs that may help in localization.—N.J. Schatz, M.D.

Contralateral Conjugate Eye Deviation in Acute Supratentorial Lesions

Tijssen CC (St Elisabeth Hosp, Tilburg, The Netherlands)
Stroke 25:1516–1519, 1994   122-96-15-8

Background.—Conjugate eye deviation (CED) can occur in patients with supratentorial stroke. It most often occurs after right-sided damage and is usually directed ipsilateral to the lesioned hemisphere. However, rare cases of contralateral CED, also called "wrong-way eyes," have been reported. Five patients with contralateral CED were reported.

Patients.—The patients were identified from a prospective study of 133 consecutive patients with CED caused by an acute supratentorial lesion. All 5 cases were associated with intracerebral hemorrhage. The lesion was located in the thalamic region in 2 cases, the frontoparietal region in 1, and the frontoparietotemporal region in 1. The remaining case was associated with subdural hematoma—a cause not previously reported. Four of the patients died. Computed tomography or autopsy revealed clinical signs of rostral brain stem dysfunction and a shift of midline structures in all patients.

Discussion.—The finding of contralateral CED is associated with hemorrhagic acute supratentorial lesions, usually in the thalamus. The prognosis is poor. The mechanism underlying contralateral CED is unknown, but it may involve impairment of the contralateral descending oculomotor pathways. From the parieto-occipital area, the descending pursuit pathway runs through the posterior limb of the internal capsule, which lies near the thalamus. The descending horizontal oculomotor pathway traverses the anterior limb of the internal capsule, diverges in the rostral diencephalon, and passes through the medial-most part of the posterior limb of the internal capsule and midbrain cerebral peduncle. Factors other than a hemispheric mass effect may be involved as well, including deep midline shifts, ventricular extension of thalamic hemorrhage, and dissection of blood around the midbrain.

▶ In this review of 133 consecutive cases of conjugate eye deviation, if the eye deviation was contralateral to the lesion in acute supratentorial lesions, then a thalamic hemmorhage was always the cause. This clinical sign is extremely important, because contralateral eye deviation has classically been believed to occur secondary to seizure. The mechanism is unclear, and the prognosis in these patients is poor.—N.J. Schatz, M.D.

Hemiachromatopsia of Unilateral Occipitotemporal Infarcts

Paulson HL, Galetta SL, Grossman M, Alavi A (Univ of Pennsylvania, Pa)
Am J Ophthalmol 118:518–523, 1994   122-96-15-9

Background.—Hemiachromatopsia, the loss of color vision in one hemifield, was first described more than a century ago. A region of the visual association cortex called the V4 has been designated as critical for color processing. The close proximity of the V4 to the inferior striate cortex in humans suggests that hemiachromatopsia may commonly occur in patients with superior quadrant field defects. The neuro-ophthalmologic and neuroanatomical findings in 2 patients were reported. In both, unilateral occipitotemporal infarcts produced inferior quadrantic achromatopsia and a superior quandrantanopia.

Patients.—The patients were a man, 56, and a woman, 76. In the first patient, neurologic assessment showed an isolated left homonymous superior quandrantanopia. Congruous left superior quadrantanopia was also evident. Although light detection and form vision were normal in the left inferior quadrant, color vision in this quadrant was profoundly disturbed. Similarly, in the second patient, light detection and form vision were normal in the left inferior quadrant, but color vision in this quadrant was markedly abnormal. This patient was unable to sort colors or name the color of objects. The infarct involved the lingual gyrus, the fusiform gyrus, and adjacent white matter.

Conclusions.—These MRI and single-photon emission CT findings suggest that color vision is encoded in the lingual and fusiform gyri. The quadrantic defect in color processing was profound in both patients, although neither was aware of it.

▶ The two patients with homonymous superior quadrantanopsias had no demonstrable disturbance to motion or light in their corresponding homonymous inferior field. The anatomical information on both MR and positron emission tomography scans convincingly demonstrates extension of the lesion to involve the lingual and fusiform gyri and does, in fact, suggest that the area for color detection and color sorting resides in this area. From a clinical point of view, testing of the homonymous inferior field in patients with homonymous superior quadrantanopsias may be of anatomical localization.—N.J. Schatz, M.D.

Neurovisual Findings in the Syndrome of Spontaneous Intracranial Hypotension From Dural Cerebrospinal Fluid Leak
Horton JC, Fishman RA (Univ of California, San Francisco)
Ophthalmology 101:244–251, 1994   122-96-15–10

Background.—Fewer than 75 cases of spontaneous intracranial hypotension have been described in the medical literature, but more cases are being recognized since the advent of MRI. The disorder occurs when CSF leaks from a defect in the spinal meninges. Patients typically have headache that lessens or resolves on lying down. They also may have nausea, vomiting, neck stiffness, vertigo, tinnitus, and hyperacusis. Visual abnormalities have not been considered an important part of the disorder.

Three Patients.—Two of the patients were seen with transient visual obscurations, and they exhibited unusual binasal visual field defects on automated perimetry. The third patient had diplopia secondary to abducens nerve paresis (Fig 15–4). The abnormalities lessened or disap-

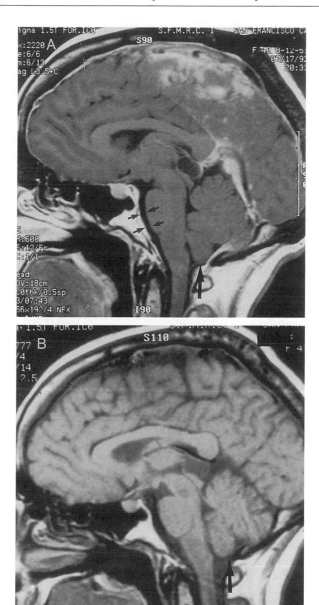

Fig 15–4.—Patient 3. **A,** T1-weighted sagittal image taken on July 17, 1992, shows gadolinium enhancement of the dura, reduction of the pontine cistern (*between arrows*), and low tonsils (*arrow*). **B,** results of a follow-up study on August 29, 1992, show expansion of the pontine cistern and a 3- to 4-mm re-ascent of the tonsils (*arrow*). (Courtesy of Horton JC, Fishman RA: *Ophthalmology* 101:244–251, 1994.)

peared after spontaneous intracranial hypotension was treated. The first two patients were treated with a blood patch, and the third by bed rest and oral hydration.

Discussion.—Intracranial hypotension most often results from CSF leakage through a dural hole made in the course of diagnostic lumbar puncture, myelography, or spinal anesthesia. Leakage of CSF causes the brain to settle in the skull base, where it exerts pressure and traction on meningeal and vascular structures. Headache, neck stiffness, and nausea result, all resolving when the patient lies flat. Neurovisual problems do occur in a substantial proportion of these patients.

▶ Headaches that lessen or resolve when the patient lies down suggest the clinical diagnosis of spontaneous intracranial hypotension. This paper discusses the other symptoms, including visual disturbances. The MRI changes of crowding of the chiasm, thickening of the dura with enhancement, and flattening of the pons are important signs that may mislead the clinician. This disorder needs clinical and radiologic attention.—N.J. Schatz, M.D.

▶ The syndrome of intracranial hypotension resulting from CSF leakage is well known, with the most widely recognized form being that which follows a lumbar puncture. Horton and Fishman remind us that this syndrome can accompany (and be a diagnostic clue to) spontaneous CSF leakage. They also point out that the syndrome of intracranial hypotension may include visual symptoms and signs, as illustrated by their 3 case reports.—R.H. Wilkins, M.D.

16 Neuro-Otology

Dizziness in Aging: A Retrospective Study of 1,194 Cases
Katsarkas A (Royal Victoria Hosp, Montreal)
Otolaryngol Head Neck Surg 110:296–301, 1994   122-96-16-1

Introduction.—There are many possible causes of postural instability, with its attendant risk of falls, in elderly patients, including multisensory deficits, drugs, and non-neurologic, nonvestibular disease. However, the problem of dizziness is so common in the elderly as to raise suspicion that it may be caused directly or indirectly by vestibular dysfunction in advanced age. A retrospective study of patients, aged 70 years or older, who were visiting a dizziness clinic for the first time, was reported.

Patients.—A total of 1,194 patients were studied, representing 12% of patients referred to the dizziness clinic over 17 years. Seven hundred fifty were women and 44 were men (mean age, 75 years). The patients had a total of 1,357 diagnoses (1.14 diagnoses per patient) related to dizziness. In 27% of the cases, the etiology was uncertain (Table 1). Paroxysmal positional vertigo was confirmed or strongly suspected in 39% of patients. Of 254 cases in which this diagnosis was confirmed, 95% were compatible with excitation of the posterior semicircular canal. No neurologic or vestibular cause could be identified in 9% of the patients. The next most common diagnoses were Meniere's disease, vestibular neuronitis, vascular episodes, and tumors (Tables 2 to 4).

Conclusions.—Among the elderly, dizziness is more common in women than men, probably because of the higher survival rate. Paroxysmal positional vertigo is a common diagnosis in these patients (39%), with there being evidence of posterior semicircular canal excitation in most cases. In many elderly patients, this condition may be diagnosed as vascular disease. Although multisensory deficits, drugs, and systemic diseases are common causes of dizziness in the elderly, vestibular function may be more prevalent in the elderly than was generally thought.

▶ Vestibular testing has become more important in our understanding of the patient with dizziness. This report of 1,194 patients older than 70 years of age suggests as many as 39% of patients have paroxysmal positional vertigo and not vertebral basilar disease, as previously suggested. Careful vestibular testing may eliminate the need for extensive evaluation and treatment of

TABLE 1.—Most Frequent Diagnoses

No. of cases (%)	Diagnosis
294 (21.67)	Uncertain
78 (5.75)	Uncertain (vestibular)
276 (20.34)	PPV, suspected
254 (18.72)	PPV, confirmed
119 (8.77)	Non-CNS, nonvestibular
86 (6.34)	Cerebrovascular disease
55 (4.05)	Meniere's disease
26 (1.92)	Bilateral low vestibular function
24 (1.77)	Vestibular neuronitis
19 (1.40)	Epidemic vertigo
19 (1.40)	Sudden unilateral hearing loss

(Courtesy of Katsarkas A: *Otolaryngol Head Neck Surg* 110:296–301, 1994.)

TABLE 2.—Less Frequent Diagnosis (I)

No. of cases (*n* = 86)	Diagnosis (vascular)
4	Ischemia, inner ear
6	Ischemia, unknown site
25	Ischemia, higher brain
3	TIAs, higher brain
30	Ischemia, brain stem
18	TIAs, brain stem

Abbreviation: TIAs, transient ischemic attacks.
(Courtesy of Katsarkas A: *Otolaryngol Head Neck Surg* 110:296–301, 1994.)

TABLE 3.—Less Frequent Diagnoses (II)

No. of cases	Diagnosis
17	Tumor
15	Head injury
13	Drop attacks
12	Sensory neuropathy
12	Cerebellar atrophy
9	Parkinson's disease
7	Recurrent vestibular neuronitis
4	Inner ear injury
4	Hemifacial spasm

(Courtesy of Katsarkas A: *Otolaryngol Head Neck Surg* 110:296–301, 1994.)

TABLE 4.—Least Frequent Diagnoses	
No. of cases	Diagnosis
3	Multiple sclerosis
3	Epilepsy
2	Inner ear fistual
2	Multisensory deficits
1	Migrane headaches
1	Syringomyelia
1	Ramsay Hunt syndrome
1	Wallenberg's syndrome

(Courtesy of Katsarkas A: *Otolaryngol Head Neck Surg* 110:296–301, 1994.)

vascular disease. Whether ischemia is a cause of paroxysmal positional vertigo in elderly patients, however is not totally resolved.—N.J. Schatz, M.D.

Age-Associated Differences in Sensori-Motor Function and Balance in Community Dwelling Women
Lord SR, Ward JA (Prince of Wales Med Research Inst, Randwick, Australia; Eastern Sydney Area Health Service, Australia)
Age Ageing 23:452–460, 1994   122-96-16–2

Objective.—There has recently been great interest in the control of balance in young and old people, including the relative contributions of the visual, vestibular, and somatosensory systems. Previous studies have demonstrated age-related declines in all the major sensory and motor inputs contributing to balance. However, it is unknown whether the rates of decline in these sensory systems vary, and also whether there are age-associated differences in the contribution of each to balance control. This issue was addressed by examination of the sensorimotor, vestibular, and visual systems in a large community population of women.

Methods.—Five hundred fifty Australian women, ranging in age from 20 to 99 years, were studied. Four hundred fourteen of the women were aged 65 years and older. Each woman underwent specific tests of visual, vestibular, sensorimotor, and balance function at a balance and gait laboratory. Balance was assessed under normal and more challenging conditions (i.e., with the research subject standing on a firm surface and then on foam, with the eyes open and, also, closed).

Results.—Significant age-related differences were noted on all sensory, motor, and balance tests. On multiple regression analyses, measures of lower limb sensation consistently contributed to balance when the women were standing on a firm surface. When the women were standing on foam with the eyes open, vision, strength, and reaction time significantly contributed to balance. When they were standing on foam with the eyes closed, vestibular function was also a significant contributor. When sway was assessed under conditions that diminished or removed the visual and peripheral sensation systems, women up to 65 years of age were more reliant on vision for balance control. For women older than 65 years, the contribution of vision decreased; thus, in the oldest women, the reduced ability of vision to supplement peripheral input led to increased sway areas. In all age groups, peripheral sensation was the most important sensory system for maintaining static postural stability.

Conclusions.—Age is significantly associated with the functioning of the visual, vestibular, and sensorimotor systems, and several of these specific "postural control systems" significantly affect balance under various conditions. Under normal conditions, lower limb sensation is the main sensorimotor factor contributing to balance; under more challenging conditions, vision, strength, reaction time, and vestibular function are important factors. Sway increases as sensory inputs are altered or diminished. Despite these associations, variance in measures of sway remains largely unaccounted for.

▶ Falls in the elderly are a serious and costly problem in health care. It is known that body sway during standing increases with age as a result of the minor degradation of vision, proprioception, and vestibular function. In this study, balance was examined in individuals standing on an unstable surface to stress the system. Sufficient power in the analysis was obtained by examining a large group of community-dwelling elderly individuals. Under these test conditions, peripheral sensation was found to be the most important sensory system in the maintenance of static postural stability. Research subjects next depended on vision to an increasing extent until the age of 65, when dependence declined. Despite careful quantification of a number of sensory measurements, this study still could not account for the degree of sway found in the elderly. Some of the shortcomings of the article include the lack of direct measurement of vestibular function, and the measurement of strength but not of flexibility. Despite these shortcomings, the study included a number of important measurements that have not been made in previous studies. The next obvious study will be one that determines the correlation of their measurements with the risk of falls.—R.J. Tusa, M.D., Ph.D.

Long-Term Results of Low Dose Intramuscular Streptomycin for Meniere's Disease
Shea JJ, Ge X, Orchik DJ (Shea Clinic, Memphis, Tenn)
Am J Otol 15:540–544, 1994   122-96-16–3

Objective.—Intramuscular streptomycin eliminates the vertigo and stabilizes hearing in patients with Meniere's disease by ablating the vestibular system. Side effects, including ataxia, wide-based gait, and oscillopsia, are reduced by partial ablation accomplished using low-dose streptomycin. The long-term effects of low-dose streptomycin treatment of bilateral Meniere's disease were studied retrospectively.

Methods.—Fourteen male patients with bilateral Meniere's disease were given 1 g of streptomycin sulfate IM twice daily 5 days per week for 2 weeks.

Results.—The patients were followed for 5–12 years. All patients had symptomatic relief. One patient had recurrent vertigo 1 year after treatment and was reperfused. Four patients had balance problems. Hearing was unchanged in 17 ears, had improved in 2 ears, and worsened in 3 ears. A hearing threshold of less than 30 dB was found in 2 ears before and after treatment, 30–60 dB in 7 ears before and 6 after, and more than 60 dB in 13 ears before and 14 after. The mean PTA of 22 ears was 58 dB before treatment and 65.5 dB after, and the mean speech discrimination scores were 61.4% before and 51.3% after.

Conclusion.—Low-dose streptomycin treatment of bilateral Meniere's disease is effective in partially ablating the vestibular function and in reducing symptoms of vertigo, stabilizing hearing, and moderating the severity of ataxia.

▶ Streptomycin appears to be an effective treatment for the symptomatic relief of patients with bilateral Meniere's disease, both in the short term and over a longer period. The low dose of streptomycin recommended in this paper resulted in efficacy without causing significant deafness or ataxia.— W.G. Bradley, D.M., F.R.C.P.

Dynamic Transcranial Doppler Assessment of Positional Vertebrobasilar Ischemia

Sturzenegger M, Newell DW, Douville C, Byrd S, Schoonover K (Univ of Washington, Seattle)
Stroke 25:1776–1783, 1994   122-96-16–4

Background.—Transient vertebrobasilar ischemia may result from either artery-to-artery embolism or hemodynamic insufficiency. Positional ischemia is most often a result of obstruction of one or both vertebral arteries. This disorder may produce specific symptoms, and it may respond very well to surgical decompression, making its accurate diagnosis important.

Objective and Methods.—The value of transcranial Doppler (TCD) sonography was examined in 14 patients suspected, on clinical grounds, of having positional vertebrobasilar ischemia of hemodynamic origin. Conventional extracranial Doppler examination and TCD were done, and the TCD transducers were then fixed to the temporal bone to monitor flow in the posterior cerebral artery (PCA) as the patients performed various head movements in sequence. Ten healthy individuals also were examined.

Findings.—Four patients with stereotypical symptoms exhibited a marked decrease in blood flow velocity in the PCA during head rotation to one side (Fig 16–1). The extent of the decrease varied, but the effect was reproducible (Fig 16–2). Angiographic studies confirmed vertebral artery obstruction on head rotation and demonstrated vascular anomalies in the

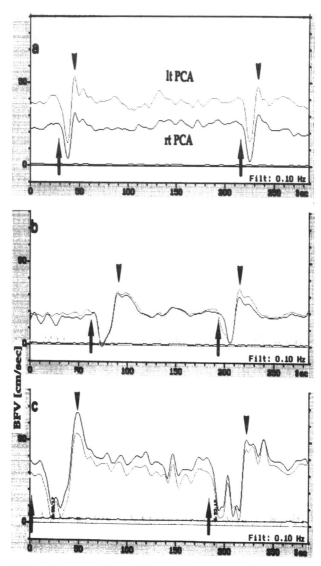

Fig 16–1.—Tracings of continuously recorded BFV in the P1 segments of left (*lt*) and right (*rt*) posterior cerebral arteries (*PCAs*) during head movements in patients in group 1 (*a,* patient 1; *b,* patient 2; and *c,* patient 3). A low-pass filter (*Filt*) (.10 Hz) was used to eliminate cluttering by pulsality. There is a marked decrease during head turning to the right (*a* and *b*) or to the left (*c*) side, with subsequent reactive hyperemia (*arrowheads*) when the head is brought back to a neutral position. This response is reproducible on each trial of head rotation. The beginning of the rotation is marked by an *arrow.* (Courtesy of Sturzenegger M, Newell DW, Douville C, et al: *Stroke* 25:1776–1783, 1994.)

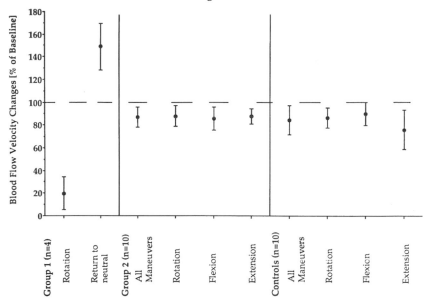

Changes of Posterior Cerebral Artery Blood Flow Velocities during Head Movements

Fig 16–2.—Graph demonstrating changes in the mean maximal blood flow velocities (BFVs) recorded in the 2 patient groups and control subjects during the performed head maneuvers. Responses in both posterior cerebral arteries are taken together and expressed as the percent change of the baseline velocities taken at rest in the neutral head position. In group 1 patients, only the values during head rotation that induced symptoms and the values of the subsequent reactive hyperemia when the head was turned back to a neutral position are shown. In group 2 patients and control subjects, the BFV changes during the different head maneuvers are shown (mean ± 2 standard deviation). (Courtesy of Sturzenegger M, Newell DW, Douville C, et al: *Stroke* 25:1776–1783, 1994.)

posterior circulation. The remaining 10 patients, whose symptoms were not stereotypical or clearly related to head motion, had only small changes in flow velocity during provocative maneuvers.

Conclusion.—Transcranial Doppler sonography is a straightforward noninvasive means of detecting hemodynamically significant compression of the vertebral artery. It may be used to select those patients with symptoms of positional vertebrobasilar ischemia who should undergo angiography.

▶ This interesting report notes that TCD was capable of showing marked decreases in posterior cerebral artery blood flow velocity during head rotation in 4 patients, suggesting hemodynamically significant vertebral artery compression that correlated with angiographic abnormalities of the posterior circulation. This group of patients was in contrast with 10 other patients who had only small changes in blood flow velocity during provocative head maneuvers and whose symptoms were more nonspecific. Unfortunately, angiography was not obtained in the latter patient group, thereby limiting the overall usefulness of the study. Larger studies in which angiography is uniformly applied will be needed to establish firm correlations. Nonetheless, these findings are provocative and suggest that TCD may contribute to the diagnosis of hemodynamically significant mechanical compression of the vertebral arteries.—M.D. Ginsberg, M.D.

17 Pain and Headache

The Effect of Systemically Administered Recombinant Human Nerve Growth Factor in Healthy Human Subjects
Petty BG, Cornblath DR, Adornato BT, Chaudhry V, Flexner C, Wachsman M, Sinicropi D, Burton LE, Peroutka SJ (Johns Hopkins Univ, Baltimore, Md; Stanford Med Ctr, Calif; Genentech Inc, South San Francisco, Calif)
Ann Neurol 36:244–246, 1994   122-96-17–1

Objective.—Nerve growth factor (NGF) plays a key role in the development and maintenance of sympathetic and sensory neurons and their neuronal extensions, as well as in the regeneration of lesioned peripheral nerves. Nerve growth factor and other neurotrophic factors have been suggested for use in treating or preventing diseases of the central and peripheral nervous systems. The safety of single doses of recombinant human NGF (rhNGF) in healthy human volunteers was assessed.

Methods.—The double-masked, randomized, placebo-controlled study included 33 men and 12 women in good health. The rhNGF was given in single IV or subcutaneous doses of 0.03 to 1.0 µg/kg. The patients were subsequently evaluated to assess the safety and tolerance of rhNGF, to determine its pharmacokinetics, and to see whether administration of rhNGF would result in antibody formation or changes in nerve conduction.

Results.—There were no life-threatening adverse effects at any dose. Mild to moderate muscle pain, mainly in the bulbar and truncal muscles, was reported by subjects receiving doses greater than 0.1 µg/kg. These myalgias varied in duration and severity in dose-dependent fashion; women appeared to be more susceptible than men. The systemic effects were earlier and more pronounced with IV than with sc administration. Hyperalgesia at the injection site occurred with sc doses. This effect lasted for up to 7 weeks and also varied in dose-dependent fashion. No subject showed antibodies to NGF.

Conclusion.—In healthy human subjects, single doses of systemically administered rhNGF cause potent and reversible biological effects. These effects—including diffuse myalgias and hyperalgesia at the site of sc injection—occur at very low doses and in dose-dependent fashion. Studies are under way to assess the effects of rhNGF on damaged peripheral nerve sensory fibers.

▶ The availability of recombinant neurotrophic factors for use in humans is opening a whole new vista for potential therapy of chronic neurologic disease.

It is also offering fascinating insights into human neurologic function. This phase I study of parenteral NGF demonstrated that patients receiving the higher doses have pain develop in the neck, throat, abdomen, and limbs. This might possibly result from the presence of *trk* receptors on small-diameter substance P–expressing dorsal root ganglion neurons. The biological significance of this is unknown at present. Studies of NGF treatment for diabetic neuropathy are in progress.—W.G. Bradley, D.M., F.R.C.P.

Oral and Genital Tardive Pain Syndromes
Ford B, Greene P, Fahn S (Columbia-Presbyterian Med Ctr, New York)
Neurology 44:2115–2119, 1994   122-96-17–2

Background.—Treatment with dopamine receptor blocking drugs may produce a range of tardive syndromes that includes dyskinetic states, dystonia, tics, and myoclonus. One case of orolingual tardive dyskinesia accompanied by pain has been reported.

Series.—Eleven further patients with severe tardive disorder were described. They were seen with tardive dyskinesias, tardive akathisia, or tardive dystonia during a period when 204 such patients were encountered. The 11 patients had chronic, painful oral or genital sensations that caused marked distress and overshadowed all other neuropsychiatric symptoms. Ten women and 1 man (mean age, 67 years) were affected.

Clinical Aspects.—Nine patients had a painful oral syndrome, whereas 2 had pain in the genital region. Eight patients had an underlying chronic anxiety state or affective disorder for which they had received neuroleptic drugs. Nine patients had been continuously exposed to neuroleptics for an average of 3.4 years. Many patients were unaware of their orofacial movements because the sensation of burning or lancinating pain was the source of unceasing discomfort. Occasionally the patients felt an urge to move in conjunction with their pain. Many patients had used various analgesics without effect. Catecholamine-depleting agents were the most effective drugs for suppressing pain, but they induced parkinsonism in 3 patients. One patient responded to α-methylparatyrosine, a dopamine synthesis inhibitor, and 2 improved when receiving propoxyphene.

Conclusion.—A specific tardive pain syndrome may complicate chronic treatment with neuroleptic drugs. With this syndrome, painful orogenital sensations overlap with other tardive symptoms.

▶ Dr. Ford and his colleagues have described a new syndrome involving severe, chronic, and painful oral or genital sensations experienced after the use of neuroleptics and associated with tardive motor disorders. Presumably, the mechanism of the tardive pain is similar to that of tardive motor phenomena, namely, an alteration of dopamine receptors. However, the location of the responsible dopamine receptors is unknown. They may well be located in the spinal cord. Dopamine fibers that orginate from cell bodies located in the caudal diencephalon and in the substantia nigra are now known to project to the spinal cord dorsal horn. In addition, dopamine receptors have been located in sites in the spinal gray matter. Moreover, behavioral studies have indicated that dopamine is involved in the regulation of the nociceptive input to the spinal cord. Basic data are needed regarding the types of dopamine receptors in the spinal cord and the alterations in their regulation produced by chronic administration of neuroleptics.—R.A. Davidoff, M.D.

'Sympathetically Maintained Pain': I. Phentolamine Block Questions the Concept

Verdugo RJ, Ochoa JL (Oregon Health Sciences Univ, Portland)
Neurology 44:1003–1010, 1994   122-96-17–3

Background.—"Sympathetically maintained pain" (SMP) is characterized by a history of physical trauma to the painful area, the presence of continuous burning pain with painful sensation to touch, and pain relief during sympathetic block. Phentolamine sympathetic block (PSB) is considered a crucial diagnostic test for SMP. However, the conflicting results in the literature question the legitimacy of prevailing concepts of the

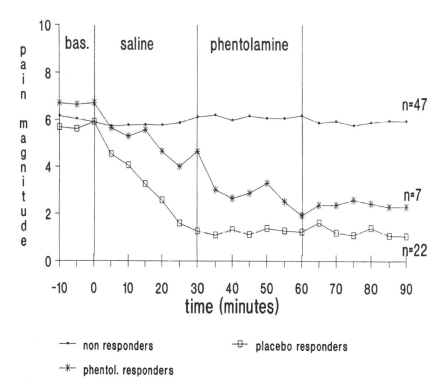

Fig 17–1.—Spontaneous pain outcome in response to phentolamine sympathetic block (protocol A: baseline, saline, and phentolamine phases). Note the pure placebo effect within 30 minutes during the saline phase in 22 of 76 patients, and the slow, steady response during the saline and phentolamine phases in 7 patients. In the 47 patients in whom saline did not induce a placebo response, the active blocker did not induce any effect. (Courtesy of Verdugo RJ, Ochoa JL: *Neurology* 44:1003–1010, 1994.)

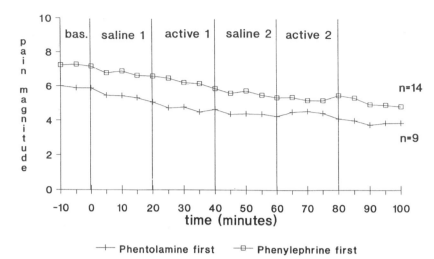

—— Phentolamine first ——   —□— Phenylephrine first

Fig 17–2.—Spontaneous pain outcome in response to phentolamine sympathetic block (protocol B) in 23 patients. Nonresponders, saline responders, and active drug responders are pooled in this graph. Note mild but significant pain relief ($P < 0.01$) progressing steadily throughout the procedure. The difference in mean pain intensity between phentolamine-first and phenylephrine-first groups is not significant ($P = 0.19$). The sequential order of active drugs made no difference in pain outcome. (Courtesy of Verdugo RJ, Ochoa JL: *Neurology* 44:1003–1010, 1994.)

pathophysiology of neuropathic pain. A total of 100 patients with chronic painful states associated with regional sensory, motor, or neurovascular symptoms were studied to clarify the meaning of a subjective pain response to PSB and the overall concept of SMP.

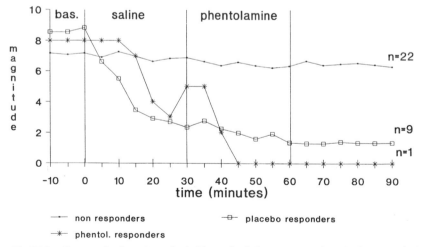

—— non responders   —□— placebo responders
—*— phentol. responders

Fig 17–3.—Outcome for dynamic mechanical hyperalgesia in response to phentolamine sympathetic block (protocol A) in 32 patients. The individual (*asterisk*) whose symptom was eventually abolished with phentolamine had initially expressed substantial placebo response followed by intervening reversal. Otherwise, the overall profile for dynamic mechanical hyperalgesia relief is similar to that for spontaneous pain response: either placebo response or no response. (Courtesy of Verdugo RJ, Ochoa JL: *Neurology* 44:1003–1010, 1994.)

Methods.—Sympathetic blocks were performed in 100 patients with "reflex sympathetic dystropy" or "causalgia". Two separate protocols were followed. In protocol A, 77 patients underwent 30 minutes of placebo infusion followed by 35 mg of phentolamine. In protocol B, 23 patients received placebo infusion, followed by double-blind infusion of 500 μg of phentolamine or phenylephrine, followed by a second placebo infusion, and finally the other active drug. A 10-point scale was used to assess the magnitude of pain and mechanical hyperalgesias; sensory and sympathetic effects were monitored as well.

Results.—In protocol A, 29% of patients reported at least a 50% reduction in pain during infusion of placebo and a 9% reduction during infusion of phentolamine (Fig 17–1). In protocol B, pain relief occurred with placebo in 17% of patients, phenylephrine in 17%, and phentolamine in 9% (Fig 17–2). Placebo infusion yielded progressive relief of pain in all "phentolamine responders" (Fig 17–3). Two patients reported relief when given phenylephrine and worsening when given phentolamine; most showed no response to either placebo or active drugs (Fig 17–4).

Conclusions.—The use of agonist or antagonist drugs to manipulate the α-1 adrenergic receptor does not appear to influence neuropathic pain. These findings question the existence of SMP, as diagnosed by sympathetic blocks without adequate controls for a placebo effect. The concept of SMP is a fallacious one; the conflicting conclusions reached by others have been interpretive in nature.

▶ See the comment following Abstract 122-96-17–4.—W.G. Bradley, D.M., F.R.C.P.

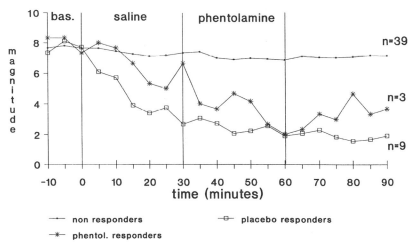

Fig 17–4.—Outcome for static mechanical hyperalgesia in response to phentolamine sympathetic block (protocol A) in 51 patients. The overall profile is similar to those for spontaneous pain and dynamic hyperalgesia responses: most patients failed to respond, and patients who responded did so through a placebo effect. (Courtesy of Verdugo RJ, Ochoa JL: *Neurology* 44:1003–1010, 1994.)

Phentolamine Sympathetic Block in Painful Polyneuropathies: II. Further Questioning of the Concept of 'Sympathetically Maintained Pain'

Verdugo RJ, Campero M, Ochoa JL (Oregon Health Sciences Univ, Portland)
Neurology 44:1010–1014, 1994   122-96-17–4

Introduction.—Many patients with "causalgia" or "reflex sympathetic dystrophy" are given a diagnosis of sympathetically maintained pain (SMP), based on relief of pain by sympathetic blockade. However, studies using standard diagnostic nerve or sympathetic blocks in patients with regional "chronic pains associated with various combinations of sensory, motor, and vasomotor phenomena" (CPSMV) have questioned the very existence of the concept of SMP. It is still possible that polyneuropathic patients with CPSMV might have a true sympathetic component underlying their pain. The possibility that such patients might have an SMP state was examined in a placebo-controlled study.

Methods.—The subjects were 14 patients with chronic painful polyneuropathies. All underwent a comprehensive clinical and laboratory evaluation, including a placebo-controlled phentolamine sympathetic block. Six patients received a 30-minute IV infusion of saline, followed by 35 mg of phentolamine. The other 8 received saline followed by a double-blind infusion of 500 µg of phentolamine or phenylephrine, a second saline infusion, and then the second active drug. The investigators used a 10-point scale to measure the magnitude of spontaneous pain and mechanical hyperalgesias every 5 minutes. They also monitored any sensory and sympathetic effects, both clinically and by quantitative thermotesting and thermography.

Results.—At least a 50% reduction in pain was reported by 5 patients, all in response to saline. None of the patients obtained pain relief with either phentolamine or phenylephrine, although all of them had signs of physiologic abnormalities reported as determinants or predictors of SMP, such as sympathetic denervation supersensitivity and hyperexcitability and sensitization of peripheral C-nociceptors.

Conclusions.—These and previous findings question the existence of SMP in patients who have post-traumatic regional pain, with or without nerve injury, who have been given a diagnosis of "reflex sympathetic dystrophy". The concept of SMP is an unfounded one, the result of a failure to provide placebo control during sympathetic blocks and failure to perform a careful neurologic evaluation in patients with chronic "neuropathic" pain.

► In a guest editorial introducing a special issue of *Muscle and Nerve* devoted to neuropathic pains, Ochoa produced telling evidence for the rejection of neuropathic pain, reflex sympathetic dystrophy, sympathetically mediated pain, and causalgia as being true entities (1). These conditions have a checkered history, with many different opinions existing with regard to their definition, nosology, and true nature. Although reflex sympathetic dystrophy has now become a very popular medicolegal field, in which many attorneys and, also, doctors are making a good living, data such as those presented by Ochoa and colleagues in Abstracts 202-95-1–1 and 202-95-1–2 make it clear that these patients are extremely strong reactors to placebos.

Ochoa and his colleagues have had a very wide experience with such patients in a national referral practice extending over many years, with the patients being put through a very rigorous quantitative battery of sensory and physiologic studies. Although some of these patients undoubtedly have organic lesions, such as neuromas in continuity, etc., many such patients show no definite changes on electrophysiologic studies. There can be changes in skin blood flow, thermography, and trophic changes that occur in such patients. There also is a possibility that chronic pain will induce a "reverberating circuit" in the dorsal horn of the spinal cord or higher levels of the nervous system that perpetuates pain. However, it is equally possible that many of these patients have a psychologically mediated pain that is either conscious or unconscious in origin. These papers behoove us to take note of the opinion of very experienced investigators, who are calling into question the existence of all these syndromes.—W.G. Bradley, D.M., F.R.C.P.

Reference

1. Ochoa JL: Essence, investigation and management of "neuropathic" pains: Hopes from acknowledgement of chaos, editorial. *Muscle Nerve* 16:997–1008, 1993.

Computed Tomography Evaluation of Patients With Chronic Headache
Dumas MD, Warwick Pexman JH, Kreeft JH (Univ of Western Ontario, London; Victoria Hosp, London, Ont)
Can Med Assoc J 151:1447–1452, 1994   122-96-17–5

Background.—Recurrent headaches are common. There is concern that an intracranial structural lesion, such as an arteriovenous malformation, aneurysm, or tumor, may be responsible for chronic headaches. A relationship between arteriovenous malformation and unilateral, complicated vascular headache, or cluster headache, has been suggested, but any such relationship is difficult to substantiate because of the low prevalence of arteriovenous malformation. It has been suggested that all patients with migraine undergo contrast-enhanced CT. This is not an easy recommendation to follow, because CT is expensive, and any strong association between migraine and arteriovenous malformation has not been substantiated. It is important to determine whether the rate of detecting a tumor, arteriovenous malformation, or aneurysm with enhanced or unenhanced CT is significant in patients with chronic headache. The cost of detecting these disorders was estimated.

Methods.—A series of 373 consecutive patients with recurrent headache (ranging from 6 months to several years) were referred for CT scanning. All patients had at least one of the following: an increased severity of symptoms or a resistance to drug therapy, a change in the characteristics or the pattern of headache, or a family history of intracranial structural lesion. Scans were either contrast enhanced with nonionic contrast medium, unenhanced, or a combination.

Results.—Of 402 scans, 14 showed minor findings that did not change patient management: 9 scans showed infarct, 2 showed cerebral atrophy, 1 showed cavum vergae, 1 showed hyperostosis frontalis interna, and 1 showed communicating hydrocephalus. There were significant lesions in 4 scans: 2 scans showed osteoma, 1 showed low-grade glioma, and 1 showed aneurysm. Only the aneurysm was treated. There was no evidence of arteriovenous malformation. The cost of 1 unenhanced scan was $82.63 (all figures are in 1991 Canadian dollars, and indicate Canadian costs); 1 enhanced scan cost $204.05. The cost per significant finding was more than $18,000. The cost of finding 1 treatable vascular lesion was $74,243.

Conclusions.—The detection rate of CT scanning in patients with chronic headache is similar to the detection rate expected in the general population, given that the neurologic findings are normal. The cost of detecting intracranial lesions is high. Because no relation was found between intracranial lesions and either severity, resistance to drug therapy, or change in headache pattern, CT is not recommended in these cases.

▶ This study from Western Ontario, Canada, is of relevance to all countries. The action to be taken, however, depends to some extent on the situation. Clearly, CT scanning is rarely beneficial or cost-effective in the group of patients who have chronic recurrent headaches for more than 6 months without neurologic signs, even when there is an increase in severity or a change in character of the headache. Nevertheless, the finding of one treatable lesion at an early stage must have some significance, and at times, management of headaches is improved with the reassurance of a negative CT scan. However, in this day and age, the use of CT scans will have to be substantiated for each patient.—W.G. Bradley, D.M., F.R.C.P.

Comorbidity of Migraine: The Connection Between Migraine and Epilepsy

Lipton RB, Ottman R, Ehrenberg BL, Hauser WA (Montefiore Med Ctr, Bronx, NY; Columbia Univ, New York; Tufts New England Med Ctr, Boston)
Neurology 44:S28–S32, 1994   122-96-17–6

Background.—Both migraine and epilepsy are chronic, episodic neurologic disorders that may involve alterations in mood, consciousness, and behavior as well as focal sensory or motor symptoms. Although there has been considerable speculation about an association between these disorders, the issue has not often been examined systematically.

Objective.—The association between migraine and epilepsy was examined using data from the Epilepsy Family Study of Columbia University. The 1,948 probands were aged 18 and older and had a lifetime history of 2 or more unprovoked seizures. Interviews were conducted with 1,423 parents and full siblings of the probands.

Findings.—Almost one fourth of the probands (24%) had a history of migraine, as did 26% of their relatives with epilepsy and 15% of relatives without epilepsy. Women were at a greater risk of having migraine than men. On multivariate analysis, the risk of migraine for probands was higher for those with partial epilepsy vs. those with generalized-onset seizures. For probands, the risk of migraine was greater when epilepsy was caused by head trauma. Probands with a positive family history of epilepsy also were at increased risk of having a history of migraine.

Implications.—These findings affirm an association between epilepsy and migraine; therefore, it is important that clinicians who see patients with either disorder are familiar with how to diagnose and treat both. For example, patients with migraine should be asked about seizures before a tricyclic drug or neuroleptic is prescribed. Physicians should be aware of drugs, such as divalproex, that are potentially useful in treating both disorders.

▶ Dr. Lipton and his colleagues have used reasonable criteria for both epilepsy and migraine, as well as effective epidemiologic analysis, to show that the risk of migraine is greater in patients with both generalized- and partial-onset seizures. A number of older reports had indicated a higher prevalence of epilepsy in patients with migraine, but many early studies were flawed by the use of poorly defined criteria for both epilepsy and migraine, and most were uncontrolled. More recent epidemiologic investigations have emphasized the independent nature of most forms of epilepsy and migraine. Our thoughts about the problem will now have to be refocused on the implications of these recent data for the diagnosis and treatment of migraine.—R.A. Davidoff, M.D.

Migraine and Major Depression: A Longitudinal Study
Breslau N, Davis GC, Schultz LR, Peterson EL (Henry Ford Health Sciences Ctr, Detroit; Case Western Reserve Univ, Cleveland, Ohio; Univ of Michigan, Ann Arbor)
Headache 34:387–393, 1994   122-96-17–7

Objective.—Recent epidemiologic studies suggesting a possible association between migraine and major depression prompted a study of this association in a random sample of 1,007 patients (age, 21–30 years) who were members of an HMO. All but 3% were available to be reinterviewed 3.5 years later.

Methods.—Psychiatric disorder was identified using the National Institute of Mental Health-Diagnostic Interview Schedule as revised to cover *Diagnostic and Statistical Manual, Third Edition, Revised* (DSM-III-R) disorders. Migraine was diagnosed according to International Headache Society criteria, which include at least 5 episodes, headache lasting longer than 4 hours, the occurrence of nausea/vomiting or photophobia/

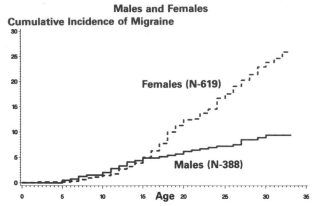

Males and Females
Cumulative Incidence of Migraine

Fig 17–5.—Lifetime (to age 33) cumulative incidence of migraine. (Courtesy of Breslau N, Davis GC, Schultz LR, et al: *Headache* 34:387–393, 1994.)

phonophobia, and at least 2 of the following: unilateral pain, pulsation, interference with daily activities, and worsening on routine physical activity.

Findings.—At age 30, the cumulative incidence of migraine was 23.8% in females and 9.4% in males (Fig 17–5). The cumulative rates of major depression at age 30 were 24.2% for females and 13.3% for males. The cumulative incidence of major depression at age 33 years was 53% in individuals with migraine and 15.9% in those without migraine (Fig 17–6), for a relative risk of 3.8. The relative risk for major depression associated with previous migraine was significantly increased in both males and females. The relative risk of migraine associated with previous major depression was 4.5 in males and 3.9 in females (Fig 17–7).

Interpretation.—An explanation for bidirectional influences of major depression and migraine on one another would require that each disorder

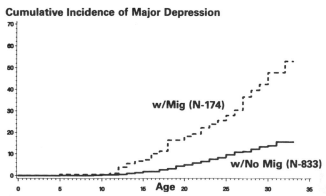

Cumulative Incidence of Major Depression

Fig 17–6.—Lifetime (to age 33) cumulative incidence of major depression in individuals with and without a history of migraines. (Courtesy of Breslau N, Davis GC, Schultz LR, et al: *Headache* 34:387–393, 1994.)

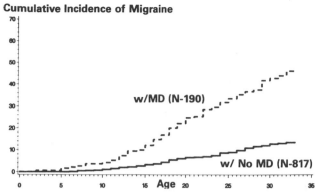

Cumulative Incidence of Migraine

w/MD (N-190)

w/ No MD (N-817)

Age

Fig 17–7.—Lifetime (to age 33) cumulative incidence of migraine in individuals with and without a history of major depression. (Courtesy of Breslau N, Davis GC, Schultz LR, et al: *Headache* 34:387–393, 1994.)

lead to the other as a result of a distinct mechanism. This is not inconceivable, but no such complex explanation is readily available. Another possibility is that comorbid cases of migraine are distinct from cases of isolated migraine.

▶ It is a well-established clinical impression that depression is frequently associated with headache, especially in individuals with a history of severe or disabling headaches. Neurologists have long realized that the relationship between depression and migraine is complex. Now, however, Dr. Breslau and her colleagues have provided the first documentation that migraine and major depression have bidirectional influences, with each affliction raising the odds for the development of the other. The present data indicate that clinicians should no longer support the outdated idea that chronic migraine pain is purely psychological in origin.—R.A. Davidoff, M.D.

A Differential Response to Treatment With Divalproex Sodium in Patients With Intractable Headache
Rothrock JF, Kelly NM, Brody ML, Golbeck A (Univ of Calif, San Diego Headache Ctr; San Diego State Univ, Calif)
Cephalalgia 14:241–244, 1994   122-96-17–8

Introduction.—Although the mechanisms that generate migraine and other primary headache syndromes are still unknown, it seems that serotoninergic cells of the midbrain dorsal raphe nuclei play a role in establishing a headache "threshold." In theory, divalproex sodium, a 1:1 mixture of valproic acid and valproate sodium, may raise the headache threshold.

Methods.—Seventy-five patients with intractable headache syndromes were divided into 3 groups: 18 with frequent migraine (FM); 43 with transformed migraine (TM); and 14 with tension type headache (TT). Fifty-eight (77%) were female. All patients were treated with divalproex sodium (500 mg twice daily).

Results.—Thirty-six patients (49%) reported a 50% or greater reduction in headache frequency. The 3 groups had significantly different treatment response rates, with patients with FM reporting the highest rate of improvement (11 of 18, or 61%); patients with TM, an intermediate rate (22 of 43, or 51%); and patients with TT, the lowest response rate (3 of 14, or 21%). Thirty-four (45%) of the 75 patients who began treatment reported side effects, and 5 reported multiple side effects. The most common side effects were gastrointestinal and chiefly involved nausea, at times profound and accompanied by vomiting.

Conclusion.—Prophylactic therapy with divalproex may be effective in selected patients with intractable headache syndromes. A response to treatment may be predicted by identifying clinically distinct headache subtypes. Given the significant 20% dropout rate among the subjects and the absence of any control group, confirmation of the efficacy of divalproex must be obtained through a prospective, placebo-controlled trial.

▶ Dr. Rothrock and his colleagues have added more evidence to the growing list of papers showing that valproate has potential in the prophylaxis of migraine and chronic daily headaches. Despite the appearance of side effects, which often are bothersome, in a substantial number of patients, the drug is rapidly becoming one of the mainstays of headache prevention. Although the mechanism of its action is unknown, valproate has at least 2 pertinent effects on neural tissue. It limits high frequency, repetitive firing of action potentials, presumably by binding to the inactive form of the sodium channel, thereby slowing the channel's recovery from inactivation. The drug also interacts with the activity of the inhibitory neurotransmitter γ-aminobutyric acid (GABA), raising levels of GABA in the brain and facilitating the postsynaptic actions of GABA. It is unclear whether the latter effect occurs at concentrations within the therapeutic range.—R.A. Davidoff, M.D.

Dihydroergotamine Nasal Spray for the Acute Treatment of Migraine
Ziegler D, Ford R, Kreigler J, Gallagher RM, Peroutka S, Hammerstad J, Saper J, Hoffert M, Vogel B, Holtz N, DiSerio F (Kansas Univ Med Ctr, Kansas City; Birmingham, Ala; Univ Hospitals, Cleveland, Ohio; Moorestown, NJ; et al)
Neurology 44:447–453, 1994   122-96-17-9

Objective.—Ergotamine tartrate, used for a long time to treat migraine, has absorption problems, significant side effects, and can lead to drug dependence, or declining effectiveness. In a double-blind, placebo-controlled, randomized study, the safety and efficacy of dihydroergotamine as a nasal spray were compared with placebo in the treatment of migraine.

Methods.—In 10 study centers, 112 patients (age, 18–65 years) who had migraine at least once a month for the past year, received either placebo nasal spray or nasal spray containing 4 mg of dihydroergotamine mesylate (DHE) administered as a 0.5-mg dose delivered twice to each nostril, with a 15-minute period occurring between dosings. The patients were asked to record their symptoms before taking the medication, and they were evaluated at 1, 2, 3, and 4 hours after taking the medication.

Results.—One hundred patients completed the study: 48 in the treatment group and 52 in the placebo group. The patients rated DHE treatment as significantly more effective than placebo treatment in relieving pain at every time point; and at relieving nausea at 2, 3, and 4 hours. Physicians also rated DHE significantly better than placebo at relieving pain and nausea. There were no significant treatment differences with respect to vomiting. Although 29% of patients taking DHE vs. 11% of those taking placebo reported adverse events, most were mild to moderate and were the result of nasal congestion, vomiting, nausea, and edema.

Conclusion.—Dihydroergotamine mesylate, administered as a nasal spray, is a safe and effective treatment for migraine.

▶ The great number of agents prescribed for the treatment of acute migraine attacks is an indication that no one particular therapy is unambiguously superior to all others. For years, ergots have been the mainstay of acute therapy. Dihydroergotamine, which has close chemical similarities to ergotamine, is a considerably safer drug to use than the parent ergot compound. It also produces little, if any, physical dependence and is reported not to cause rebound phenomena. It also has the advantage that it is a long-lasting agent. At present, dihydroergotamine is only available for parenteral use. However, as this study indicates, administration by the nasal route is safe, well tolerated, and effective. Nasal dihydroergotamine can easily be manufactured by some local pharmacists, and it may be released by the Food and Drug Administration in the future. It is already available in several European countries. It should be a valuable addition to our therapeutic armamentarium.—R.A. Davidoff, M.D.

Elevated Cerebrospinal Fluid Levels of Substance P in Patients With the Fibromyalgia Syndrome
Russell IJ, Orr MD, Littman B, Vipraio GA, Alboukrek D, Michalek JE, Lopez Y, MacKillip F (Univ of Texas, San Antonio; Pfizer Central Research, Groton, Conn; Armstrong Laboratory, Brooks Air Force Base, San Antonio, Texas)
Arthritis Rheum 37:1593–1601, 1994   122-96-17–10

Introduction.—The musculoskeletal pain typical of fibromyalgia syndrome (FMS) may be related to increased CSF levels of substance P (SP), an 11–amino acid peptide that plays a role in the neurotransmission of pain from the periphery to the CNS. To further examine this potential relationship, concentrations of SP were measured in CSF obtained from patients with FMS and normal control subjects. An attempt was made to correlate SP levels and clinical measures in FMS.

Methods.—The 32 patients with FMS had a mean age of 49.6 years; 26 were women. Fifteen controls and 13 patients were white; 15 controls and 19 patients were Hispanic. Because of the difficulty in recruiting controls who were willing to undergo a lumbar puncture, patients and controls differed in age and sex: only 17 of the 30 controls were women, and the group had a mean age of 36.6 years. Scores on the Health Assessment Questionnaire indicated substantial physical dysfunction among patients with FMS.

Results.—Measurements of SP in CSF differed significantly, with mean concentrations of 42.8 fmol/mL in the FMS group and 16.3 fmol/mL in the control group. Regression models showed that age and sex did not contribute significantly after adjustment for ethnicity, and group mean values for CSF SP remained significant after adjustment for ethnicity. Overall, whites exhibited higher mean CSF SP levels than did Hispanics. The differences in CSF SP between patients and controls remained significant when the younger controls and older patients were omitted from analysis, leaving 21 patients and 22 controls of comparable mean age. No correlation was found between the clinical variables and psychological profiles of patients and SP levels.

Conclusion.—As reported in previous studies, patients with FMS had CSF SP levels that were three-fold higher than those of normal controls. It is possible that patients with FMS have a lower-than-normal pain threshold, the result of biochemical interactions between serotonin and SP. The significance of increased SP is uncertain, however, and measurements of CSF SP are not currently recommended for diagnostic purposes.

▶ Fibromyalgia, although a condition with criteria laid down by the American College of Rheumatology, remains a somewhat uncertain syndrome. That chronic sleep deprivation can give an almost identical syndrome not only supports investigation of sleep hygiene in such patients, but it also raises the possibility that FMS has many origins. This study demonstrating apparently increased levels of substance P in the CSF raises as many questions as it answers. One possible explanation is that chronic pain syndromes raise the CSF level of SP and, therefore, this is a result and not a cause of FMS. This study, however, *does* prompt the further scientific evaluation of patients with fibromyalgia as a result of the hypotheses generated from such research.—W.G. Bradley, D.M., F.R.C.P.

18 Spinal Disorders

The Treatment of Acute Low Back Pain: Bed Rest, Exercises, or Ordinary Activity?
Malmivaara A, Häkkinen U, Aro T, Heinrichs M-L, Koskenniemi L, Kuosma E, Lappi S, Paloheimo R, Servo C, Vaaranen V, Hernberg S (Finnish Inst of Occupational Health, Helsinki; Natl Research and Development Ctr for Welfare and Health, Helsinki; City of Helsinki Occupational Health Care Ctrs, Finland)
N Engl J Med 332:351–355, 1995   122-96-18-1

Purpose.—Two competing strategies—bed rest and back extension exercises—are commonly prescribed for patients with low back pain. Experts disagree as to which treatment is best for this extremely common and expensive problem. In a randomized, controlled trial, the 2 treatments were compared with usual activity for their effectiveness and cost.

Methods.—The subjects were 186 employees of the city of Helsinki who were evaluated at the city's occupational health centers for acute, nonspecific low back pain. The patients were randomized, in roughly equal numbers, into 3 groups. One group was assigned 2 days of bed rest and another to perform light back mobilizing exercises; the third group was told to continue ordinary activities as tolerated. The outcome and costs of the 3 groups were evaluated at 3 and 12 weeks.

Results.—At both assessments, the control group demonstrated better recovery than either the bed rest or the exercise group. In terms of duration of pain, pain intensity, lumbar flexion, subjective ability to work, Owestry back disability index, and lost work days, the ordinary activity group was favored to a significant degree. Patients in the bed rest group had the longest recovery times. There were no significant differences in cost between the 3 groups.

Conclusions.—In patients with acute low back pain, simply maintaining ordinary activity as tolerated leads to quicker recovery than either bed rest or back mobilization exercises. The advantages of ordinary activity are remarkably consistent across outcome variables. If widely used in clinical practice, this approach would likely yield considerable cost savings.

▶ This paper describes a randomized, controlled study of 2 days' bed rest vs. light back mobilizing exercises vs. continued ordinary activities, as tolerated in a group of subjects with acute low back pain in Helsinki, Finland. The outcome is clear, demonstrating significantly better outcomes in the patients who were instructed to remain at work and undertake activities as their pain allowed. It is clear that patients with acute low back pain but without neurologic signs should be urged to remain at work.—W.G. Bradley, D.M., F.R.C.P.

▶ This is an important study because it establishes, in a fairly homogeneous patient population, that bed rest (although only for 2 days) and back-mobilization exercises have no advantage in the acute care of patients with nonspecific low back pain.—R.H. Wilkins, M.D.

Dorsal Ramus Irritation Associated With Recurrent Low Back Pain and Its Relief With Local Anesthetic or Training Therapy
Sihvonen T, Lindgren K-L, Airaksinen O, Leino E, Partanen J, Hänninen O (Univ Hosp of Kuopio, Finland)
J Spinal Disord 8:8–14, 1995   122-96-18–2

Introduction.—Nerves leave the spinal cord as motor primary and sensory rootlets and join to the nerve root before leaving the spinal canal. After leaving the root canal, the nerve root branches into the ventral and dorsal roots. The dorsal ramus innervates the back muscles and other posterior structures; it sometimes becomes irritated, resulting in the dorsal ramus syndrome. The medial branch, which innervates the multifidus muscle and contains pain fibers, is especially prone to entrapment. The effects of segmental anesthesia and back muscle exercise in patients with low back pain associated with dorsal ramus neuropathy were described.

Patients.—Twenty-one patients had recurrent low back pain, all with current low back symptoms and recurrent diffuse referred symptoms in the lower extremities. None had any distinct neurologic deficiencies on clinical testing, and radiologic studies showed no abnormalities of the nerve roots or spinal canal. However, electroneuromyography showed damage to the medial branch of the dorsal ramus, demonstrated as fibrillations and positive sharp waves in the multifidus muscle. There was no evidence of more proximal ventral nerve root damage in the spinal cord or at the nerve route origin.

Treatment.—Nine patients were sent to the rehabilitation unit for back muscle activation and coordinative, muscle-strengthening training therapy. Exercise therapy started with isometric back muscle activation and gradually proceeded to more dynamic exercise. The remaining 12 patients received injection therapy. Injections of 10% lidocaine, 4–5 mL, and betmethasone acetate, 5 mg, were directed to the dorsal ramus region near the laminar bone in the affected segment.

Results.—All patients reported the disappearance of local back pain and referred symptoms after injection. The pain-free period varied widely, from 2 days to 1 year. After injection treatment, the patients were able to begin training and muscle therapy; they were less afraid of using the back than before. Seven of 9 patients in the exercise group reported freedom from pain and went back to their usual work. After treatment, all but one patient in the injection group had clear changes in kinetic back muscle function. The surface electromyography (EMG) pattern from the low back muscles during lumbar-pelvic rhythm normalized, eccentric back muscle activity was reduced, the extension-flexion ratio of the mean maximum microvolt level of surface EMG increased, and flexion relaxation improved.

Conclusions.—The diagnosis and treatment of dorsal ramus irritation in patients with low back pain were reported. Symptoms can be relieved by either local anesthetic injection or training therapy. Electroneuromyography studies are recommended in patients with low back pain whose radiologic findings are not consistent with typical nerve root impingement but who have referred pain. The diagnosis of dorsal ramus irritation requires the demonstration of segmental denervation in the multifidus muscle using a sufficiently long EMG needle.

▶ The major conundrum of acute and chronic low back pain is what causes it. Most patients do not have evidence of an acute disk prolapse or of other proposed etiologies. It has now been well demonstrated that a rapid return to normal activity, with back strengthening exercises, is the best therapy for this syndrome. This paper suggests that a nerve entrapment syndrome of the medial branch of the dorsal ramus of the segmental nerve is responsible for the back pain, and that injection of local anesthetic and corticosteroid can relieve the entrapment and pain, thereby producing more rapid mobilization. The observation of fibrillations and positive sharp waves on EMG in the paraspinal muscles is interesting but not totally convincing. It would have been instructive to have included a group receiving placebo injection to determine whether the medications or the placebo effect of injection was responsible for the apparent therapeutic effect. The return of the patient to back muscle training exercises was the positive outcome of this study.— W.G. Bradley, D.M., F.R.C.P.

Long-Term Results of Cervical Epidural Steroid Injection With and Without Morphine in Chronic Cervical Radicular Pain
Castagnera L, Maurette P, Pointillart V, Vital JM, Erny P, Sénégas J (Hôpital Pellegrin, Bordeaux, France)
Pain 58:239–243, 1994   122-96-18–3

Background.—Cervical epidural cortical steroid injection (CESI) has been proposed as a treatment alternative for patients experiencing cervical radicular pain (CRP). It has also been suggested that co-administration of morphine and corticosteroid produces better long-lasting pain relief than that produced by each drug alone in patients with recurrent low-back pain. The short-, mid- and long-term effectiveness of a single CESI administered with or without morphine was investigated in patients with chronic CRP who were not in need of surgery.

Patients and Methods.—Twenty-four patients experiencing CRP of noncompressive and nonmalignant origin for more than 12 months were included in a prospective, randomized study. A C7-D1 18-gauge needle was used to inject the cervical epidural space with an increasing volume of isotonic saline solution to intensify radicular pain. A maximum of 10 mL was injected. Fourteen patients were then randomly assigned to the corticosteroid group (group S), and they received an equivalent volume of .5% lidocaine together with triamcinolone acetonide, 10 mg/mL. The remaining 10 patients were assigned to the corticosteroid plus morphine group (S + M group). These patients received the same combination as those in the S group plus 2.5 mg of morphine sulphate. Anthropometric data were comparable between groups. Pain relief was defined as the percentage of pain decrease measured via a visual analogue scale on day 1 and at months 1, 3, 6, 8, and 12 after CESI.

Results.—In groups S and S + M, the mean volume injected in the epidural space was 6.6 and 6.3 mL, respectively. This volume produced intensified pain in 21 of 24 patients. A better transient improvement was noted in the S + M group the day after CESI treatment. However, long-term results did not differ between groups (Fig 18–1). Success rates of 78.5% and 80% were noted in groups S and S + M, respectively, providing pain relief of 86.8% and 86.9%, respectively. Pain relief remained stable during a mean follow-up of 43 months.

Conclusions.—Patients with chronic CRP unrelated to a compressive or malignant origin and not requiring surgery can benefit from a single CESI

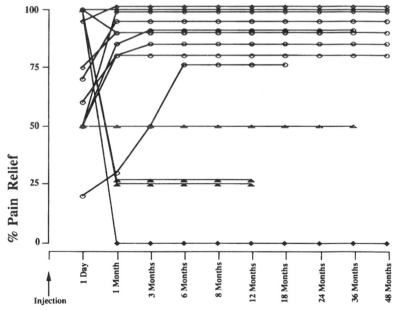

Fig 18–1.—Evolution of short- and long-term pain relief in each patient in group S. *Open diamond,* complete; *open circle,* excellent; *open triangle,* good; *filled triangle,* fair; *filled diamond,* none. (Courtesy of Castagnera L, Maurette P, Pointillart V, et al: *Pain* 58:239–243, 1994.)

when medical treatment proves ineffective. This treatment alternative leads to long-lasting pain relief in 70.8% of patients, without the addition of morphine.

▶ This small but carefully designed French study indicates that, in appropriately selected patients, epidermal injection of corticosteroids can decrease chronic CRP over the course of months to years. The addition of morphine to the injection added only some short-term relief, which was not worth the side effects. The origin of the pain in these patients was idiopathic and was presumed to be "irritation." The authors point out that a true placebo group, receiving needle insertion but no injection, would have allowed a firmer conclusion about whether the corticosteroids were themselves useful; however, "unfortunately the Ethics Committee did not allow us to use such a method." The problems in interpreting this potentially important study without the inclusion of a placebo group are relevant to current polemics against the use of placebos in clinical trials in the United States.—J.P. Blass, M.D., Ph.D.

Bilateral Distal Upper Limb Amyotrophy and Watershed Infarcts From Vertebral Dissection
Pullicino P (State Univ of New York, Buffalo)
Stroke 25:1870–1872, 1994   122-96-18–4

Introduction.—Motor neuron deficits sometimes occur in patients with vertebral artery disease. The pathogenesis of these deficits is unknown. A case of bilateral distal upper extremity atrophy in a patient with right vertebral artery dissection was reported, including the MRI findings.

Case Report.—Man, 39, awoke after a night of heavy drinking with sudden vertigo, chest and bilateral arm pain, and bilateral arm weakness. Examination revealed marked weakness of grasp, no finger extension or abduction, and no triceps strength bilaterally. Magnetic resonance imaging showed an infarct in the distribution of the right posterior inferior cerebellar artery, without involvement of the medulla. Magnetic resonance angiography demonstrated the typical peripheral eccentric hyperintensity of dissection of the right vertebral artery. Subsequently, the patient experienced wasting of the muscles innervated by the sixth cervical to first thoracic spinal cord segments. On repeat MRI scanning 6 weeks later, there were bilateral focal hyperintensities in the region of each anterior horn, extending from the middle to the lower part of the cervical spinal cord (Figs 18–2 and 18–3). Recanalization of the right vertebral artery with irregular margins was documented at 2 months after the stroke; by 3 months, the patient had achieved only minimal functional recovery.

Discussion.—A disabling bilateral amyotrophy of the upper extremities may result from unilateral vertebral artery dissection. The symmetric, bilateral focal hyperintensities of the anterior cervical spinal cord documented in this case are compatible with watershed infarction. The lower

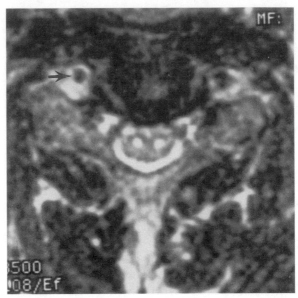

Fig 18–2.—A T2-weighted MR axial scan at the C-5 level 6 weeks after the stroke, showing spinal cord containing symmetrical focal hyperintensities in the region of the anterior horns. The right vertebral artery (*arrow*) is seen to be smaller than the left vertebral artery and is surrounded by hyperintensity compatible with a chronic hematoma, characteristic of a dissection. (Courtesy of Pullicino P: *Stroke* 25:1870–1872, 1994.)

motor neuron injury appears to have resulted from this watershed infarction, which involved both anterior horns.

▶ Spinal cord vascular disease is more frequently recognized at autopsy than diagnosed clinically, probably indicating that the infarct is asymptomatic in most instances. Striking cases, such as that described by Pullicino, are rare. This paper highlights the at-risk nature of the blood supply of the

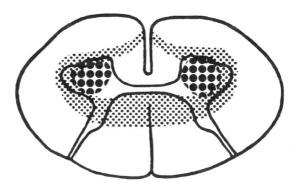

Fig 18–3.—Diagram of the blood supply to the cervical spinal cord (adapted from Turnball IM, Breig A, Hassler O: *J Neurosurg* 24:951–965, 1966), showing a peripheral area supplied by branches of the plial artery plexus separated by a border zone (*small dots*) from the central anterior spinal artery territory. The *large dots* show the locations of the presumed infarcts. (Courtesy of Pullicino P: *Stroke* 25:1870–1872, 1994.)

anterior horns of the spinal cord, particularly in the cervical region. Although vertebral artery dissection was responsible for this case, it is possible that compression of the anterior spinal artery resulting from cervical spondylosis may rarely produce a similar syndrome.—W.G. Bradley, D.M., F.R.C.P.

19 Sleep Disorders

Effect of Octreotide, a Somatostatin Analog, on Sleep Apnea in Patients With Acromegaly
Grunstein RR, Ho KKY, Sullivan CE (Univ of Sydney, Australia; Garvan Inst of Med Research, Sydney, Australia; Saint Vincent's Hosp, Sydney, Australia)
Ann Intern Med 121:478–483, 1994   122-96-19–1

Background.—Octreotide is a new long-acting somatostatin analogue. Preliminary studies have reported that, in patients with acromegaly, the drug may reduce sleep apnea by decreasing upper airway soft-tissue swelling and increasing upper airway dimensions. In an open-label prospective study, the effect of octreotide on sleep apnea and measures of hormonal activity was further defined.

Patients and Methods.—Nineteen patients with acromegaly and sleep apnea and a mean age of 50 years were evaluated. The patients received octreotide in total dosages of 100 µg, 200 µg or 500 µg, administered in a stepwise incremental design over a 6-month period. Sleep studies and measured indices of hormonal activity, including levels of insulin-like growth factor (IGF-1) and growth hormone, were performed at baseline and at 6 months.

Results.—A 50% reduction in the respiratory disturbance index was noted after 6-month treatment with octreotide compared with baseline (19 events vs. 39 events per hour, respectively). A 40% decrease was also observed in total apnea time after the treatment period vs. before (15.1% vs. 27.6% of total sleep time, respectively). Improved indices of oxygen desaturation, sleep quality, and subjective sleepiness were also noted. Although a parallel decrease was seen for mean levels of growth hormone and IGF-1, no correlation was found between the reduction in the total amount of sleep time spent in apnea and the reduction in growth hormone levels. At 6 months of treatment, a similar residual respiratory disturbance index was noted for patients who improved, regardless of whether biochemical remission had occurred.

Conclusions.—In patients with sleep apnea and acromegaly, octreotide treatment leads to improved indices of the severity of sleep apnea. However, sleep apnea can persist despite normalization of growth hormone levels, and it may improve dramatically even when only partial biochemical remission occurs. In this study, 10 of 14 patients still met polysomnographic criteria for sleep apnea after 6 months of treatment. Such patients need to be carefully evaluated and may require more definitive treatment, such as nasal continuous positive airway pressure.

▶ Numerical measures of sleep apnea can be shown to be reduced with octreotide and other medications. The work presented in this article increases the available experience with the relationship of hormones to sleep and breathing. It also highlights the importance of objective evaluation to assess therapeutic responses accurately. More than 70% of patients with moderate-to-severe sleep apnea that was treated with octreotide for 6 months had persistent sleep apnea. In cases of acromegaly with sleep apnea, objective comparison of treatment alternatives, such as nasal continuous positive airway pressure or combined therapy, may be warranted.—B. Nolan, M.D.

Sleep Cycles and Alpha-Delta Sleep in Fibromyalgia Syndrome
Branco J, Atalaia A, Paiva T (Hosp de Santa Maria, Lisboa, Portugal)
J Rheumatol 21:1113–1117, 1994   122-96-19–2

Background.—An alpha-wave intrusion in non–rapid eye movement (NREM) sleep has been observed during nocturnal sleep electroencephalography in many patients with fibromyalgia syndrome (FMS). Alpha intrusion in NREM sleep probably causes nonrefreshing sleep, which is also common in FMS. The delta and alpha activity and alpha–delta ratio across sleep cycles of patients with FMS was examined in a prospective study.

Methods.—Night-long polysomnography recordings were performed in 10 patients with FMS and in 14 healthy control subjects. Conventional electroencephalogram (EEG) frequency bands were automatically computed using spectral analysis. Integrated and normalized values for alpha and delta power were calculated for each sleep cycle, and the evolution of these activities across successive sleep cycles was studied.

Results.—Patients with FMS had a higher percentage of wake and 2 NREM sleep and markedly lower 4 NREM and REM sleep compared with controls. Delta decay across sleep cycles was different in patients with FMS; alpha activity was greater and declined. In contrast, controls were persistently low throughout their sleep. The alpha-delta ratio increased progressively in successive sleep cycles in patients with FMS but not in controls.

Conclusion.—The frequency of subjective sleep disturbances is high in FMS. These disturbances include an increased incidence of alpha EEG NREM sleep and abnormal sleep cycle organization. Additional studies are needed to uncover the functional significance of the alpha EEG NREM anomaly.

▶ The debate as to whether sleep disturbances in FMS are the cause or the effect of the syndrome prompted me to select this paper, despite the drawbacks of the study. This study has limitations, some of which the authors acknowledge, that should be kept in mind when assessing their results. The authors compared alpha power and slow-wave sleep measures for a group of patients who met criteria for FMS and insomnia and had a mean age that was 18 years older than that of a group of apparently unmatched controls. Effectively, the authors compared older insomniacs who had pain with younger healthy asymptomatic subjects. Interpretation of the results was further limited by nonidentification of the patient group's medication status.

Slow-wave sleep in NREM stages 3 and 4 diminishes with age in the absence of any particular disease. Alpha–delta sleep may be seen with various medications and has been reported in a number of other disorders. Unfortunately, more than 20 years of interest, study, and suggested hypotheses for a casual effect of sleep disruption in FMS have not provided a convincing answer, and the controversy continues.—B. Nolan, M.D.

20 Neuroimaging

Initial Clinical Experience in MR Imaging of the Brain With a Fast Fluid-Attenuated Inversion-Recovery Pulse Sequence
Rydberg JN, Hammond CA, Grimm RC, Erickson BJ, Jack CR Jr, Huston J III, Riederer SJ (Mayo Clinic and Found, Rochester, Minn; Univ of Minnesota, Minneapolis)
Radiology 193:173–180, 1994   122-96-20–1

Purpose.—T2-weighted spin-echo (SE) MRI has been used in the evaluation of many diseases. However, some diseases (such as multiple sclerosis) have signal strengths of intermediate intensity, requiring both T2-weighted and proton density–weighted images for reliable evaluation. Fluid-attenuated inversion-recovery (FLAIR) is a technique in which tissue abnormalities are projected as the brightest object in the image. Although FLAIR has enhanced images not seen with conventional T2-weighted imaging, the long acquisition times required have limited its use. A technique with increased efficacy, fast FLAIR, was evaluated and compared with conventional T2-weighted SE imaging in patients with brain abnormalities.

Methods.—Two techniques—sequential interleaving and use of increased numbers of phase encodings per repetition (RARE)—were incorporated to develop a fast FLAIR sequence that would provide 36 contiguous sections in 5 minutes. The resulting images were then compared with images obtained using conventional T2-weighted SE. A total of 41 patients with brain abnormalities underwent imaging. Images obtained with each technique were evaluated using quantitative (lesion-to-background contrast; lesion-to-background contrast/noise ratio [C/N]; lesion-to-CSF contrast; and lesion-to-CSF C/N and qualitative criteria (lesion conspicuity, lesion detectability, and image artifact).

Results.—Fast FLAIR imaging resulted in lesion-to-background contrast 4 times that of first-echo SE. The C/N performance of fast FLAIR also surpassed that of first-echo imaging. A higher lesion-to-background contrast was also observed with fast FLAIR as compared with second-echo SE. As was expected, lesion-to-background C/N was poorer (approximately 12%) with fast FLAIR as compared with second-echo SE. Fast FLAIR resulted in lesion-to-CSF contrast approximately 38 and 75 times that of first- and second-echo SE, respectively. Lesion-to-CSF C/N with fast FLAIR was also greater than with first- and second-echo SE (2.26 and 3.3 times greater, respectively). Qualitative assessment showed fast FLAIR to be comparable or superior to T2-weighted SE imaging for all evaluations

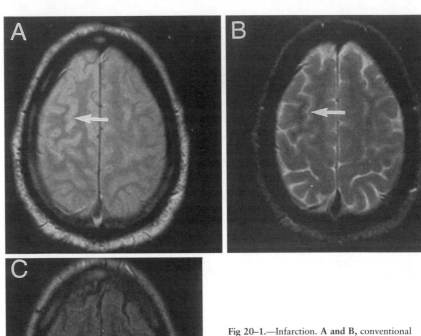

Fig 20–1.—Infarction. **A and B,** conventional SE images (2,350/30, 80) do not show the lesion. C, fast fluid-attenuated inversion-recovery (FLAIR) image (11,000/145/2,600). *Arrow* indicates infarct. Increased signal intensity was also visible on previous caudal fast FLAIR section. (Courtesy of Rydberg JN, Hammond CA, Grimm RC, et al: *Radiology* 193:173–180, 1994.)

of lesion detection and in all but 3 evaluations for lesion conspicuity. The T2-weighted SE imaging was found to be superior to fast FLAIR for overall image artifact. However, no difference was found between the 2 techniques in interference of image interpretation. When assessing images from individual patients, infarction in 1 patient was visible only with fast FLAIR and not with any T2-weighted SE images (Fig 20–1). Imaging with fast FLAIR also resulted in better lesion definition in 1 patient with multiple sclerosis as compared with SE imaging (Fig 20–2). In another patient with small vessel ischemia, fast FLAIR showed increased lesion conspicuity, and it also revealed an additional lesion undetected by conventional SE images (Fig 20–3).

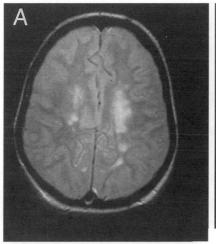
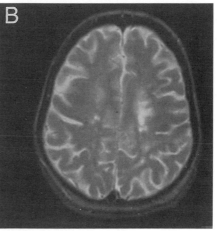
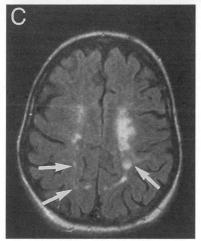

Fig 20–2.—Multiple sclerosis. A and B, conventional SE image (2,350/30, 80). C, fast fluid-attenuated inversion-recovery (FLAIR) image (11,000/145/2,600). Fast FLAIR image gives much better lesion definition than either T2-weighted SE image, especially in the parietal white matter of the brain (*arrows*). (Courtesy of Rydberg JN, Hammond CA, Grimm RC, et al: *Radiology* 193:173–180, 1994.)

Conclusions.—Incorporation of 2 techniques—sequential interleaving and RARE—resulted in improved efficacy of FLAIR imaging. These changes resulted in a fast FLAIR sequence that could image 36 contiguous 5-mm-thick sections in a very short period (5 minutes 8 seconds), a 13-fold improvement. Lesion-to-background contrast was significantly improved with fast FLAIR compared with first- or second-echo SE. Lesion conspicuity and detectability were also rated higher with fast FLAIR. Although studies with more patients are needed to fully evaluate the potential of the fast FLAIR technique, these results have shown fast FLAIR to be superior to conventional SE imaging for detection of brain abnormalities.

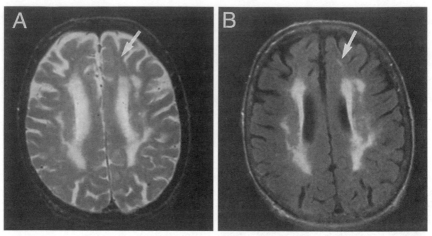

Fig 20–3.—Small-vessel ischemia. A, conventional SE image (2,300/30, 80). B, fast fluid-attenuated inversion-recovery (FLAIR) image (11,000/145/260) shows increased lesion conspicuity in white matter of left lobe. Fast FLAIR image also depicts an additional lesion in left frontal lobe (*arrow*) not seen on either SE image. (Courtesy of Rydberg JN, Hammond CA, Grimm RC, et al: *Radiology* 193:173–180, 1994.)

▶ The ability to use an MR pulse sequence that nulls signal from CSF yet simultaneously allows abnormalities to be detected as high signal has distinct advantages over routine SE and fast SE images. A sequence called FLAIR (fluid-attenuated inversion-recovery) accomplishes this, and as a result, many lesions (e.g., MS plaques and ischemic changes) are better seen. The exceptionally long TRs required for conventional FLAIR imaging made it not generally useful for clinical practice. However with the incorporation of multiecho averaging into FLAIR, the excessive time factor is no longer an issue. The basic question is when one should use the fast FLAIR technique, and although more widespread experience is necessary, patients suspected of a stroke or multiple sclerosis would be candidates. In the latter situation, it would be particularly useful in the follow-up lesions after treatment.—R.M. Quencer, M.D.

Subcortical Low Intensity in Early Cortical Ischemia
Ida M, Mizunuma K, Hata Y, Tada S (The Jikei Univ, Tokyo, Japan)
AJNR 15:1387–1393, 1994   122-96-20–2

Introduction.—In patients with cerebral infarction, T2-weighted MR images usually show an increase in signal intensity in the focus of infarction. The 9 patients who were reported, however, had early cortical ischemia and proton density–weighted and T2-weighted images showing low intensity in the subcortical white matter. Several possible causes of this finding were discussed.

Patients and Methods.—Two of the patients—a 3-year-old girl and a 4-year-old boy—had moyamoya disease. The remaining 7 patients had cortical infarction and ranged in age from 39 to 85 years. Initial MRI was done within 3 days of onset in 2 cases and from 4 to 21 days of onset in 7 cases. Six follow-up MRI examinations were performed in 4 patients. Imaging was performed at 1.5 tesla, and multisection, spin-echo proton density– and T2-weighted images were obtained in all cases.

Results.—All 9 cases exhibited high intensity to isointensity in the cortex and low intensity in the adjacent subcortex on the proton density– and T2-weighted images. The T1-weighted images showed no significant signal abnormalities in the subcortex. In all 6 patients studied with gadolinium, T1-weighted images demonstrated gyriform enhancement in the affected cortex. On follow-up MRIs, the subcortical low intensity remained low in 2 patients in the chronic stage and changed to high intensity in the remaining 2 patients. Five cases studied with CT of the brain exhibited neither hemorrhage nor calcification—both possible causes of reduced signal intensity—in the affected cortex or subcortex.

Conclusion.—The reduction of signal intensity on the proton density– and T2-weighted images seen in the subcortical white matter in these patients with early cortical ischemia may have resulted from production of free radicals caused by hypoxia or ischemia and iron accumulation caused by disruption of the axonal transportation. The phenomenon of subcortical low intensity in acute or subacute infarction does not appear to be rare and is an important diagnostic sign. Clearing of the subcortical low intensity did not indicate a better clinical prognosis.

▶ Because of the importance of diagnosing cerebral infarction and distinguishing it from other brain lesions, it is important to recognize all the radiologic signs associated with cerebral infarction. Although this paper describes only 2 cases studied in the acute phase of stroke (less than 3 days after onset), future investigations should be directed toward determining whether this finding of low signal intensity on T2-weighted images in the subcortical region could be a helpful adjunctive sign in hyperacute stroke (within the first 4 to 6 hours of onset). The accumulation of free radicals or a deficiency in iron transport in the subcortical region accounts for this T2-shortening effect, and as this paper demonstrates, there is resolution of this finding over time. Future imaging in acute infarction should be directed toward techniques that detect the earliest signs of infarction, such as diffusion imaging.—R.M. Quencer, M.D.

Magnetic Resonance Imaging and Dynamic CT Scan in Cervical Artery Dissections
Zuber M, Meary E, Meder J-F, Mas J-L (Hôpital Saint-Anne, Paris)
Stroke 25:576–581, 1994   122-96-20–3

Background.—The typical MRI picture of arterial dissection is a narrowed eccentric signal void surrounded by a semilunar signal hyperintensity on T1- and T2-weighted images. However, the sensitivity of MRI for diagnosing cervical dissection has not been well-documented. Therefore, the sensitivity of routine 0.5-tesla MRI in detecting a typical picture of

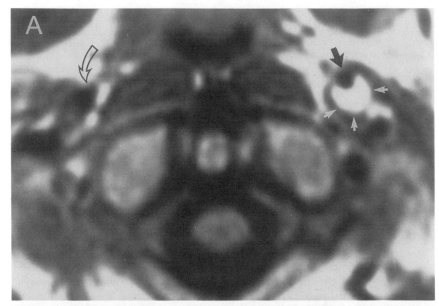

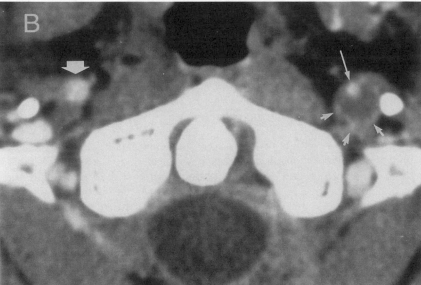

Fig 20–4.—Left internal carotid artery dissection (stenotic type). A, axial T1-weighted (repetition time, 500 ms; echo time, 20 ms) MRI: an eccentric signal void (*large arrow*) surrounded by a semilunar hyperintensity (*small arrows*) (typical MRI picture). The *curved arrow* indicates a normal right internal carotid artery. B, dynamic CT scan at the same level: an eccentric contrast enhancement (corresponding to residual lumen) (*long arrow*) surrounded by a relative hypodensity as compared with the muscle (corresponding to a mural hematoma), itself surrounded by a thin annular enhancement (*small arrows*) (typical dynamic CT scan picture). The *thick arrow* indicates a normal right internal carotid artery. (Courtesy of Zuber M, Meary E, Meder J-F, et al: *Stroke* 25:576–581, 1994.)

cervical artery dissection and the value of dynamic CT scans in providing evidence of dissecting hematoma were determined.

Methods.—Fifteen consecutive patients underwent a standardized 0.5-tesla spin-echo MRI protocol with axial slices. All had angiographically proved extracranial internal acrotid or vertebral dissections. Twelve patients also had dynamic CT scanning at the dissection site suggested by angiography.

Findings.—Eighty percent of the patients had a typical MR picture of cervical artery dissection in 68% of the dissected vessels. The sensitivity of MRI was 78% in internal carotid dissections, 60% in vertebral dissections, and 85% in stenotic-type dissections. These sensitivities were higher than for occlusive or aneurysmal-type dissections. The dynamic CT scan demonstrated mural hematoma in 92% of the patients and 80% of the dissected vessels (Fig 20–4).

Conclusions.—Routine 0.5-tesla MRI with axial slices is sensitive for diagnosing dissection. However, in about one fifth of the patients with cervical artery dissection, MRI will demonstrate no typical abnormality. Dynamic CT scans are sensitive for confirming the presence of the mural hematoma but needs to be directed by previous angiography.

▶ Judging the patency of extracranial cervical vessels with MRI, by virtue of the intraluminal signal, can at times be difficult. For instance, slow flow in a narrowed but patent carotid artery can demonstrate increased signal and, therefore, mimic thrombosis; however, seeing an eccentric flow void adjacent to a high signal within a vessel is strongly suggestive of vascular dissection (see Figure 20–4A). Dynamic CT (postcontrast, rapid image acquisition) through a dissection gives nearly a mirror-image picture, i.e., the patent lumen is bright (contrast filled) and the thrombus is dark (see Figure 20–4B). In either situation, follow-up angiography is warranted. With the newest CT technology in which volume images are obtained (spiral or helical CT), reformatted sagittal and/or coronal images depict well vascular dissection in an angiographic-like format.—R.M. Quencer, M.D.

▶ Zuber and associates evaluated the sensitivity of 0.5-tesla MRI and dynamic CT for the diagnosis of cervical arterial dissection. Nine internal carotid artery dissections and 10 vertebral artery dissections were studied. The routine MRI protocol used would have allowed the diagnosis of dissection in only 80% of the patients. Likewise, a typical dynamic CT scan of dissection was found in only 80% of the dissected vessels. Neither method was as sensitive as angiography for the diagnosis of cervical arterial dissection.—R.H. Wilkins, M.D.

Hypertrophic Olivary Degeneration: MR Imaging and Pathologic Findings

Kitajima M, Korogi Y, Shimomura O, Sakamoto Y, Hirai T, Miyayama H, Takahashi M (Kumamoto Univ, Japan; Kumamoto Municipal Hosp, Japan)
Radiology 192:539–543, 1994   122-96-20–4

Introduction.—Hypertrophic olivary degeneration (HOD) is defined as transsynaptic degeneration subsequent to lesions in the "Guillain-Mollaret triangle." It is a unique morphologic type of transsynaptic degeneration because of its association with hypertrophy of degenerated neurons. Although several reports have described the characteristic MRI findings of HOD, there have been no systematic studies of this issue. The MRI findings of HOD caused by hemorrhage were described and correlated with the pathologic findings.

Methods.—Eleven patients with posthemorrhagic HOD underwent MRI scanning. Eight patients had pontine tegmental hemorrhages (THs), and 3 had cerebellar hemorrhages in the dentate nuclei. The scans were performed 3 weeks to 49 months after the hemorrhagic ictus. Pathologic correlations were performed using specimens from a patient who died of brain stem hemorrhage.

Findings.—Ipsilateral HOD resulted from involvement of the central tegmental tract, whereas contralateral HOD resulted from involvement of the dentate nucleus or superior cerebellar peduncle. Only those patients with TH involving the superior cerebellar peduncle showed bilateral olivary changes. Patients with bilateral THs had HOD limited to the dominant bleeding side, the result of the lateral position of the central tegmental tract. Patients scanned 3 weeks after the ictus showed hyperintense areas of the oliva; hypertrophy was seen at 5 to 15 months. Pathologic examination revealed vacuolar degeneration of neurons and hypertrophy of astrocytes with gliosis.

Conclusions.—Very early posthemorrhagic changes in the oliva may be depicted by MRI. The MRI findings in cases of HOD are well correlated with the pathologic staging. Atrophy after HOD may appear much later than previously suspected.

▶ Magnetic resonance imaging is now clarifying in life what previously could only be recognized as a pathologic snapshot in time: HOD. This paper provides an excellent temporal dissection of the development of HOD, which appears to result from lesions of the central tegmental tract, ipsilateral to the HOD. I have seen one such case in a physician who had a unilateral pontine TH and, approximately 1 year later, the MRI changes of HOD. That patient has a progressive syndrome of ataxia, and bulbar and unilateral limb weakness that is still difficult to understand. Palatal myoclonus has been described in some patients with this condition. This article concentrates on comparing the imaging and pathologic studies. A study reviewing the clinical features would be most welcome.—W.G. Bradley, D.M., F.R.C.P.

MRI in Subacute Combined Degeneration

Murata S, Naritomi H, Sawada T (Natl Cardiovascular Ctr, Osaka, Japan)
Neuroradiology 36:408–409, 1994   122-96-20–5

Introduction.—Patients with vitamin B_{12} deficiency may have subacute combined degeneration, a condition chiefly affecting the posterior and lateral columns of the spinal cord. It results in dysesthesias and disordered deep sensation in the lower legs.

Case Report.—Man, 66, was admitted with numbness and tingling in both legs 13 years after total gastrectomy for gastric cancer. He also had a history of pulmonary tuberculosis. Numbness and tingling had first developed in the toes 3 months before admission. The patient was unable to walk with his eyes closed. Tendon reflexes were increased in the legs, and positional and vibratory sensation and proprioception were markedly impaired below the knees. The patient walked unsteadily with a wide-based gait and had a positive Romberg sign. A macrocytic, hyperchromic anemia was documented. The serum vitamin B_{12} was less than 50 pg/mL. Abnormal high signal in the posterior column at the T9–11 level was demonstrated on MRI. Short somatosensory evoked potentials could not be elicited in the legs. Cyanocobalamin was administered by IM injection with oral methylcobalamin. The patient's gait became normal within a month, and repeated MRI after 10 weeks no longer showed abnormal signal in the posterior column.

Discussion.—The spinal lesions of subacute combined degeneration are characterized by demyelination and, later, less marked axonal degeneration. Disappearance of high-signal lesions after treatment in this patient suggests that they represented demyelination.

▶ The ability to define intrinsic alterations in cord parenchyma secondary to a non–mass-producing lesion is effectively demonstrated in this case report of dorsal column disease in subacute combined degeneration. Although unproven, it is most probable that the high signal on T2-weighted images represents demyelination. The mechanism by which remyelination is induced by injections of vitamin B_{12} is not clear. This case adds to our differential diagnosis of focal well-defined signal abnormalities within the spinal cord; certainly, in the absence of a history, multiple sclerosis would have been a prime consideration because of the location of the signal abnormality in the face of a normal-sized cord.—R.M. Quencer, M.D.

Friedreich's Ataxia: MR Findings Involving the Cervical Portion of the Spinal Cord
Mascalchi M, Salvi F, Piacentini S, Bartolozzi C (Universita' di Pisa, Italy, Universita' di Firenze, Florence, Italy)
AJR 163:187–191, 1994   122-96-20–6

Objective.—Friedreich's ataxia is the most common of the spinocerebellar progressive ataxias. Its features include loss of myelinated fibers and neuronal loss in the spinal ganglia and Clarke's column accompanied by atrophy of the upper portion of the spinal cord. The usefulness of MRI examination of the cervical spinal cord in the differential diagnosis of Friedreich's ataxia was examined.

Methods.—Magnetic resonance imaging of the cervical spinal cord was performed in 10 patients with Friedreich's ataxia and in 14 control patients with other forms of ataxia, including corticocerebellar and cerebellar–brain stem atrophy. The anteroposterior (AP) diameter of the spinal cord at C3 was measured on axial images, and all images were examined for possible intramedullary signal abnormalities.

Results.—The AP diameter of the spinal cord at C3 was decreased in 9 patients with Friedrich's ataxia, but it was normal in all of the controls. Thinning and intramedullary signal changes consistent with degeneration of white matter tracts in the lateral and posterior columns was seen on the sagittal and axial images of 9 patients with Friedreich's ataxia, but in none of the controls.

Conclusion.—Magnetic resonance imaging of the cervical spinal cord is useful in the differential diagnosis of progressive ataxia of uncertain clinical type.

▶ The presence of cord atrophy in association with high signal abnormalities on T2-weighted images in the dorsal and lateral columns raises a number of diagnostic possibilities in addition to Friedreich's ataxia. Most common, of course, is multiple sclerosis; however, in cases of MS of the cord, there may be cord swelling when the symptoms are acute. Although this may, at first glance, mimic an intramedullary tumor, localization of high signal and enhancement in the lateral and dorsal columns speak strongly for MS or any disease that affects primarily the white matter. In the differential diagnosis, metabolic abnormalities such as vitamin B_{12} deficiency (subacute combined degeneration), AIDS myelopathy, viral/postviral myelitis, and radiation changes all must be considered. Therefore, although the findings described in this study, are not diagnostic of Friedreich's ataxia, this entity is clearly part of the aforementioned differential diagnosis.—R.M. Quencer, M.D.

Cross-References

For further information, see also the following relevant Neurosurgery articles:

CEREBROVASCULAR OCCLUSIVE DISEASE

122-96-31–2
122-96-31–6
122-96-31–7

EPILEPSY

122-96-33–1
122-96-33–2
122-96-33–4

SPINAL DISORDERS

122-96-35–3

PERIPHERAL NERVE DISORDERS

122-96-37–1
122-96-37–2
122-96-37–5
122-96-37–6

PAIN

122-96-41–1

NEUROSURGERY

Robert H. Wilkins, M.D.

The Evolution of Organized Neurological Surgery in the United States*

CARL H. HAUBER, J.D., C.A.E., AND CHRIS A. PHILIPS

In this "nation of associations," organizations are frequently established to serve the common interests of their constituencies. The periodic emergence of associations serving the neurosurgical community is a matter of historical record. However, little attention has been paid to the reasons why these neurosurgical associations have come into being. Because little has been published documenting the developmental phases of these associations, the research for this study has concentrated on the personal correspondence of the founders, as well as on the minutes and the historical records of the organizations themselves. The results demonstrate a definite pattern in the sequence of events that has led to the establishment of five national neurosurgical organizations over the past 75 years. All of them were designed to pursue the same general goals. Yet, each was conceived by its designers to fulfill unmet needs of the surgeons that it was established to represent. It is postulated that the definable pattern of these events provides a sound basis for predicting a reoccurrence of the phenomenon in the future. The conspicuous absence of several prominent academic and research societies from these discussions is not meant to reflect upon the value of these organizations to their respective constituencies. This study is limited to the evolutionary "chain" of organizations devoted to the specialty as a whole, which have, to one extent or another, played a part in the development of policies and activities that have influenced the neurosurgical specialty since its inception. Other national, regional, and special interest societies continue to serve defined elements of the specialty and could be the subject of a similar historical summary.

Key words: The American Academy of Neurological Surgeons, The American Association of Neurological Surgeons, Congress of Neurological Surgeons, The Harvey Cushing Society, The Neurosurgical Society of America, The Society of Neurological Surgeons.

The integral role played by volunteer associations among the established scientific disciplines was never more clearly demonstrated than at the October 1919 meeting of the American College of Surgeons, at which neurological surgery was declared to exist as a surgical specialty. Those surgeons in attendance who were most interested in this work decided that formal meetings for the exchange of pertinent information should be arranged without delay (25). This phenomenon, common to all legitimate scientific disciplines, provided immediate reinforcement for the newest of surgical specialties. It was a spontaneous and quite natural response for these surgeons to join together and seek fulfillment of common needs,

---

*Reprinted with permission from *Neurosurgery* 36:814–826, 1995.

which could be satisfied through group interaction. In the words of Harvey Cushing, who first envisioned this organized effort, the initial needs were to" ... discuss our problems and compare results...." Thus, a handful of surgeons committed themselves to pursue Cushing's suggestion, without thought to the fact that they were intuitively following a pattern, which, although not uncommon throughout the western world, has had a profound impact on sociopolitical development in the United States. With the decision to join together, they took the first steps to form a voluntary association in the country that has long been referred to as "the nation of associations," a social phenomenon that has led to the existence of a gigantic complex of volunteer institutions that perform many of the functions that are strictly reserved for the government elsewhere in the world (4, 7, 9, 10).

Years passed before neurological surgery showed all the essential elements of an established surgical specialty: 1) recognition by the American Medical Association in 1937 of a system of formal postdoctoral education unique to the specialty (11), 2) establishment of the American Board of Neurological Surgery in 1940 (2), and 3) proliferation of residency programs after World War II (27, 28). In contrast, the development of the association structure was rapid and, not unlike those individuals who made up its nucleus, forceful.

THE SOCIETY OF NEUROLOGICAL SURGEONS (EST. 1920)

On March 19, 1920, only 5 months after the October 1919 meeting of the American College of Surgeons commonly accepted the formal genesis of the neurosurgical specialty in the United States, 11 interested surgeons (mostly educators) met at the Peter Bent Brigham Hospital in Boston, with Cushing as host. During the course of this clinical meeting, The Society of Neurological Surgeons was formed. Ernest Sachs recorded the founders as: Alfred Adson, Charles Bagley, Harvey Cushing, Charles Dowman, Charles Frazier, Samuel Harvey, Gilbert Horrax, Dean Lewis, Jason Mixter, Ernest Sachs, and Edward Towne (26). In his history of the first 50 years of The Society of Neurological Surgeons, A. Earl Walker notes that Cushing and Bagley invited Walter Dandy to join, but strained relationships between Dandy and both Frazier and Cushing caused him to decline (3).

The first formal meeting of The Society of Neurological Surgeons (November 26, 1920) was also convened in Boston. The first officers of the Society were Harvey Cushing, President, and Ernest Sachs, Secretary. Dean Lewis became the first Vice President the next year (3, 26). The original purposes of the Society, as set forth in its first adopted bylaws, were: 1) the development of the field of neurosurgery, and 2) the education of the medical profession, particularly the surgeons, in the idea that neurological surgery requires a special training in addition to that of the general surgeon (26).

The format of the meetings (semiannual until 1932 and annual thereafter) remained essentially unchanged until the early 1950s. This change to one meeting per year may have been influenced by the emergence of The Harvey Cushing Society in 1932, which is discussed in the next section. Prominent members took their turns hosting The Society of Neurological Surgeons meetings, which focused on morning operative clinics conducted by the host, then afternoon sessions at which scientific papers were delivered by members of the host institution. Those attending consisted of Society members and the guests whom they sponsored. From among these guests, new members were chosen. As the membership grew, the hosted operative clinic format became impractical and gave way to oral presentations of a growing selection of scientific papers. However, long before this time, the limited meeting format and the restricted access to membership (only open to prominent academicians in the neurosurgical community and limited to 45 members [26]) left a growing number of surgeons without access to these vital activities. In 1931, The Society of Neurological Surgeons consisted of only 29 members. History was to repeat itself.

THE HARVEY CUSHING SOCIETY (EST. 1931)

Mounting concerns over the lack of a forum, much like that which the original founders of The Society of Neurological Surgeons sought in 1919, caused a group of 23 younger neurosurgeons to gather in Boston on May 6, 1932, to formally establish a second organization, which became known as The Harvey Cushing Society. Once again, legitimate common needs motivated a body of professionals to band together. However, unlike that of its precursor, the genesis of this organization was not spontaneous. Considerable discussion preceded its formal emergence, as those who were to be identified with this effort dealt with their concerns over the reaction that might be expected from their "seniors" who comprised The Society of Neurological Surgeons.

The fascinating dialogue and circumstances leading to the formation of this new society are well documented in a collection of original letters bound into two volumes, the first of which is entitled *Notes of the History of the Founding of The Harvey Cushing Society, 1930–1931* (22). These volumes contain the letters between William P. Van Wagenen, R. Glen Spurling, R. Eustace Semmes, and Temple Fay that outline the philosophy and goals of their new society. For example, in his June 24, 1931, letter to Van Wagenen, Spurling describes the need for a new society:

> The present society has only about two vacancies left, and that will bring their membership up to thirty-five [*sic*]. If they get beyond that number, the society will lose much of its charm and usefulness, because, as you undoubtedly realize, the small society is far more desirable from every point of view. Assuming that to be the case, there are, I figure, about 20 men who are doing neuro-surgery exclusively and are doing a good job of it, who will not be included in the membership of the old society for many years to come. In other words, it seems to me that there is a real need and place for another society, not with the idea of making it a stepping stone to the old society, but organized along the lines that would make it desirable to remain independent in its own right. (22)

The letters between the prospective organizers over the next several months often emphasized their beliefs that the new society was not to compete with The Society of Neurological Surgeons and was to allow the potential for neurosurgeons to be members of both societies. The July 17, 1931 letter to Spurling from Fay captures the essence of the philosophy of the new society and reflects how it is organized to this day:

> I am distinctly of the feeling that if this society is organized certain fundamental principles should be established, to avoid some of the difficulties encountered in the older society. I would far rather see a group of younger men organized to meet regularly, in a round table discussion of problems confronting the neurosurgeons, with a definite program assigned, similar to that carried on in the Association for Research in Nervous and Mental Diseases, than to gather each year at some clinic to see the host, 'strut his stuff,' to the envy or unfair criticism of those attending the meeting. I have felt that such a society would have its own place, irrespective of the older men, and would contribute more, in the end, if many of its members were assigned one year in advance, portions of the problem that required unbiased and fair analysis. Such a meeting could make a joint report, after it had heard the evidence from all sides, which could clarify many of the disputed points now under consideration, and advance in an orderly manner towards constructive additions to our neurological knowledge. (22)

Fay clearly recognized the historical need for the personal observation of surgical procedures, as these early neurosurgeons concentrated on the development and refinement of their surgical techniques. He also recognized that there was an emerging need to encourage independent research and developmental efforts by neurosurgeons and proposed that a new society could satisfy these needs by providing a forum for them to discuss their work and report on their results. Fay described this need as follows:

> The most important phase of our problem rotates around investigation and advancement in the fields of neurosurgery, with the fundamental needs of establishing methods of early diagnosis and postoperative treatment, directed toward the protection of the patients, and a decrease in mortality. Such a program could be undertaken with a "clinic" as a minor factor. If such a society is organized, I believe it should stand on its own merits, the members feeling sufficient pride in its own maintenance, so that [subsequent] membership in the older society would be unnecessary, or at least no added advantage. With the dedication of the younger society's activities toward the advancement of research problems, there would be no reason to confuse the two groups. (22)

Never were more visionary thoughts expressed during the period leading up to the formation of The Harvey Cushing Society.

A meeting was held on October 10, 1931, at the Hotel Raleigh in Washington, D.C., with Fay, Semmes, Spurling, and Van Wagenen in attendance. It was at this meeting that they decided that this new society was to encompass the disciplines of neurosurgery, medical neurology, neurophysiology, neuropathology, and roentgenology (29). They compiled a list of 36 physicians who would be encouraged to attend an organizational meeting for this new society.

Perhaps the most important decision the founders made was to consult Cushing about these plans. Less than a week after the organizational meeting, Van Wagenen visited "the Chief" and outlined plans for the new society. He discussed this visit in an October 15, 1931, letter to Spurling:

> All told he was very much in favor of the idea as presented to him. He said that he had felt for a number of years that the old society had become too gastronomically inclined to be of much use. I believe that he also will allow us to use his name in connection with the society. (22)

Plans for the new society progressed, and, with Cushing's endorsement, most of those who were initially approached in connection with founding membership were quick to accept. In a great show of generosity and patriarchal pride in these plans that were made by so many of his past residents, Cushing offered to provide the facilities for the first meeting. This may have been the singular event that insured the acceptance of this new society, for no further notations fearing the displeasure of the "old society" are found in the letters. However, the format of this initial meeting resembled The Society of Neurological Surgeons meetings much more than it resembled the original concepts of its founders!

The first meeting of the new society was held on May 6, 1932, in Boston. Dr. Cushing welcomed 23 of the charter members, saying that he felt like an obstetrician bringing a new and protesting offspring into existence. He also cautioned them to remember that in 10 years' time, another group would be coming along that would look upon the present one as "senile and antiquated" (5).

The following officers were elected: William P. Van Wagenen, President; Glen Spurling, Vice-President; and Tracy Putnam, Secretary/Treasurer. After much discussion and many interesting suggestions, the name "The Harvey Cushing Society" was adopted. The single purpose of The Harvey Cushing Society, as stated in its first bylaws, was to promote the advancement of the various fields of organic neurology. Despite the lofty goals of The Harvey Cushing Society founders, and the genuine effort to broaden the scientific scope of the Society's meetings, membership was limited to just 35 at the outset (to include not only neurosurgeons but other neuroscientists, as aforementioned). The membership limit was increased to 50 in 1936, resulting in heated discussions the next year about "retiring" active members after 7 years to preserve the youth and integrity of the Society. Despite all of this, the number of members remained at fewer than 40 for several years. In fact, it took only 7 short years for The Harvey

Cushing Society to find itself facing the very same challenge that brought it into existence, the disinclination to recognize and respond to the needs of the discipline to which it had devoted itself. In its initial form, The Harvey Cushing Society took its place alongside The Society of Neurological Surgeons as another inaccessible club.

THE AMERICAN ACADEMY OF NEUROLOGICAL SURGEONS (EST. 1938)

In his history of the first 50 years of the Academy (23), Byron C. Pevehouse notes that the self-imposed limitation on total membership by both of the existing societies (as detailed in the previous sections) resulted in a growing number of neurological surgeons who were unable to participate in organized activities, except as invited guests. The specialty was simply growing faster than either organization desired to expand its membership.

The tendency of The Harvey Cushing Society not to respond to the needs of the younger element of the specialty clearly surfaced at the Society's Seventh Annual Meeting in Memphis, in 1938, where the leadership, including President Temple Fay, suggested that these young neurosurgeons might best solve their own problem by forming a third neurosurgical society. At the time, it was estimated that some 25 neurological surgeons in the United States were without organization affiliations. Several individuals (Spencer Braden, Dean Echols, Joseph Evans, William S. Keith, Frank Mayfield, Francis Murphey, and John Raaf) took the suggestion of a new society to heart and immediately convened an organizational meeting (April 22, 1938, in Memphis), at which they agreed to establish the third neurosurgical society. Cincinnati was selected as the site of the First Annual Meeting, to be convened the next October.

At that first meeting (October 28, 1938), the new organization was named The Academy of Neurosurgery (somewhat a misnomer, as it was not intended to limit the membership to academicians), and the following officers were elected: Dean H. Echols, President, and Francis Murphey, Secretary/Treasurer. The name was later changed to The American Academy of Neurological Surgery.

Distinguishing this association somewhat from those preceding it, the organizers of the Academy decided that scientific attainment was not the only important factor to be considered in the selection of new members and that the interpersonal qualities of the candidates were to be assessed as well. This call for social compatibility among peers seems to reflect fundamental concerns among the "outsiders" of the time and suggests that the "private club" image of the established societies weighed heavily in the shaping of the Academy. The organizers even considered a plan similar to that which caused so much controversy among The Harvey Cushing Society leaders just 2 years before, suggesting that active membership be limited to 10 years to make room for younger members, insuring perpetuation of the Academy and avoiding the need for a fourth society. This suggestion was finally rejected by the Academy's leaders, just as it had been by the leaders of The Harvey Cushing Society.

Pevehouse reports that, at the Eighth Annual Meeting of the Academy (September 1946), as many as 20 invited guests were present. Only 4 new members were elected to membership, raising the total to 43. Serious discussions ensued regarding the many fine young neurosurgeons who wanted to become members. Lengthy discussions during this meeting, and again at the Ninth Annual Meeting in 1947, are said to have detracted from the usual positive tenor of Academy meetings. Interestingly, it was at the Tenth Annual Meeting of the Academy that Mayfield launched his first effort to resolve the multi-association conundrum, which had become a source of ongoing frustration to members and nonmembers alike. His concept envisioned combining the three associations into a single national body. After considerable discussion, the matter was referred to the Academy's Executive Committee for study.

With all the discussion and expressions of frustration, in the final analysis, a solution to finding a niche for the growing number of young neurosurgeons eluded the organized community. Simply stated, the members of the three existing societies placed a greater value on the professional and social intimacy that their limited numbers provided than they placed on any sort of obligation to assist their juniors along the path of professional growth. Thus, less than a decade after the Academy was established, a new generation of neurosurgeons who could not find a place in the existing societal structures was faced with forming its own group to satisfy these needs.

THE NEUROSURGICAL SOCIETY OF AMERICA (EST. 1948)

It was Arthur Morris who, acting upon conversations with R. Eustace Semmes (one of the founders of The Harvey Cushing Society), decided to discover whether there was sufficient interest among other unaffiliated neurosurgeons to support the formation of yet another neurosurgical society. The response was encouraging and resulted in a meeting of the 17 founders who were listed in *The Neurosurgical Society of America: 25th Anniversary Volume* (Claude Bertrand, Joseph F. Dorsey, Carl J. Graft, C. Douglas Hawkes, Lew Helfer, Thomas J. Holbrook, Everett F. Hurteau, Harry P. Maxwell, William F. Meacham, Arthur Morris, William B. Patton, Frank J. Otenasek, George E. Roulhac, Edward B. Schlesinger, I. Joshua Spiegel, Charles E. Troland, and Jack I. Woolf). The first elected officers were: Arthur Morris, President; Frank Otenasek, Vice President; Jack Woolf, Recording Secretary; Edward Schlesinger, Corresponding Secretary; and I. Joshua Spiegel, Treasurer. Joseph F. Dorsey, C. Douglas Hawkes, and George Roulhac were elected Councilors (21). The new society was originally named The Neurosurgical Society of North America, in deference to Canadian founder Bertrand and an anticipated Canadian constituency.

This new society was the first to structurally commit to a youthful membership, originally limiting active membership to neurological surgeons under age 45 and requiring transfer to a senior category of membership when members reached that age. In later years, when the first members became subject to this restriction, the bylaws were changed to allow them to continue in active membership!

This Society did not distinguish between academicians and private practitioners. Instead, it placed strong emphasis upon members *and* their families, encouraging the attendance of wives and children at annual meetings and selecting meeting locations conducive to this sort of involvement. According to *The Neurosurgical Society of America: 25th Anniversary Volume*, it was equally clear that the approach to the Annual Scientific Program was to be less formal and unfettered by tradition:

> The tradition of frank, searching but friendly discussion of the papers in depth was inaugurated and set a useful pattern for the future. The usefulness of a society geared to sharing mutual problems, unhampered by conventional constraints on candor and debate was immediately apparent. (21)

Although The Neurosurgical Society of America had established a permanent and useful niche in the organizational milieu of neurosurgery, it certainly was not seen by the neurosurgical community as a solution to the problem of providing universal access to significant organizational activities and relationships among colleagues. This Society was to be the fourth and the last of the series of "limited access societies" that, at their origin, seemingly offered the final solution to the "insiders versus outsiders" problem that had plagued neurosurgery since it was first recognized that The Society of Neurological Surgeons was not destined to be the ultimate forum for all neurosurgeons.

A New Era for Organization

The post-World War II years witnessed unprecedented growth in the numbers of neurological surgeons and major repositioning in neurosurgery's organizational complex. The Harvey Cushing Society, which had limited membership to Board-certified neurological surgeons just 2 years after the American Board of Neurological Surgery was established in 1940 (29), gradually emerged as the principal forum for both discussion and publication of important developments in neurological surgery. However, Board certification would prove to be the next (and perhaps the final) arbitrary obstacle to accessing the organizational relationships that virtually every neurological surgeon has insisted on since the specialty emerged.

CONGRESS OF NEUROLOGICAL SURGEONS (EST. 1951)

Only 2 years after The Neurosurgical Society of America was founded, an important chapter in the history of organized neurosurgery unfolded. An association was formed with no ostensible limitations to membership among neurosurgeons. All neurosurgeons were welcome, including those who were youthful or experienced, those who were Board certified or non-Board certified, and those from any country of origin. This new association envisioned, as the key to protecting its liberal membership philosophies, a firm policy to limit the age of its leadership to 45 years. Unlike the more drastic measure originally taken by The Neurosurgical

Society of America (to limit the age of all active members to 45 years), this innovative concept stood the test of time and remains in effect today (8).

The origin of the Congress of Neurological Surgeons can be traced to the September 1950 meeting of a group of neurological surgeons at Sea Island, GA, then to a Chicago meeting on February 6, 1951, which resulted in the distribution of invitations to attend a formational meeting the next May in St. Louis. Twenty-two neurosurgeons attended. The following purposes were agreed upon: 1) to study and discuss the principles of neurological surgery, 2) to study developments in scientific fields allied to neurological surgery, and 3) to honor living leaders in the field of neurological surgery. The first officers were: Elmer C. Schultz, President; Carroll A. Brown, Vice President; and Bland W. Cannon, Secretary. The "Congress," as it was to become known, convened its First Annual Meeting in Memphis on November 15, 1951. During its 1st year in existence, membership grew to nearly 70 active members, which was larger than the active membership of any other neurosurgical organization except The Harvey Cushing Society, a remarkable testimonial to the genuine need for such an organization.

The Era of Parallelism: The Cushing and the Congress

In the years that followed, The Cushing Society (with its annual meeting in the spring) and the Congress (convening its annual meeting each fall) both thrived. The Cushing Society concentrated on communicating significant scientific developments in both its annual meeting program and its principal publication, *The Journal of Neurosurgery* (6, 12, 28). The Congress maintained a decidedly didactic format, inviting selected leaders in the field to discuss their work and making every practical effort to encourage young neurosurgeons and neurosurgical residents to participate, thus exposing these young professionals to a broad range of practical philosophies and techniques. In 1977, the establishment of the official journal of the Congress, *Neurosurgery* (30), allowed for broader dissemination of information in this dimension.

Although The Cushing Society continued to wrestle with the fact that a significant element of the specialty was not qualified to join its ranks, its leaders would not compromise the Board certification prerequisite. Even concepts of provisional membership were consistently rejected. Despite the organizational complexities that can be traced to this restrictive philosophy, it must be observed that the insistence upon Board certification as the hallmark of neurosurgical practice has had a profound impact on the quality of neurosurgical care delivered in the United States. Moreover, this philosophy is supported, without reserve, by all established neurosurgical societies, including the Congress, which has contributed significantly to preparing young neurological surgeons for that "final step" in their career preparation, the Oral Board Examination.

As the years passed and these two organizations continued to develop in parallel, another significant factor emerged. When younger neurosurgeons became Board certified and joined The Cushing Society, they did not drop out of the Congress. Instead, most maintained membership in both organizations, attesting to the valuable role that each has played in the professional lives of contemporary neurological surgeons.

A National Spokesman for Neurosurgery

It was in 1962 that Hendrick J. Svein, then Secretary of The Cushing Society, raised the issue that was first touched upon by Frank H. Mayfield at The American Academy of Neurological Surgeons meeting in 1948, that of forming a single organizational voice for the neurosurgical community (29). Although Mayfield originally suggested combining the three existing associations, Svein threw the gauntlet down before The Harvey Cushing Society:

> During the last several years I have occasionally had some misgivings and doubts as to whether or not The Harvey Cushing Society is fulfilling its obligations to its members. These misgivings and doubts can be pretty well summarized by asking the question, should neurosurgery in this country have an official spokesman: if so, who? Should The Harvey Cushing Society not be a bit more imaginative, a bit more aggressive, and provide a bit more in the way of leadership? There are many areas and problems which directly involve neurosurgery and neurosurgeons in this country in which I think The Harvey Cushing Society should interest itself and serve as an official spokesman. (29)

Mayfield was to become President-elect of The Cushing Society the next year. Later, he was to reflect upon his strategy:

> The educational and social experiences derived from membership in The Harvey Cushing Society were consuming, but I continued to be concerned by its failure to deal with [this] important problem. The post of President-Elect, with the assurance that I would become President, appeared to me to provide the opportunity to address this issue. (29)

And so he did address the issue, gathering his political forces and diplomatically paving the way for this major step in the organizational listing of the neurosurgical specialty (29). Two years later, at the end of his term as The Cushing Society President, and with all of his plans carefully laid, he used his Presidential Address to issue what was to become known as the "Mayfield Proclamation:"

> ... by rather common agreement among neurosurgeons within the United States, and I think throughout the world, The Harvey Cushing Society has in fact become the representative organization for neurosurgeons within the United States. ... with the approval of the Board of Directors of The Harvey Cushing Society, I, Frank H. Mayfield, President, do hereby proclaim The Harvey Cushing Society, Inc. to be in fact the official organization representing the neurological surgeons of the United States ... (13)

Mayfield went on to suggest that the name not be changed but that an appropriate subtitle be added. The Cushing Society's Articles of Incorporation were amended just one year later (May 1966) to add "The American Association of Neurological Surgeons," in parentheses after the official name. That same year, the bylaws of The Cushing Society were amended to realign the Board of Directors in such a way as to provide representation from the other four national neurosurgical societies (The American Academy of Neurological Surgeons, the Congress of Neurological Surgeons, The Neurosurgical Society of America, and The Society of Neurological Surgeons).

In 1967, the transition continued. The name, The Harvey Cushing Society, was changed to the name the society maintains today: "The American Association of Neurological Surgeons, founded in 1931 as The Harvey Cushing Society," soon to become known as "AANS."

THE AMERICAN ASSOCIATION OF NEUROLOGICAL SURGEONS

The bylaws were amended in 1967, this time in reaction to an appeal from the Canadian Neurosurgical Society, reminding AANS leadership that this society was designed to represent all neurological surgeons on the North American continent, that membership was not exclusively available to those certified by the American Board of Neurological Surgery, but was equally available to certificants of the Canadian Royal College of Physicians and Surgeons (Neurosurgery). Furthermore, the Canadian Society stressed that the Canadian constituency of the AANS was of sufficient size when compared with the memberships of any association in the United States except the Congress of Neurological Surgeons. A representative of the Canadian Neurosurgical Society was added to the AANS Board of Directors. That same year, the Chairman of the AANS Membership Committee was removed from the Board of Directors in favor of a Board member-at-large, once again underlining the effort of the AANS leadership to equitably represent the interests of all members of the specialty, whatever their chosen affiliation (or lack thereof).

In the years that ensued, the sociopolitical distinction between the AANS and the Congress, on the one hand, and the other more narrow-interest neurosurgical societies, on the other hand, became progressively more clear. At the same time, this "grass roots" element became more and more vocal, principally through the forum made available by a Joint Socio-Economics Committee (JSEC), one of four operational committees maintained conjointly by the AANS and the Congress. These activities continued to intensify as the JSEC met twice each year (at the AANS and the Congress annual meetings). Through deliberations of state delegates, resolutions were framed and presented to the two parent organizations for consideration. Finally, these and related activities resulted in some profound changes in the AANS structure as state representatives sought a greater voice in the national affairs of neurosurgery. The following summary of this evolution, extracted from the official records of the AANS, was first cataloged by Byron C. Pevehouse (24).

In 1976, the AANS bylaws were amended to add two members-at-large to the Board of Directors, bringing the total to three. These three Board members were each assigned to represent a region of the United States (Eastern, Mid-country, and Western). Not satisfied with this solution, the JSEC suggested that the three Board members-at-large be replaced by four Board members, each representing one of four geographical quadrants, defined by the JSEC as Northeast, Southeast, Northwest, and Southwest. In 1977, the AANS bylaws were once again amended, reflecting this suggestion. The Board, now comprised of five officers, the two most recent past-presidents, five neurosurgical society representatives, and four quadrant representatives, was the largest ever to manage the AANS. This Board configuration remained unchanged until 1980, when a strong backlash occurred, bringing into question the advisability of allowing the majority of the AANS Board of Directors (9 of 16) to be selected by either another neurosurgical society or a joint committee.

Again, the bylaws were amended, eliminating all nine of these special interest positions on the Board of Directors and adding an equal number of Board members-at-large, to be elected by the general membership. The most senior of the two past-presidents were also eliminated, reducing the size of the Board to 15 members. This "nationalized" concept was to last only 3 years, when members of the former JSEC, now the Joint Council of State Neurosurgical Societies, sponsored an amendment to the AANS bylaws reinstituting directorship for the four regional quadrants and stipulating that the nominees be selected by the state delegates from each quadrant.

Over the next decade, the bylaws were amended several times; each successive amendment provided a more equitable balance between the AANS Nominating Committee, other organized "power bases," and the grass roots membership. This delicate balance was further enhanced by a carefully constructed nominating protocol, later supplemented by nomination procedural requirements that were levied upon the quadrants to ensure that individual members were provided every opportunity to participate in the nominating process.

The final composition of the Board of Directors, as it exists today (five officers, one past-president, five members-at-large, and four quadrant members), was supplemented in 1992 by the addition of a non-voting liaison from the Young Neurosurgeons Committee, established that same year (14). Involvement of young neurosurgeons in the leadership of the AANS vaulted from desirable to essential when the AANS bylaws were amended to provide voting membership for a "provisional" class of membership designed to encompass those individuals who have completed their residencies and who are fulfilling practice requirements before taking their Oral Board examinations.

Organized Neurosurgery Today

The years that came after the Mayfield Proclamation were truly evolutionary in terms of taking organized neurosurgery out of the hands of a few dynamic individuals and projecting the decision-making process well out into the neurosurgical community. The AANS Board of Directors was undoubtedly cognizant of the axiom that association leaders who feel directly answerable to their constituencies will reflect that obligation in their decision-making processes. Those leaders who sense a freedom from this link tend to demonstrate a propensity to do as they see fit. Irrespective of their commitment and their sincerity, it is inevitable that association leaders who take this latter course may be remembered for their valor and their panache but not for their sensitivity and their responsiveness to the members who must rely upon elected leaders to ensure that they are not forgotten in the heat of battles that are fought in their names!

During the years of rapid evolution experienced by the AANS, the relationship between the two major neurosurgical associations (the AANS and the Congress) has cycled several times between harmony and uncomfortable truce, with the other neurosurgical societies remaining essentially uninvolved. Problems, for the most part, can be traced to strong individuals (and groups of strong individuals) among the respective leaderships who were inclined toward less-than-positive interpretations of the actions of their counterparts.

Although precious time and resources have been wasted on these political skirmishes, the parallel relationship of the AANS and the Congress has fared quite well in terms of reflecting the fundamental needs of the neurosurgical community. In fact, the element of competition can be seen as a driving motivation to both organizations, with the AANS leaders feeling closely scrutinized in their judgments and evaluated on the results and the Congress leaders striving to attain a position of greater parity in key scientific, educational, and sociopolitical areas of interest.

The Joint Committees, another phenomenon of the parallel structure, were designed to serve the specialty in four key operational areas. In addition to the socioeconomically oriented forum discussed previously, the AANS and the Congress have provided for Joint Committees in the areas of education, government-related activities, and the assessment of substances and devices. Although these joint efforts have minimized duplication of effort and costly parallel operations in some key areas, they have had a tendency to operate somewhat independently of their parent organizations. It would be unfair to blame this condition on the Joint Committees. To the contrary, the examination of official records from both parent organizations demonstrates (with important exceptions) that the Joint Committees were left without defined charges and specific directions, designed to take maximum advantage of their substantial capabilities. The results of Joint Committee activity, although often productive and of notable value to the specialty, were not part of any "master plan" conceived by the AANS and the Congress to bring these substantial resources to bear on the highest priority challenges facing the specialty at any given point in time. In fact, until the strategic planning activities of the parent organizations are more closely coordinated, it will be difficult to realize the potential of these joint operational arms.

To further complicate matters, the activities generated by these Joint Committees were reported separately to the parent organizations, resulting in independent deliberations and decisions. Inevitable inconsistencies required subsequent resolution, a cumbersome and time-consuming process, frequently taking months to accomplish, and even prompting a notable element of independent activity at the Committee level. This condition presented a formidable obstacle to AANS efforts to fulfill its "national spokesman" role and ultimately prompted a decisive reaction from throughout organized neurosurgery.

By mutual agreement among the established neurosurgical societies, the Liaison Committee was established, consisting of the presidents and presidents-elect of the AANS, the Congress, The Canadian Neurosurgical Society, the Academy, The Neurosurgical Society of America, and The Society of Neurological Surgeons. This Liaison Committee met in April 1976 at the AANS Annual Meeting (20). Only the Canadian Society was not in attendance. The AANS was represented by Richard DeSaussure (outgoing President), Lester Mount (incoming President), Charles Drake (President-elect), and Donald Dohn (Secretary); the Congress representatives were Robert Ojemann (President), Bruce Sorenson (President-elect), and David Kelly (Secretary); the Academy was represented by William Sweet (President-elect); The Neurosurgical Society of America representatives were George Ehni (President) and Shelley Chou (President-elect); and The Society of Neurological Surgeons was represented by William Collins (Secretary). The purpose of the meeting was to deal with a general concern over the need to ensure that the neurosurgical specialty would be heard as a single voice and not through random opinions being expressed without prior consensus among applicable leaders. Apparently, the greatest concern lay in unauthorized testimony and statements on the Washington scene. Other problems involved the overlap in committee work and the negative effect that could result from a lack of harmony in such activities. The difficulty in coordinating other Joint Committees (in addition to the Washington Committee) was voiced, and discomfort was expressed over the lack of budget controls. It was clear that the organized neurosurgical community was not at all comfortable with the manner in which the national spokesman role, delegated to the AANS in 1965, was being diluted. The Committee called upon the AANS and the Congress, along with their Joint Committees, to find a solution to this problem.

Soon thereafter, the presidents and secretaries of the AANS and the Congress met in New York City (18). After considerable discussion, it was agreed that regularly scheduled joint meetings of the AANS and the Congress officers should be convened for the purpose of ensuring that organized surgery would speak with a single voice that reflected previously agreed-upon policies.

The first meeting of the Joint Officers convened in October 1976 at the Congress annual meeting in New Orleans. Although the parent organizations vested no decision-making authority in this joint meeting process, understanding and coordination between the two broadly based associations improved markedly. However, as the years have passed, demands upon organized medicine (including neurosurgery) have increased exponentially, as has the flow of important information throughout the specialty and between the AANS and the Congress. By the mid-1980s, the Joint Officers had become as much a "bottleneck" in the communications flow as it was a solution to the problem of coordinating these important activities.

In 1991, AANS President James T. Robertson convinced the AANS Board of Directors that, if the Congress was to continue to share equally in the critical decision-making process that supported the national spokesman role, then it should share equally in the substantial costs related to all of these activities (16). Robertson envisioned the Congress as an equal "stakeholder" in all of neurosurgery's support facilities, most of which are owned by the AANS. He suggested that the AANS Board of Directors and the Congress Executive Committee could together direct the Joint Officers, who would, in turn, be empowered to manage and coordinate all operational activities in support of the neurosurgical specialty. The Congress leaders decided that they did not want to undertake this responsibility. Instead, their alternative solution was that the Joint Officers be delegated the authority to manage the Joint Committees (including the Joint Council of State Neurosurgical Societies, formerly JSEC) and such other joint activities that the two parent organizations deemed appropriate. They, in turn, agreed that the AANS President would chair all Joint Officers meetings thereafter and that tie votes of the Joint Officers would be decided by the AANS President. These latter provisions were designed to preserve the national spokesman role of the AANS within the new structure, while at the same time providing the younger Congress leaders maximum participation in the deliberations on issues affecting the specialty. This concept was adopted by the Joint Officers (19) and later by the AANS Board of Directors (15) and the Congress Executive Committee (17).

At this writing, the new Joint Officers concept has been in effect for 4 years. In that short time, it has been demonstrated that the decision-making process could be streamlined without further complicating the national spokesman role.

The Future of Organized Neurosurgery

Over the years, many well-meaning individuals (and groups) have brought forth "solutions" to the somewhat ungainly parallel structure within which organized neurosurgery has continued to function. There were those who would form an "umbrella organization." Others would merge the AANS and the Congress into a single organization. Some would be content to simply dissolve one of the organizations altogether. However, these are not three distinct suggestions at all. They encompass a single concept, variously described, to seek compatibility with as many interests as possible within the specialty. Why then, when a national survey (1) of neurosurgeons demonstrated that a substantial majority of the neurosurgical community would favor a single organization, has some formal amalgamation not occurred? Is it because the ultimate structure has not yet been conceived or that the perfect compromise has not yet been negotiated? The solution does not lie in structures and compromises. The Harvey Cushing Society was not formed by some structural genius. Nor was the Congress of Neurological Surgeons the product of diplomatic prowess. These key organizations each emerged in their own time, because the fundamental needs of neurosurgeons were not being met, which resulted in an element of unified action to seek a solution. Yet, as we have shown, The Harvey Cushing Society did not remain static after the Congress came into being. Instead, it entered an unprecedented period of development. After 15 years of parallel activity, it was The Cushing Society/AANS, a somewhat unwieldy organization, but nonetheless operational in all essential areas, that the neurosurgical community finally accepted as the overall organizational catalyst.

It is noteworthy that, with all its complexities, the current sociopolitical structure has survived nearly 30 years, much of this during the most difficult, frustrating, and demanding times ever faced by organized medicine in the United States. It has adapted to change and has gained steadily in its responsiveness and effectiveness. If this positive pattern ends, if the present association structure becomes unresponsive to the fundamental needs of its constituency as a whole, then it will be changed, just as surely as it changed in 1931, 1938, 1948, 1951, and 1965.

The true challenge that the leaders of neurosurgery face today is to concentrate all resources at their disposal upon the contemporary challenges facing the specialty (and its patient population). If they do so, then internal (structural) change will be ongoing, positive, and taken in stride, not drastic and regressive.

Above all, it must be remembered that these associations are social phenomena in the purest sense. They belong to their members, not to their leaders. They are manifestations of the neurosurgical community as a whole, not the products of a few visionary individuals' decisions. The genuine visionaries, history repeatedly confirms, are those who can recognize and articulate the true will of the community *as a whole* and thereby initiate an effective response. The day when these fundamental truisms are forgotten will be the day that history begins to repeat itself once again.

Acknowledgments

The contributions of neurosurgeons and others to the historical materials collected by the Archives of The American Association of Neurological Surgeons provided an excellent basis for the research performed in the development of this document, and, to them, we are indeed grateful.

References

1. American Association of Neurological Surgeons Strategic Planning Survey: 1990. Park Ridge, IL, AANS National Office.
2. Mahaley MS, Kline DG (eds): *The American Board of Neurological Surgery: Fifty Years of Service to American Neurosurgery.* Houston, American Board of Neurological Surgery, 1990, p 1.
3. Boldrey EB: *The Society of Neurological Surgeons 1920–1970.* The Society of Neurological Surgeons, 1970, pp 11, 43.
4. Bradley JF: *The Role of Trade Associations and Professional Business Societies.* University Park, PA, Pennsylvania State University Press, 1965, pp 17–45.
5. Brown HA: The Harvey Cushing Society: Past, present, future—The 1958 AANS Presidential Address. *J Neurosurg* 15:587–601, 1958.
6. Bucy PC: *Journal of Neurosurgery:* Its origin, development. *J Neurosurg* 28:1–12, 1964.

7. Caruso F: *Tocqueville Speaks*. Englewood, CO, Association Insite, Inc., 1991.
8. *Congress of Neurological Surgeons: Informational Brochure*. Congress of Neurological Surgeons, 1988, ed 2, pp 9.
9. de Tocqueville AC: *Democracy in America*. George Lawrence Translation. New York, Harper & Row, 1966.
10. Hausknecht M: *The Joiners: A Sociological Description of Voluntary Association Membership in the United States*. New York, Bedminster Press, 1966.
11. Journal of the American Medical Association: Hospitals approved for residencies in specialties. *JAMA* 109:693–712, 1937.
12. Laws ER: The binding influence of the *Journal of Neurosurgery* on the evolution of neurosurgery. *J Neurosurg* 81:317–321, 1994.
13. Mayfield FH: A proclamation: the 1965 AANS Presidential Address. *J Neurosurg* 23:129–134, 1965.
14. Minutes. American Association of Neurological Surgeons Board of Directors Meeting, Chicago, IL, November 16–18, 1990. Park Ridge, IL, AANS National Office.
15. Minutes. American Association of Neurological Surgeons Board of Directors Meeting, San Francisco, CA, April 9–11, 1992. Park Ridge, IL, AANS National Office.
16. Minutes. American Association of Neurological Surgeons Board of Directors Meeting, Chicago IL, November 22–24, 1992. Park Ridge, IL, AANS National Office.
17. Minutes. Congress of Neurological Surgeons Executive Committee Meeting, Washington, D.C., January 18, 1992. Minutes are held by the Secretary of the Congress of Neurological Surgeons.
18. Minutes. Joint Officers of the AANS CNS Meeting, New Orleans, LA, October 26, 1976. Park Ridge, IL, AANS National Office.
19. Minutes. Joint Officers of the AANS CNS Meeting, Rosemont, IL, January 25, 1992. Park Ridge, IL, AANS National Office.
20. Minutes. Liaison Committee (Presidents, Presidents-Elect of the Representative Societies) Meeting, San Francisco, CA, Wednesday, April 7, 1976. Park Ridge, IL, AANS National Office.
21. *The Neurosurgical Society of America: 25th Anniversary Volume—1948–1973*. The Neurosurgical Society of America, 1973, p 28.
22. *Notes of the History of the Founding of The Harvey Cushing Society 1930–1931*. Park Ridge, IL, AANS Archives, vol 1.
23. Pevehouse BC: *An Epitome of the History of The American Academy of Neurological Surgery*. The American Academy of Neurological Surgery, 1988, p 1.
24. Pevehouse BC: A history of the structure, membership of the Board of Directors, American Association of Neurological Surgeons (Harvey Cushing Society) (1960–1987), in: *Guide to The American Association of Neurological Surgeons*: The American Association of Neurological Surgeons, Park Ridge, IL, 1993, pp 15.
25. Sachs E: *Fifty Years of Neurosurgery: A Personal Story*. New York, Vantage Press, 1958, p 68.
26. *The Society of Neurological Surgeons 1920–1960*. The Society of Neurological Surgeons, 1960, p 1.
27. Walker AE: *A History of Neurological Surgery*. Baltimore, Williams & Wilkins, 1951, pp 456–457.
28. Walker AE: Leaders in neuroscience, in Udvarhelyi GB, Uematsu S (interviewers): *AANS Archives, Interviews 78 and 79*. Park Ridge, IL, AANS Archives, 1991 (video interview).
29. Wilkins RH: *History of the American Association of Neurological Surgeons, 1931–1981*. Chicago, American Association of Neurological Surgeons, 1981, pp 9, 10, 12, 35, 43.
30. Wilkins RH: Birth of a journal: The origin and early years of *Neurosurgery*. *Neurosurgery* 10:820–826, 1982.

21 Patient Management

Prospective Double-Blind Placebo-Controlled Randomized Trial on the Use of Ranitidine in Preventing Postoperative Gastroduodenal Complications in High-Risk Neurosurgical Patients
Chan K-H, Lai ECS, Tuen H, Ngan JHK, Mok F, Fan Y-W, Fung C-F, Yu W-C
(The Univ of Hong Kong)
J Neurosurg 82:413–417, 1995   122-96-21–1

Background.—The H_2-receptor blockers are used extensively in patients undergoing neurosurgery to prevent stress-related gastroduodenal lesions. The efficacy of cimetidine in preventing gastroduodenal bleeding has only been proved in patients with severe head injury; the usefulness of H_2-receptor blockers for prophylaxis of gastroduodenal lesions in patients with nontraumatic neurosurgical disease is unknown. The efficacy of ranitidine in preventing postoperative gastroduodenal lesions in high-risk patients with nontraumatic neurosurgical disease was determined.

Methods.—In a standard, double-blind trial, 101 patients with nontraumatic neurosurgical lesions with 2 or more risk factors randomly received ranitidine (50 mg every 6 hours) or placebo and then underwent emergency neurosurgery. Postoperatively, serial gastroduodenal endoscopy documented the occurrence of complications. An overt symptomatic complication was defined as bleeding requiring transfusion or surgery.

Results.—Of the 101 patients, 52 received ranitidine and 49 received placebo. A total of 30 patients had overt gastroduodenal bleeding; 9 of these had received ranitidine and 21 had received placebo. The risk factors independently significant in predicting symptomatic gastroduodenal lesions were (1) use of placebo; (2) gastric pH less than 4; and (3) high daily volume of gastric output. Ranitidine significantly decreased the incidence of overt gastroduodenal bleeding compared with placebo.

Conclusions.—Ranitidine is effective in preventing postoperative overt stress-related gastroduodenal bleeding in high-risk patients with nontraumatic neurosurgical disease. Identification of the parameters that predict symptomatic bleeding may alert neurosurgeons to use aggressive means at an early stage to prevent bleeding. Prophylaxis for stress ulceration should be targeted at patients at high risk for these lesions developing.

▶ The authors have demonstrated that the prophylactic administration of ranitidine reduces the incidence of gastroduodenal (GD) complications in high-risk patients after neurosurgical operations performed on an emergency basis. The specific risk factors, determined by the authors in a previous study, were a preoperative Glasgow Coma Scale score less than 9, inappropriate secretion of antidiuretic hormone, major postoperative complications requiring reoperation, age 60 years or older, and pyogenic CNS infection. In this study, patients with 2 or more of these risk factors were considered to be at high risk for postoperative GD lesions developing.

Endoscopic examination of the stomach and duodenum was performed in all patients within 12 hours of surgery. A nasogastric tube was passed into the stomach after endoscopy, and its drainage was assessed periodically. Follow-up endoscopy was performed if there was evidence of gastrointestinal bleeding or abdominal pain.

Of the 49 patients given ranitidine, 10 had no endoscopic abnormalities, 30 had asymptomatic lesions without bleeding, and 9 had symptomatic lesions with bleeding. The corresponding numbers for the 52 patients given the placebo drug were 7, 24, and 21.—R.H. Wilkins, M.D.

22 Neurosurgical Technique

Efficacy of Prophylactic Antibiotics for Craniotomy: A Meta-Analysis
Barker FG II (Univ of California, San Francisco)
Neurosurgery 35:484–492, 1994   122-96-22–1

Background.—The efficacy of antibiotics for prophylaxis in shunt surgery has recently been examined in a meta-analysis. The new technique of cumulative meta-analysis was applied in a recent study to determine whether prophylactic antibiotics are effective for craniotomy.

Methods and Findings.—Ten studies were reviewed, 8 of which met the inclusion criteria for the meta-analysis. Antibiotics were superior to placebo at the $P < 10^{-8}$ level. Tests for the homogeneity-of-effect size among the individual studies demonstrated similar effects of antibiotic therapy among studies, even though the randomization methods and antibiotic regimens used varied. There was no significant difference between antibiotic regimens that did and did not cover gram-negative organisms or between single- and multiple-dose regimens. The cumulative meta-analysis also indicated that this conclusion could have been reached confidently by 1988, with only 4 of the 8 studies. The studies published after these 4 did not significantly change the conclusions drawn.

Conclusions.—Meta-analysis is a powerful tool for evaluating the combined findings of multiple clinical studies. Future research should compare proposed new antibiotic regimens with regimens already known to be effective, rather than with placebo.

▶ Much has been written about the use of antibiotics to prevent postoperative wound infections in patients undergoing neurosurgical operations. However, there have been relatively few scientific studies of this important topic. Barker has analyzed the results of 8 such scientific investigations of the efficacy of prophylactic antibiotics in preventing craniotomy wound infections; he concludes that antibiotic prophylaxis reduces the rate of wound infection rate in craniotomies by approximately fourfold.—R.M. Wilkins, M.D.

A Guide to Placement of Parietooccipital Ventricular Catheters: Technical Note

Howard MA III, Srinivasan J, Bevering CG, Winn HR, Grady MS (Univ of Iowa, Iowa City; Univ of Washington, Seattle)

J Neurosurg 82:300–304, 1995   122-96-22-2

Background.—Accurately placing parieto-occipital ventricular catheters can be difficult. The catheter tip needs to lie in the ipsilateral frontal horn to minimize the morbidity of the procedure and lengthen the duration of shunt function. A posterior ventricular guide (PVG) for placement of parieto-occipital catheters was described.

Ventricular Guide.—In the PVG, a simple mechanical assembly, an adjustable catheter guide tube is oriented along a line intersecting a fixed target point. The guide tube and target point are coupled mechanically so that a catheter passed through the guide tube with a rigid stylet has the optimal orientation toward the target point. The lightweight aluminum guides can be used on all patients, regardless of head circumference (Fig 22–1). Before each use, the guides are sterilized by autoclave.

Patients and Outcomes.—Thirty-eight patients underwent ventriculo-peritoneal shunting with the assistance of the guide. Postoperative CT

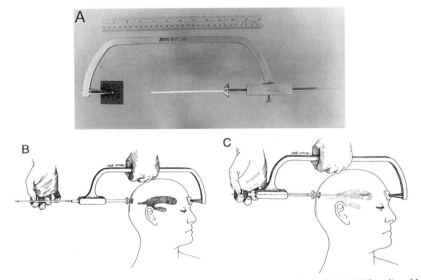

Fig 22–1.—A, photograph depicting elements of the posterior ventricular guide (PVG). The adjustable catheter guide tube is inserted into the main assembly and secured by tightening the guide screw, and the modified square cautery cleaning pad is secured to the frontal target site. During catheter placement, the conical nosepiece of the main assembly rests on the frontal target site. The adjustable catheter guide tube is in position and a ventricular catheter has been passed through the tube using a metal stylet. The catheter follows a straight trajectory toward the frontal target site (**A**). **B** and **C**, schematic drawings showing the guide technique. The PVG is positioned for right occipital catheter placement, and the adjustable guide tube is positioned close to the burr hole so that the catheter is visible as it exits the guide tube and enters the brain (**B**). The surgeon has passed the stylet and catheter through the tube and into the ipsilateral lateral ventricle. Note the straight trajectory of the ventricular catheter toward the frontal target site (**C**). (Courtesy of Howard MA III, Srinivasan J, Bevering CG, et al: *J Neurosurg* 82:300–304, 1995.)

scanning showed that 92% had accurate catheter placement. By contrast, a retrospective review of free-hand posterior catheter placement showed good catheter position in only 51%. The use of the guide increased procedure time by less than 5 minutes. No complications were associated with it.

Conclusions.—The PVG is a valuable asset in parieto-occipital shunt procedures and will help minimize the morbidity associated with this common neurosurgical procedure. It enabled accurate catheter placement in 92% of the patients.

▶ This seems to be a simple, yet accurate, technical development. In view of the fact that ventricular catheter placement by the parieto-occipital route has been used for so many years, I am surprised that no one has produced such a guide until now.—R.H. Wilkins, M.D.

Transcranial Approach to the Orbit: Microsurgical Anatomy
Natori Y, Rhoton AL Jr (Univ of Florida, Gainesville)
J Neurosurg 81:78–86, 1994   122-96-22–3

Objective.—An anatomical study was done in 15 adult cadaver heads to explore 3 intraorbital routes to the orbital apex and optic nerve that can be reached microsurgically via a fronto-orbital craniotomy.

Medial Approach.—An approach directed through the space between the superior oblique muscle and the levator and superior rectus muscles exposes the optic nerve from the globe to the optic canal. This is the most direct operative approach to the apical part of the optic nerve, and it is used for lesions located superomedial to the nerve.

Central Approach.—The levator muscle is retracted medially, and the superior rectus muscle is retracted laterally. The frontal nerve may be retracted either medially with the levator muscle or laterally with the superior rectus muscle; the former maneuver carries less risk of injury to the frontal nerve. The central approach is the shortest and most direct route to the midpart of the intraorbital segment of the optic nerve. This technique may be used for biopsy of the optic nerve.

Lateral Approach.—The optic nerve is approached between the lateral rectus muscle, which is retracted laterally, and the superior rectus and levator muscles, which are retracted medially. This approach provides the widest working space. If the superior ophthalmic vein and connective tissue hammock are dissected free rather than being retracted medially with the levator muscle, a good view is afforded of the deep apical region. Dividing the annulus of Zinn between the superior and lateral recti exposes the deep apical area where it joins the superior orbital fissure.

▶ This is another detailed and well-illustrated microanatomical study with clinical relevance from the valuable series produced by Dr. Rhoton and his colleagues.—R.H. Wilkins, M.D.

Tissue Expansion in Neurosurgical Reconstructive Technique: Case Report

Rotondo M, Parlato C, Iaccarino C, Scrocca A (Second Univ of Naples, Italy; Univ of Reggio Calabria, Italy)
Surg Neurol 43:201–204, 1995   122-96-22–4

Background.—The term "expansion of skin" originated in 1957, when Neumann attempted to reconstruct an ear by serially inflating a rubber balloon that was placed under the temporal skin. The technique then remained unused for 19 years until another report surfaced. In the 1980s, there were numerous reports on the use of tissue expanders in head and neck surgery.

Case Report.—Man, 23, had a scalp laceration, depressed skull fracture, and a dural tear after a traffic accident. An initial repair failed, resulting in necrosis of the scalp and a CSF leak. These deficits were corrected, and a silicone tissue expander was placed in an adjacent subgaleal pocket. After 10 days and at 5-day intervals, saline was injected percutaneously until there was expansion of the overlying skin. Expansion was carried out for 30 days with 250 mL of saline. The tissue expander was removed, and the skin flap was used to create an acceptable cosmetic result.

Conclusion.—The use of a tissue expander produces a pericranial flap of appropriate size that also has acceptable anatomical, functional, and cosmetic features. These features remain unchanged with tissue expansion. There may be other conditions that could benefit from the use of tissue expansion.

▶ The tissue expansion technique that is now being used by plastic surgeons may be of value in certain situations to provide sufficient skin for the closure of defects in the scalp or in the skin overlying the spine.—R.H. Wilkins, M.D.

Intraoperative Monitoring of the Vagus Nerve During Intracranial Glossopharyngeal and Upper Vagal Rhizotomy: Technical Note

Taha JM, Tew JM Jr, Keith RW, Payner TD (Univ of Cincinnati, Ohio; Mayfield Neurological Inst, Cincinnati, Ohio)
Neurosurgery 35:775–777, 1994   122-96-22–5

Background.—Intracranial section of the glossopharyngeal nerve and the upper vagal rootlets for the treatment of vagoglossopharyngeal neuralgia may cause dysphagia, vocal cord paralysis, or irritating cough in 10% to 20% of patients. To minimize this complication, a technique of intraoperative monitoring of the vagus nerve for preservation of the recurrent laryngeal nerve during thyroid surgery, as described by Lipton and McCaffery, was used in a man, 43, who was undergoing intracranial rhizotomy for vagoglossopharyngeal neuralgia.

Surgical Technique.—The patient was prepared for intraoperative electrophysiologic monitoring of the left vagus nerve. A response needle electrode was inserted lateral to the ipsilateral vocal fold near the arytenoid muscles. After surgical exposure, the rootlets of the vagus nerve were stimulated rostrally to differentiate the motor and sensory components of the nerve. Counting from rostral to caudal, the first, second, and fourth rootlets that were unresponsive to stimulation were sectioned.

Outcome.—At the time this report was prepared, the patient had been free of pain for about 1 year after the operation and had shown no signs of dysphagia, hoarseness, or irritating coughing.

Conclusion.—During intracranial sectioning of the glossopharyngeal nerve and the upper rootlets of the vagus nerve in this patient, intraoperative monitoring of the vagus nerve allowed preservation of a rostral vagal rootlet, which, if sectioned, could have caused dysphagia or vocal cord paralysis; sectioning of sensory rootlets; and sectioning of the fourth rostral rootlet, which might have otherwise been preserved. Intraoperative monitoring of the rostral vagal rootlets is an important technique for minimizing the complications of upper vagal rhizotomy.

▶ The authors describe an apparently useful method for avoiding the hoarseness and dysphagia that sometimes accompany intracranial rhizotomy of the upper rootlets of the vagus nerve as part of the treatment of vagoglossopharyngeal neuralgia. In follow-up correspondence in the same journal, Stechison cited his experience with this technique, dating back to 1992. He mentioned a study he had performed in 16 patients, comparing the results of recordings from endoscopically placed vocal fold electrodes with those from a method of percutaneous laryngeal electrode insertion (1).—R.H. Wilkins, M.D.

Reference

1. Stechison MT: Intraoperative monitoring of the vagus nerve during intracranial glossopharyngeal and upper vagal rhizotomy: Technical note. *Neurosurgery* 36:1238, 1995 (letter).

Intraoperative Digital Subtraction Angiography: A Review of 112 Consecutive Examinations

Derdeyn CP, Moran CJ, Cross DT, Grubb RL Jr, Dacey RG Jr (Washington Univ, St Louis, Mo)
AJNR 16:307–318, 1995   122-96-22–6

Background.—Potential advantages of intraoperative angiography all relate to timing. Information gained from intraoperative study can lead to modifications at an initial operation that can prevent complications or eliminate the need for a second operation. Recent technologic advances have made high-quality examinations possible, but there have been few reports of the technical success, accuracy, and safety of intraoperative

TABLE 1.—Frequency of Detection of Unexpected Residual Nidus

Study	Number of Exams	Residual Nidus
Bauer, 1984	11	3
Hieshema, 1987	12	2
Martin, 1990	48	5
Barrow, 1992	39	6
Present study	18	3
Total	128	19(16%)

(Courtesy of Derdeyn CP, Moran CJ, Cross DT, et al: *AJNR* 16:307–318, 1995.)

angiography in patients with neurovascular disease. The effects of intraoperative angiography on neurosurgical treatment were examined, as were the technical success, accuracy, and safety of such angiography.

Methods.—Medical records of 112 consecutive procedures in which intraoperative angiography was performed during neurosurgery were reviewed. Also reviewed were the results of conventional postoperative angiograms after 28 of the 112 procedures.

Results.—A portable digital subtraction angiography unit was used for all patients. There were 18 studies performed after resection of an arteriovenous malformation; in 3 patients, an unsuspected residual nidus was identified and resected (Table 1), and in 2 patients undergoing staged resections of arteriovenous malformations, the intraoperative angiogram altered therapy. There were 66 studies performed after aneurysm clipping; in 5 patients, clinically significant changes were made in surgical therapy (Table 2). There were 28 examinations after carotid endarterectomy; 3 led to revision. There were 2 complications of angiography; 1 led to a permanent neurologic deficit. The complication rate for stroke was 1.5%. Two examinations were not completed because of technical reasons, and 2 false negative examinations were identified on postoperative studies. In 1 patient with a normal intraoperative study after carotid endarterectomy, the repaired internal carotid artery thrombosed after surgery.

Discussion.—Intraoperative angiography can be easily performed and can show potentially important abnormities. Findings support routine use of this technique in arteriovenous malformation surgery and in complicated aneurysms. The use of this technique is not supported in routine carotid endarterectomy.

TABLE 2.—Frequency of Aneurysm Clip Replacement or Other Change in Therapy

Study	Number of Exams	Change in Therapy
Bauer, 1984	33	7
Martin, 1990	57	5
Barrow, 1992	62	7
Present study	66	6
Total	218	25(11%)

(Courtesy of Derdeyn CP, Moran CJ, Cross DT, et al: *AJNR* 16:307–318, 1995.)

▶ The authors have reconfirmed the value of intraoperative angiography in patients undergoing surgery for an arteriovenous malformation or an aneurysm. In contrast, intraoperative angiography after carotid endarterectomy did not seem valuable; in this study, it was not clear whether the abnormalities detected would have caused any postoperative complications if not repaired, and the sole neurologic complication after carotid endarterectomy occurred despite a normal intraoperative study.—R.H. Wilkins, M.D.

Cranioplasty With the Medpor Porous Polyethylene Flexblock Implant
Couldwell WT, Chen TC, Weiss MH, Fukushima T, Dougherty W (Univ of Southern Calif, Los Angeles)
J Neurosurg 81:483–486, 1994   122-96-22-7

The Implant.—The Medpor Surgical Implant is made of high-density polyethylene microspheres that are sintered together to create a framework of interconnected pores in which vessels and soft tissue may grow and in which bone may form. It is a very stable and flexible implant that has been approved for use in humans requiring cosmetic cranioplasty. It is available in block form or in preformed anatomical shapes.

Implant Placement.—The Medpor Flexblock implant may be fashioned with scissors or a scalpel to fit any shape of cranial defect up to 8 cm in size. The best fit is achieved by drawing a pattern of the defect on a paper template and transferring this to the implant surface. The conical undersurface of the implant permits it to be flexed to fit any contour. The Flexblock implant costs about the same as a methyl methacrylate cranioplasty kit. The operating time is less than that for conventional alloplast cranioplasty.

The Flexblock implant was used for cranioplasty in 25 patients with small to medium-sized cranial defects, most often resulting from temporal craniectomy. Excellent cosmetic results were achieved in all patients, including 3 in whom the implant served to reconstruct the lateral orbital ridge. The median follow-up was 9.5 months. No implant-related complications occurred. No infection developed in 2 patients in whom the implant was placed adjacent to an open frontal sinus.

Conclusion.—The Medpor Flexblock implant is a safe and cosmetically excellent option for use in cranioplasty when a small or medium-sized defect is present.

▶ Many materials have been used for cranioplasty. Couldwell and his colleagues describe their experience with a type of polyethylene that is porous and flexible; their initial impression is favorable. For coverage of cranial defects smaller than 8 cm in diameter, they found the Medpor Flexblock implant to be "a safe, cosmetically equivalent alternative to standard methyl methacrylate cranioplasty while ease of implantation shortens operation time."—R.H. Wilkins, M.D.

Application of Purified Bone Morphogenetic Protein (BMP) Preparations in Cranio-Maxillo-Facial Surgery: Reconstruction in Craniofacial Malformations and Post-Traumatic or Operative Defects of the Skull with Lyophilized Cartilage and BMP

Sailer HF, Kolb E (Univ Hosp Zürich, Switzerland)
J Craniomaxillofac Surg 22:191–199, 1994   122-96-22–8

Background.—The use of purified bone morphogenetic protein (BMP) preparations in compromised cranio-maxillofacial reconstructions in which titanium implants are used has been reported. More recently, the results of a novel treatment that incorporates BMP were reported.

Methods.—A stacked composite of lyophilized cartilage strips interspersed with BMP layers was used in 5 patients having craniofacial reconstruction. Two adults had late post-traumatic defects with depressions, 1 adult had a fresh donor site craniectomy defect, and 2 children had complicated defects incurred in the repair of synostotic malformations caused by Apert's syndrome in one and Crouzon's syndrome in the other. In the 3 adult patients, the plywood-like composite paste was used alone to fill the defects and indentations. In the 2 children, the composite paste was used in combination with autologous bone struts to rebuild the cranium.

Results.—Use of the lyophilized cartilage strips and BMP combination induced early bone formation. The reconstructed areas became clinically solid after a few months. Progressive calcification starting in the BMP layers was sometimes already visible on CT scans after just a few weeks. No resorption of the implants was seen during a mean follow-up of 10 months.

Conclusions.—The application of lyophilized cartilage strips treated with BMP for craniofacial reconstruction considerably accelerates the calcification and ossification process compared with lyocartilage alone.

▶ The authors describe an interesting technique for skull reconstruction that uses both lyophilized bank cartilage and BMP (which is purified from fresh bovine bone obtained from the femoral diaphysis of 4- to 8-week-old calves). This method does not require the harvesting of the patient's own bone or cartilage, and it has the potential for more rapid reossification of cranial defects than standard grafting techniques allow.—R.H. Wilkins, M.D.

23 Neurosurgical Complications

Relative Risks of Ventriculostomy Infection and Morbidity
Paramore CG, Turner DA (Durham VA Med Ctr, NC)
Acta Neurochir (Wien) 127:79–84, 1994   122-96-23–1

Background.—Patients with increased intracranial pressure commonly undergo ventricular catheter placement. Catheter infection is an important complication. It is thought to result from either contamination at the time of catheter insertion, in which case the time the catheter was in place would have little effect on the risk of infection, or from contamination after insertion, in which case duration would have an important influence on risk.

Methods.—This retrospective study evaluated the frequency of infectious and noninfectious complications of ventricular catheter placement in 161 patients in an attempt to determine whether routine catheter replacement is warranted. The patients underwent a total of 253 catheter placements over a 3-year period. A total of 220 placements in a subgroup of 135 patients were reviewed to focus on infectious complications.

Findings.—The overall infection rate was just over 4%. However, there was an exponential increase in daily infection hazard over time, to a maximum of 10% by the sixth day the catheter was in place. There was nearly a 6% risk of noninfectious complications, frequent ones including hemorrhage and misplacement severe enough to require new catheter placement. By the fifth day of catheter insertion, the daily hazard of infectious and noninfectious risk was comparable.

Conclusions.—These retrospective data support the hypothesis that infection of ventricular catheters occurs because of catheter contamination after infection and the recommendation that catheters should be changed after 5 days. Confirmation of this hypothesis will require prospective studies of the daily risk of CSF infection. Such studies could also determine whether antibiotic prophylaxis could reduce the risk of infectious complications.

▶ This study addresses an important question. Should a ventriculostomy catheter be replaced after a certain interval (to minimize the occurrence of associated infection), or should it be kept in place for the entire time it is needed (to avoid the complications of replacing the catheter such as intracerebral hemorrhage)? Several previous studies have addressed this question, as reviewed by the present authors. In 1993, Winfield et al. (1) found in their retrospective study of 212 intracranial pressure (ICP) monitors that there was no relation between the duration of ICP monitoring and the rate of daily infection during a monitoring period of 1 to 2 weeks, and they concluded that the decision to continue ICP monitoring can be based solely on the clinical necessity for further monitoring rather than on concerns for monitor removal to prevent infection. In contrast, Paramore and Turner found in this study that the daily infection hazard increased exponentially with time, and they agreed with Mayhall et al. (2) that catheters should be routinely replaced after 5 days to avoid a significant risk of infection.—R.H. Wilkins, M.D.

References

1. Winfield JA, Rosenthal P, Kanter RK, et al: Duration of intracranial pressure monitoring does not predict daily risk of infectious complications. *Neurosurgery* 33:424–431, 1993.
2. Mayhall CG, Archer NH, Archer-Lamb V, et al: Ventriculostomy-related infections. *N Engl J Med* 310:553–559, 1984.

Timing of Postoperative Intracranial Hematoma Development and Implications for the Best Use of Neurosurgical Intensive Care
Taylor WAS, Thomas NWM, Wellings JA, Anthony Bell B (Atkinson Morley's Hosp, London)
J Neurosurg 82:48–50, 1995   122-96-23–2

Introduction.—Hematomas that develop after neurosurgical procedures are detected by close nursing observation. The use of intensive care beds for this purpose may make fewer beds available for emergency admissions.

Objective.—The pattern of hematoma formation was studied in 2,305 patients who underwent burr-hole freehand or stereotactic biopsy, craniotomy, or posterior fossa surgery either electively or on an emergency basis during a 5-year period.

Findings.—Fifty patients (2.2%) had a postoperative hematoma. Those undergoing emergency procedures were most often affected. There were 26 extradural, 22 intracerebral, and 2 subdural hematomas. All but 6 of the 50 patients deteriorated clinically within 6 hours of surgery (Fig 23–1). Nineteen patients had their hematomas evacuated 24 hours or longer after initial surgery. Only 55% of 38 patients who initially had elective surgery made a good recovery. The final outcome could not be related to the time of either clinical deterioration or reoperation.

Conclusions.—Patients who regain their baseline neurologic status 6 hours after neurosurgery may safely be transferred out of intensive care. Such a policy seems warranted for patients having biopsy or elective craniotomy.

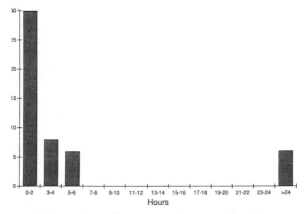

Fig 23–1.—Bar graph showing the time from intracranial surgery to clinical deterioration in 50 patients who had postoperative hematoma develop. (Courtesy of Taylor WAS, Thomas NWM, Wellings JA, et al: *J Neurosurg* 82:48–50, 1995.)

▶ In recent years, there has been an effort to control the costs of medical care in the United States, one aspect of which has been to lower the costs of inpatient treatment. Many tests and treatments that formerly were performed in the hospital are now being done in a less expensive outpatient setting. Patients who are admitted to the hospital are now staying for shorter periods, and there has been a trend toward less invasive surgical procedures. This study by Taylor and associates is important in this context of cost reduction.—R.H. Wilkins, M.D.

Postoperative Mutism in Neurosurgery: Report of Two Cases
Crutchfield JS, Sawaya R, Meyers CA, Moore BD III (MD Anderson Cancer Ctr, Houston)
J Neurosurg 81:115–121, 1994   122-96-23–3

Background.—Mutism describes a state in which a conscious patient is unwilling or unable to speak. There are many possible causes, including trauma, epilepsy, tumors, and stroke: surgery is an uncommon cause. When postoperative mutism occurs, it is usually transient. The authors report 2 patients with mutism immediately following brain surgery and discuss the neural circuitry that may have been involved in this complication.

Patients.—The patients were a 46-year-old man and a 7-year-old boy in whom mutism developed immediately following bifrontal craniotomy for a parasagittal meningioma and suboccipital craniectomy for a posterior fossa medulloblastoma, respectively. The adult patient could not speak immediately after surgery and the following day displayed motor apraxia. This patient could carry on brief conversations and read short sentences by the second day, and he recovered considerably by day 13. He had mild dysphasia that resolved by 6 months. He had no problems with apraxia or expressive speech at 16 months.

The child could speak the day after surgery but on the second day, he had stopped speaking. He also had upper limb dysmetria and truncal ataxia. He could say simple words at 7 weeks and soon began to speak spontaneously, often in a whisper. He could initiate speech by the second month, and at 3 months he spoke fluently but with slight dysarthria. Although receptive vocabulary was intact, the patient still had some dysnomia. This problem was unchanged at 21 months, although the dysarthria was almost completely gone.

Discussion.—Two patients with mutism after brain surgery are described. This complication likely resulted from transient injury to the supplementary motor cortex in the adult patient and to the dentate nuclei in the child. There are pathways connecting these 2 areas via the ventrolateral nucleus of the thalamus, lesions of which can cause mutism. Although uncommon and usually transient, mutism is a possible complication of brain operations that interrupt neurologic pathways involving the thalamic ventrolateral nucleus.

▶ It is easy to understand why a patient might exhibit dysphasia or aphasia after an operation in the midportion of the dominant cerebral hemisphere. What has been harder to explain have been those cases of mutism or speech disturbance following operations involving other areas of the brain, such as the cerebellum. In this paper, Crutchfield and his associates review the subject and focus the reader's attention on the connections between the dentate nucleus of the cerebellum and the contralateral ventrolateral nucleus of the thalamus, and the connections between this thalamic nucleus and the ipsilateral supplementary motor area. They conclude that some of the instances of postoperative mutism, such as the 2 presented in their paper, result from bilateral disruption of elements of the dentatothalamocortical pathways.—R.H. Wilkins, M.D.

Hearing Loss After Neurosurgery: The Influence of Low Cerebrospinal Fluid Pressure

Walsted A, Nielsen OA, Borum P (Gentofte Univ Hosp, Denmark; Glostrup Hosp, Denmark)
J Laryngol Otol 108:637–641, 1994   122-96-23–4

Background.—In patients undergoing neurosurgery, decreases in volume and pressure in the CSF may affect hearing. The extent and cause of any hearing loss after neurosurgery were systematically evaluated in a prospective study.

Patients and Methods.—Thirty-two patients (age, 19 to 72 years) who underwent neurosurgery and 32 control patients (age, 19 to 73 years) who had surgical procedures that did not involve opening or puncturing the dura mater were evaluated. Of the 32 neurosurgical patients, 20 underwent removal of an intracranial tumor; six had an operation for normal CSF pressure hydrocephalus; two for an intracranial aneurysm; and four had surgery for epilepsy. The 32 control patients had a middle ear procedure (11), other otologic operation (10), thyroid surgery (8), or parotid surgery (3). Patients were asked about existing audiologic symptoms, and all underwent preoperative assessments, including otoscopy, pure tone audiometry, speech audiometry, and tympanometry. All patients underwent 2 postoperative tests scheduled between days 1 and 3 and days 4 and 7. Any new subjective symptoms, including hearing loss, fullness, tinnitus, and dizziness or nausea, were reported at this time.

Results.—Seventeen patients who underwent neurosurgery had a significant hearing loss during the first postoperative week. The threshold shift toward worse hearing was more common at frequencies of 125, 250, and 500 Hz, but it was also noted at 4 and 8 kHz. In the entire neurosurgery group, 49 significant threshold changes showing worse hearing at the first postoperative audiometry were noted compared with only 6 in the control patients. Among the neurosurgery group, 2 patients reported subjective postoperative symptoms of nausea, 3 experienced dizziness, 3 had fullness in the ears, 8 reported decreased hearing, and 9 had a new symptom of tinnitus develop. Only 1 patient in the control group reported subjective symptoms, which were comprised of a sensation of occlusion in the ears, confirmed by audiometry and tympanometry. The latter patient was among those in the control group who had experienced a significant threshold decrease.

Conclusions.—In patients undergoing neurosurgery, the mechanism of hearing loss results from a decrease in pressure and/or volume of the CSF, which is reflected within the perilymphatic fluid and is similar to a transitory endolymphatic hydrops. Further studies that can help clarify the pathophysiologic mechanisms leading to hearing loss after CSF leakage are needed.

▶ Neurosurgeons are accustomed to testing the hearing of patients before and after the removal of cerebellopontine angle tumors. However, few carefully assess hearing after supratentorial operations. If a patient undergoing such a procedure complains of a unilateral or bilateral decrease of auditory acuity in the immediate postoperative period, it is expected to be temporary, and it is usually ascribed to transient impairment of the patency of one or both eustachian tubes, caused by such things as a nasopharyngeal and oropharyngeal trauma from endotracheal intubation. These authors invoke another possible explanation, i.e., that a decrease in the pressure and/or volume of the CSF causes a decrease in perilymphatic fluid pressure, which in turn is reflected as a temporary decrease in auditory acuity that tends to recover within a week. I agree with the authors that further studies are needed to clarify this relationship (and to prove the possible etiologic association of decreased CSF pressure or volume and reduced auditory acuity in neurosurgical patients).—R.H. Wilkins, M.D.

24 Skull Base Lesions

Infiltration of the Carotid Artery by Cavernous Sinus Meningioma
Kotapka MJ, Kalia KK, Martinez AJ, Sekhar LN (Univ of Pittsburgh, Pa)
J Neurosurg 81:252–255, 1994   122-96-24–1

Background.—Intracranial meningiomas infiltrate surrounding structures such as the calvaria and dural sinuses, as well as the brain itself. In cases of meningioma that has not invaded the wall of the carotid artery, complete tumor removal may be achieved with careful dissection from the carotid artery. However, if the tumor has infiltrated the wall of the carotid artery, complete removal may necessitate sacrificing the artery. In a retrospective review, it was determined whether cavernous sinus meningiomas invade the carotid artery.

Methods.—The histopathology of 19 consecutively treated patients with carotid arteries sacrificed during removal of a meningioma involving the cavernous sinus was reviewed. Patients were selected for carotid artery resection based on preoperative MRI studies, showing complete encasement of the artery. Carotid artery reconstruction was planned based on the results of preoperative balloon test occlusion with blood flow determinations.

Findings.—There was no pathologic evidence of malignant tumor in any patient. Forty-two percent had infiltration of the carotid artery by meningioma. Focal involvement of the adventitia of the carotid artery wall was observed in 5 patients, and the vessel was infiltrated up to the tunica muscularis in 3. The tumor did not invade the tunica muscularis in any patient.

Conclusions.—Meningiomas of the cavernous sinus can infiltrate the internal carotid artery. To completely resect these lesions and effect a surgical cure, the carotid artery may need to be sacrificed, with or without reconstruction.

▶ These authors provide unique and valuable documentation that benign meningiomas involving the cavernous sinus frequently infiltrate the adventitia of the internal carotid artery, a fact that has both therapeutic and prognostic implications.—R.H. Wilkins, M.D.

Outcome of Aggressive Removal of Cavernous Sinus Meningiomas

DeMonte F, Smith HK, Al-Mefty O (MD Anderson Cancer Ctr, Houston; Univ of Mississippi, Jackson; Univ of Arkansas, Little Rock)
J Neurosurg 81:245–251, 1994
122-96-24–2

Background.—Despite recent advances in the surgical treatment of the cavernous sinus, meningiomas in that area are still difficult to treat. Aggressive surgical removal of cavernous sinus meningiomas is thought to be appropriate, because the extent of removal is presumed to be inversely associated with the rate of recurrence. The outcome of aggressive removal of cavernous sinus meningiomas was investigated.

Methods and Findings.—Forty-one patients with histologically benign meningiomas involving the cavernous sinus underwent aggressive surgery in the past 10 years. Total removal was achieved in 31 patients (76%). Twelve patients were followed up for more than 5 years. Ten had total tumor removal, only 1 of whom had a recurrence. The other 2 patients had subtotal removal, showing symptomatic and radiologic evidence of regrowth 3 and 4 years after surgery. Preexisting cranial nerve deficits improved in 14% of the patients, remained the same in 80%, and permanently worsened in 6%. Seven patients had a total of 10 new cranial nerve deficits. Four of these involved the nerves subserving ocular motor function. In the 25 patients with a seeing eye ipsilateral to the tumor, extraocular muscle function did not worsen. No visual worsening occurred in this group. Two patients died 4 months after surgery. The causes of death were severe delayed vasospasm and hypothalamic infarction in 1 and myocardial infarction in the other. Another patient died 9 days after surgery from a pulmonary embolus. Three cases of cerebral ischemia occurred—1 transient, lasting less than 24 hours, and 2 related to injury of the middle cerebral artery, resulting in residual hemiplegia. Other complications were nonfatal pulmonary emboli, CSF leaks, exposure keratitis, acute hypothyroidism, and cerebral edema.

Conclusions.—In most patients, complete resection of cavernous sinus meningiomas can be achieved with acceptable levels of mortality and morbidity. Increasing evidence indicates that the rate of recurrence is reduced.

▶ DeMonte et al. give an honest account of what can currently be accomplished by a group experienced in the resection of meningiomas invading the cavernous sinus. Such resection remains a difficult surgery with significant morbidity. This experienced surgical team has a 7% mortality rate. Dr. Al-Mefty and others who have pioneered in operations of this sort have certainly expanded the indications for, and benefits of, skull base surgery. However, accurate outcome assessments such as this one are necessary to establish exactly what has been achieved so far, and to serve as a baseline for further refinements and advancements.—R.H. Wilkins, M.D.

Base of Skull Chordoma: A Correlative Study of Histologic and Clinical Features of 62 Cases

O'Connell JX, Renard LG, Liebsch NJ, Efird JT, Munzenrider JE, Rosenberg AE (Massachusetts Gen Hosp, Boston)
Cancer 74:2261–2267, 1994   122-96-24-3

Introduction.—Chordoma is among the most common of the skull base neoplasms. Its slow, progressive growth causes varied signs and symptoms. The location of the tumor usually makes complete surgical resection impossible. Therefore, patients are usually treated with combined partial resection and radiation therapy. The prognosis is generally poor, but the factors predicting relative outcome have not been established. A retrospective evaluation examined the clinical and pathologic factors that predicted survival.

Methods.—The records of 62 patients with skull base chordomas treated with postoperative radiation therapy between 1979 and 1990 were examined. Histologic features, tumor extent and volume, age, and sex were noted, and their association with disease progression and mortality were analyzed.

Results.—During a follow-up of 20–158 months, 29 patients had disease progression and 21 patients died of the chordoma. With univariate analysis, female gender, preradiation tumor necrosis of more than 10%, and prominent nucleoli strongly predicted shorter survival. With multivariate analysis, female gender significantly predicted disease progression. Female gender, preradiation tumor necrosis of more than 10%, and tumor volume larger than 70 mL independently predicted shortened survival when controlling for age, mitoses, nucleoli, pleomorphism, vascular invasion, and chondroid elements.

Discussion.—Female gender, tumor volume, and tumor necrosis in initial biopsy specimens are significant predictors of 2 patient outcomes: survival and local failure. These findings can be used to classify prognostic groups of patients with skull base chordoma. The combination of the dramatic gender-based difference in survival and the trend toward shorter survival in postmenopausal women compared to premenopausal women and men suggest that sex hormones play a role in the biological behavior of chordomas.

▶ This investigative group from Massachusetts General Hospital has had considerable experience with treating skull base chordomas. The reported series of 62 patients received treatment (after surgical confirmation of the diagnosis) with combined photon and proton irradiation. Despite this state-of-the-art management, 21 of the patients died of their disease. The median survival for female patients was 86 months, whereas that for male patients was 158 months. The authors have clarified prognostic factors for this disease, but, clearly, there is room for further improvement with regard to treatment.—R.H. Wilkins, M.D.

Experience in Charged Particle Irradiation of Tumors of the Skull Base: 1977–1992

Castro JR, Linstadt DE, Bahary J-P, Petti PL, Daftari I, Collier JM, Gutin PH, Gauger G, Phillips TL (Univ of Calif, Berkley; Univ of Calif, San Francisco)
Int J Radiat Oncol Biol Phys 29:647–655, 1994   122-96-24–4

Background.—In patients with primary neoplasms of the skull base or extending to the skull base from the nasopharynx and paranasal sinuses, the presence of critical normal structures in those areas compromises the use of surgical and standard radiotherapeutic techniques. The use of heavy charged particles, such as protons and helium and neon ions, in the treatment of these tumors can deliver equivalent tumor doses from 15% to 35% higher than those that can be delivered by standard x-ray techniques, with corresponding improvements in local control and survival. A 15-year experience with the use of charged particles to irradiate tumors of the skull base was reported.

Patients.—Two hundred twenty-three patients received this type of treatment from 1977 to 1992 for tumors either arising in or extending to the skull base. Twenty-two percent had lesions that had recurred after previous surgery or radiotherapy. The lesions arose in the skull base in 126 patients, most commonly chordoma, chondrosarcoma, and paraclival meningioma. Nineteen patients in this group had tumors of other histologies, such as osteosarcoma or neurofibrosarcoma. Thirty-one patients had primary or recurrent nasopharyngeal carcinoma extending to the skull base. Forty-four had major or minor salivary gland tumors, mainly adenocarcinomas, and 22 had squamous carcinomas of the paranasal sinuses, extending to the cranial base (Table 1).

Results.—Charged particle irradiation delivered high doses, with a mean of 65 Gy-equivalent, to the tumors, with relative sparing of normal tissues in the area. Improvements in local control and survival were apparent. At a median follow-up of 51 months, Kaplan-Meier 5-year local control rates were 85% for patients with meningioma, 78% for those with chondrosarcoma, 63% for those with chordoma, and 58% for those with other sarcomas (Table 2). For patients with tumors arising in the skull

TABLE 1.—Patient Information

	No.
Tumors arising in skull base	
Chordoma	53
Chondrosarcoma	27
Meningioma	27
Sarcoma	19
Total	126
Tumors invading skull base	
Primary or recurrent squamous carcinoma of the nasopharynx	31
Major or minor salivary gland tumors	44
Squamous carcinoma of the paranasal sinuses	22

(Courtesy of Castro JR, Linstadt DE, Bahary J-P, et al: *Int J Radiat Oncol Biol Phys* 29:647–655, 1994.)

TABLE 2.—Results in 126 Patients with Tumors Arising in the Skull Base
Treated With Charged Particles

	%
Kaplan-Meier 5 year local control	
Meningioma	85
Chondrosarcoma	78
Chordoma	63
Other Sarcoma	58
Kaplan-Meier 5 year survival	
Meningioma	82
Chondrosarcoma	83
Chordoma	75
Other Sarcoma	71

(Courtesy of Castro JR, Linstadt DE, Bahary J-P, et al: *Int J Radiat Oncol Biol Phys* 29:647–655, 1994.)

base, Kaplan-Meier survival was 77% at 5 years and 62% at 10 years (Fig 24–1). Improvements in survival were noted in the overall series as well (Fig 24–2).

Conclusions.—Charged-particle radiotherapy is an effective means of controlling tumors of the skull base, especially those that arise in the skull base. Complication rates are acceptable as long as patients have not previously received significant amounts of radiation. Local control, sur-

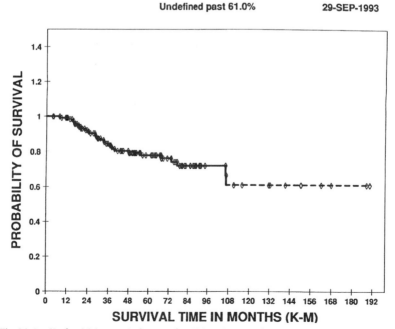

Undefined past 61.0%   **29-SEP-1993**

Fig 24–1.—Kaplan-Meier survival curve for 126 patients with tumors arising in the skull base (1977–1992). (Courtesy of Castro JR, Linstadt DE, Bahary J-P, et al: *Int J Radiat Oncol Biol Phys* 29:647–655, 1994.)

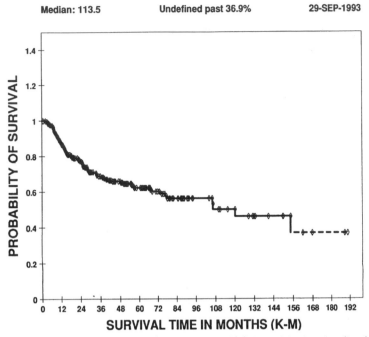

Fig 24–2.—Kaplan-Meier survival curve for 223 patients with lesions arising in or invading the skull base that were treated with charged particles (1977–1992). (Courtesy of Castro JR, Linstadt DE, Bahary J-P, et al: *Int J Radiat Oncol Biol Phys* 29:647–665, 1994.)

vival, and complications rates continue to improve as advances are made in MRI tumor localization, 3-dimensional treatment planning, and beam delivery.

▶ This group at the Lawrence Berkeley Laboratory has had a unique experience with charged-particle therapy. In this report, the authors document the value of this form of treatment for tumors involving the base of the skull.—R.H. Wilkins, M.D.

25 Pituitary Disorders

Pituitary Magnetic Resonance Imaging in Normal Human Volunteers: Occult Adenomas in the General Population
Hall WA, Luciano MG, Doppman JL, Patronas NJ, Oldfield EH (Natl Inst of Neurological Disorders and Stroke, Bethesda, Md; The Clinical Ctr, NIH, Bethesda, Md)
Ann Intern Med 120:817–820, 1994   122-96-25-1

Objective.—The prevalence of focal pituitary lesions consistent with adenoma was determined in 100 normal persons 18 to 60 years of age. Magnetic resonance images of the pituitary fossa were acquired in the coronal and sagittal planes, before and after the intravenous administration of gadolinium-diethylenetriaminepentaacetic acid.

Observations.—All 3 reviewers agreed that a normal pituitary was present in 59 of the 100 subjects. At least 1 reviewer found a site of abnormal signal intensity in the pituitary in 21 subjects before contrast administration. Seven others had focal areas of reduced signal. After contrast injection, 41 sites of abnormal signal intensity were found in 34 subjects, 10 of whom had changes interpreted as representing pituitary adenoma in the view of at least 2 of the reviewers. These 10 patients all had normal endocrine studies.

Patient Review.—Of 50 patients with Cushing's disease who had an adenoma identified operatively, 56% had focal areas of low signal intensity on MRI after contrast administration. In 4 instances, however, the site of the adenoma was incorrectly read on the MRI study.

Conclusions.—Approximately 10% of normal adults have MRI changes in the pituitary that are consistent with pituitary adenoma. Most of these adneomas remain asymptomatic and need not be treated.

▶ Through autopsy studies, it has been known for some years that a significant percentage of the population have asymptomatic pituitary adenomas. Estimates of the prevalence of asymptomatic pituitary adenomas have varied from 1.5% to 27%, depending on the thoroughness of the search and the criteria for identifying an adenoma. In the present study, Hall and his colleagues have performed a similar assessment using MRI rather than autopsy examination and conclude that about 10% of "normal" adults have changes suggestive of pituitary adenoma.—R.H. Wilkins, M.D.

Immediate Recovery of Pituitary Function After Transsphenoidal Resection of Pituitary Macroadenomas

Arafah BM, Kailani SH, Nekl KE, Gold RS, Selman WR (Case Western Reserve Univ, Cleveland, Ohio; Univ Hosps of Cleveland, Ohio)
J Clin Endocrinol Metab 79:348–354, 1994   122-96-25–2

Introduction.—Patients with pituitary macroadenomas that do not secrete PRL commonly have mild hyperprolactinemia along with hypopituitarism. This association suggests that hypopituitarism may result from compression of portal vessels. If this is so, hypothalamic control over pituitary function should return immediately after adenomectomy.

Methods.—This hypothesis was tested by evaluation of pituitary function before and after transsphenoidal adenomectomy in 26 ACTH-deficient patients. Twenty-three subjects with normal adrenal and thyroid function served as controls. The ACTH-deficient patients received glucocorticoids, which were withdrawn 36 hours after surgery. All subjects underwent twice-daily measurement of ACTH, cortisol, and PRL.

Results.—In controls, ACTH and PRL levels increased within hours after surgery, returning to baseline over 4 days. The hypopituitary patients showed a 50% decrease in PRL levels within hours of adenomectomy, and this decrease persisted until discharge. In 65% of the hypopituitary patients, ACTH levels increased within hours; all of these patients had normal adrenal function by the time they were discharged. The remaining patients required cortisol replacement for low ACTH levels.

Conclusions.—In patients with pituitary macroadenomas that do not secrete PRL, hypopituitarism appears to be reversible and to result primarily from compression of the portal vessels and the resulting interruption in delivery of hypothalamic hormones. However, hypopituitarism persists in some patients, suggesting that ischemic necrosis of the anterior pituitary can limit recovery.

▶ In this clinical investigation, Arafah et al. show that pituitary function can be improved by the resection of a macroadenoma. What is surprising is that improvement occurs within hours after the operation. This nice piece of work also indicates the technical skill of the neurosurgeons involved.—R.H. Wilkins, M.D.

Treatment of Invasive Growth Hormone Pituitary Adenomas With Long-Acting Somatostatin Analog SMS 201-995 Before Transsphenoidal Surgery

Lucas-Morante T, García-Uría J, Estrada J, Saucedo G, Cabello A, Alcañiz J, Barceló B (Clínica Puerta de Hierro, Madrid, Spain)
J Neurosurg 81:10–14, 1994   122-96-25–3

Objective.—The value of administering the long-acting somatostatin analogue SMS 201–995 (octreotide) before transsphenoidal surgery was examined in 10 previously untreated acromegalic patients having active disease and invasive tumors.

Patients.—The 9 women and 1 man studied had a mean age of 41 years. Acromegaly had developed over an average of 5.2 years before being diagnosed. All patients were considered to be severely affected. The mean 24-hour growth hormone (GH) level was 93 µg/L, and GH was not adequately suppressed by oral glucose in the 7 patients studied.

Treatment.—Patients received octreotide subcutaneously in a dose of 100 µg every 8 hours for 6 weeks before performing transsphenoidal surgery. Tumor volume was estimated from coronal and axial CT scans.

Results.—The activity of acromegaly decreased throughout the treatment period. Levels of GH decreased significantly to an average of 45 µg/L after 2 weeks of treatment, at which time the level of insulin-like growth factor–I also had decreased significantly. Six patients had a decrease in tumor volume, which averaged 30%. There were no side effects from octreotide therapy. Six of the 10 patients had all gross tumor tissue removed and were endocrinologically cured.

Conclusion.—A majority of these patients had relatively small tumors, and preoperative administration of octreotide had no clear effect on the operative results.

▶ The authors found that preoperative administration of the long-acting somatostatin analogue SMS 201-995 to 10 acromegalic patients for 6 weeks improved the symptoms of acromegaly in all patients, decreased the mean levels of both GH and insulin-like growth factor–I by about half, and resulted in average tumor shrinkage of 30% in 6 of the 10 patients. However, the effects of GH, insulin-like growth factor–I, and tumor size reached a plateau by 2 weeks. Only pretreatment tumor size was of predictive value with respect to the surgical outcome.—R.H. Wilkins, M.D.

Perioperative Management and Surgical Outcome of the Acromegalic Patient With Sleep Apnea
Piper JG, Dirks BA, Traynelis VC, VanGilder JC (Univ of Iowa Hosps and Clinics, Iowa City)
Neurosurgery 36:70–75, 1995   122-96-25–4

Introduction.—Sleep apnea is a rare complication of acromegaly that disposes patients to perioperative airway compromise. How the disorder responds to transsphenoidal resection of the pituitary tumor is unclear. Patients with sleep apnea were reviewed, and postoperative objective and subjective improvement of their sleep disorders was documented.

Patients.—Four acromegalic patients with significant sleep apnea underwent transsphenoidal resection of a growth hormone–secreting pituitary tumor. Sleep apnea had been present for as long as 26 years before surgical treatment, long before more obvious manifestations appeared. One patient also was obese. The mean hourly number of apneic and hypopneic episodes was 58. Three of the patients were surgically treated for sleep apnea before their tumors were resected. All 3 patients underwent tracheostomy, one of which followed uvulopalatopharyngoplasty.

Outcome.—The mean plasma somatomedin C level decreased from 855 ng/mL preoperatively to 229 ng/mL after pituitary surgery. Symptoms of sleep apnea, which initially were moderate to severe in all patients, consistently lessened after resection of the pituitary tumor. Cine CT studies of the airway, obtained postoperatively in 2 patients, showed no obstruction. Two patients were weaned from tracheostomy, and the other patient, who was morbidly obese, improved symptomatically.

Discussion.—If there is any question of the adequacy of the airway in an acromegalic patient with sleep apnea syndrome, tracheostomy should be done before pituitary surgery. The sleep apnea generally improves within 2 months of tumor resection, and it sometimes resolves completely.

▶ Louis Pasteur noted that in the fields of observation, chance favors only the mind that is prepared. Occasionally, a neurosurgeon is faced with an unusual circumstance and has an opportunity to contribute to medical knowledge (not necessarily in the field of neurosurgery), if he or she recognizes that opportunity and acts on it. This report is an example of such an occurrence.—R.H. Wilkins, M.D.

Changes in the Immunophenotype of Recurrent Pituitary Adenomas
Mindermann T, Kovacs K, Wilson C (Univ of California, San Francisco; Univ of Toronto)
Neurosurgery 35:39–44, 1994   122-96-25–5

Background.—There have been only 2 reported cases of a pituitary adenoma that changed phenotype between its initial resection and recurrence. The frequency of such cases among 1 series of patients was examined.

Methods.—The charts of 1,023 patients were reviewed. All had pituitary adenomas that were treated surgically between 1984 and 1992 at 1 center. Sixty-five patients had either surgery for or clinical evidence of tumor recurrence.

Findings.—Of these 65 patients, 5 (7.7%) had tumors that changed phenotype. The ratio of women to men was 4:1. The mean age at onset was 33.2 years. Changes in hormone production and hormone release occurred after a mean of 6.4 years. All 5 tumors were invasive, and 4 were macroadenomas at some point. Two patients had more than one operation for tumor recurrence. Three had silent or symptomatic pituitary apoplexy, and 3 had sellar irradiation before the changes in phenotype occurred. Therefore, the behavior of these tumors is apparently aggressive.

Conclusions.—The complete immunostaining of primary and recurrent pituitary adenoma was advocated so that additional data on their clinical course can be collected. It is unclear whether phenotypic changes in pituitary adenomas have any implications for treatment.

▶ The authors document that a pituitary adenoma occasionally (7.7% in their series) can change phenotype between the time of its initial resection and the time of retreatment for recurrence (6.4 ± 3.4 years later). This phenomenon raises questions about the origin of pituitary adenomas and the mechanisms that cause this uncommon change of phenotype.—R.H. Wilkins, M.D.

Radiation Therapy for Pituitary Adenoma: Treatment Outcome and Prognostic Factors
Tsang RW, Brierley JD, Panzarella T, Gospodarowicz MK, Sutcliffe SB, Simpson WJ (Princess Margaret Hosp, Toronto)
Int J Radiat Oncol Biol Phys 30:557–565, 1994   122-96-25–6

Introduction.—Radiation therapy (RT) is an established treatment for pituitary adenoma, although no randomized, controlled trials have assessed the efficacy of RT after initial surgical decompression. Recent reports of RT-induced brain tumors prompted a reexamination of the clinical indications for postoperative RT in patients with pituitary adenoma. Factors predicting tumor recurrence were investigated to identify high-risk patients who should receive RT.

Methods.—The records of 160 patients with a diagnosis of hormonally inactive pituitary adenoma who were treated with RT during a 14-year period were examined. Of the 160 patients, 128 received postoperative RT, 3 received RT without surgery, and 29 had tumor recurrences after previous surgery and were treated with surgery and RT in 20 cases and RT alone in 9 cases. Outcome measures for analysis included recurrence-free survival and disease- or treatment-specific mortality rates.

Results.—The 10- and 15-year local tumor control rates were 87% and 83%, respectively, for the whole study population. The 10- and 15-year local tumor control rates were 91% and 88%, respectively, for the 128 patients receiving postoperative RT for initial management and 78% and 72%, respectively, for the 29 patients treated with RT for tumor recurrence (Fig 25–1). The overall survival rates were 81% and 70%, and the cause-specific survival rates were 93% and 89% at 10 and 15 years, respectively. Age and radiation field size were significant prognostic factors, with age younger than 30 years and older than 60 years and field sizes greater than 60 cm^2 predicting increased risk of tumor recurrence. Hypopituitarism could be attributed to RT alone in up to 23% of the patients, and hypopituitarism was weakly associated with higher radiation doses.

Discussion.—Although postoperative RT caused few acute side effects, the risk of hypopituitarism was increased with RT. In addition to initial data regarding tumor grade, tumor size, suprasellar extent, and the com-

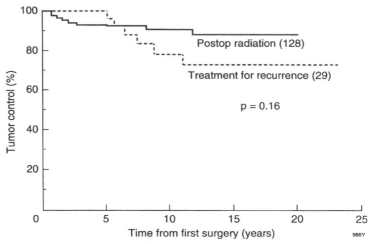

Fig 25–1.—Actuarial tumor control rate for 128 patients receiving surgery and postoperative radiation therapy as initial treatment (*solid line*) compared with the 29 patients treated for recurrence (*dashed line*). (Courtesy of Tsang RW, Brierley JD, Panzarella T, et al: *Int J Radiat Oncol Biol Phys* 30:557–565, 1994.)

pleteness of surgical removal, age, and radiation field size distinguish high- from low-risk patients. It may be feasible to delay RT in young patients after gross excision of small tumors.

▶ Although this was not a prospective, randomized study, the authors reaffirm the value of RT, especially postoperative RT, for hormonally inactive pituitary adenomas.—R.H. Wilkins, M.D.

26 Acoustic Tumors

Facial Myokymia Due to Acoustic Neurinoma
Kiriyanthan G, Krauss JK, Glocker FX, Scheremet R (Univ Hosp, Freiburg, Germany)
Surg Neurol 41:498–501, 1994   122-96-26–1

Background.—Facial myokymia (FM) is characterized by involuntary and usually unilateral wormlike, rippling movements of the facial muscles. Clinical and electrophysiologic findings of unequivocal FM caused by acoustic neurinomas are rare. A patient with FM caused by acoustic neurinoma was described.

Case Report.—Woman, 62, was evaluated for a 13-year history of progressive left-sided hearing loss and gradual progression of involuntary, rippling, wormlike movements of the left facial muscles. Neurologic examination also revealed mild paresis of the left lower facial muscles, hypesthesia of the left side of the face, and diminution of the left corneal reflex. A tumor situated in the left cerebellopontine angle was revealed on a CT scan. Typical double and triple discharges, with a frequency of 10–25 Hz, were recorded from the left orbicularis oculi muscle during electrophysiologic examination, verifying the diagnosis of FM. The tumor, which arose from the eighth cranial nerve, was completely removed using microsurgical techniques. The displacement of the trigeminal, facial, and lower cranial nerves and the brain stem by the tumor was pronounced. The facial nerve came apart during tumor removal; an end-to-end anastomosis was performed. Histopathologic examination of the tumor showed a highly regressive acoustic neurinoma. Postoperative recovery was uneventful. The patient had postoperative facial nerve paralysis, and the FM was no longer evident. The postoperative CT scan was unremarkable. At 6-week follow-up, left-sided anacusis and left facial nerve paralysis were observed. All other symptoms had resolved.

Conclusions.—Facial myokymia may be triggered by changes at 1 of the various sites along the course of the motor axons of the facial nerve. In patients with persistent and unilateral FM, the differential diagnosis should include the possibility of a posterior fossa tumor, which, although rare, could be an acoustic neurinoma.

▶ Although a vestibular schwannoma can stretch the adjacent facial nerve considerably as it grows, it ordinarily does not cause obvious facial weakness. It can, on rare occasion, cause hemifacial spasm ipsilateral to the tumor. (At least 2 cases have been described in which a tumor has caused contralateral hemifacial spasm, presumably by shifting the brain stem.) A phenomenon even more rare than ipsilateral hemifacial spasm is the occurrence of ipsilateral FM in association with an acoustic tumor, as documented by the authors.

There has been some confusion in the medical literature about the definition of FM, its etiology and pathophysiology, and its significance. Cherington and associates have noted that facial myokymia "...almost always is associated with an intramedullary brainstem lesion.... The various brainstem lesions...that have been reported with facial myokymia are: pontine glioma, multiple sclerosis,...and pontine tuberculoma" (1). However, the term *facial myokymia* has also been applied to benign fine flickering or quivering movements of individual facial muscle bundles, usually around the eyelids (2). In reports about FM, it is important to define not only the appearance of the facial movements, but also their electromyographic features. Kiriyanthan and colleagues have done this in the abstracted paper.— R.H. Wilkins, M.D.

References

1. Cherington M, Sadler KM, Ryan DW: Facial myokymia. *Surg Neurol* 11:478–480, 1979.
2. Blair RL, Berry H: Spontaneous facial movement. *J Otolaryngol* 10:459–462, 1981.

Management of the Small Acoustic Neuroma: A Decision Analysis
Telian SA (Univ of Michigan, Ann Arbor)
Am J Otol 15:358–365, 1994   122-96-26–2

Objective.—Gadolinium contrast–enhanced MRI may be able to detect small acoustic neuromas before they cause significant symptoms. Particularly if the finding is an incidental one, surgeon and patient alike may wonder whether the tumor requires any treatment. A computerized clinical decision analysis was done of the decisions facing physicians involved in the treatment of small acoustic neuromas.

Methods.—The model looked at the decisions encountered in the management of 5- to 15-mm acoustic neuromas. The decision tree created was designed to be flexible enough to consider tumor size, hearing level, and the patient's feelings about unilateral hearing loss and facial paralysis (Fig 26–1).

Findings.—Surgery at the time of diagnosis appeared to be appropriate if the tumor was expected to grow, at least unless the patient had a short life expectancy. This decision was unaffected by expected variations in surgical proficiency and patient risk aversion, especially for the smaller tumor sizes. The tumor's likelihood of growth appeared to be the most important variable.

Conclusions.—In deciding whether to operate on a patient with a small acoustic neuroma, the critical factor appears to be the likelihood that the

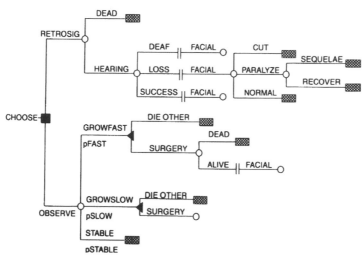

Fig 26–1.—Decision tree. *Filled squares* represent decision nodes; *open circles,* chance nodes; *cross-hatched boxes,* terminal nodes where utility functions are calculated; and *filled triangles,* Boolean nodes where either the patient dies of unrelated causes before requiring surgery or the tumor grows to a predetermined size when surgery is mandatory. At each chance node, there is a probability that this outcome will occur. This is illustrated in the *OBSERVE* subtree (e.g., *pFAST* is the probability that the tumor will grow at a fast rate). For simplicity of illustration, subtrees that appear repeatedly (e.g., *FACIAL* for facial nerve outcome) are truncated except for 1 instance. (Courtesy of Telian SA: *Am J Otol* 15:358–365, 1994.)

tumor will grow. Further studies of the growth rate of small acoustic neuromas, e.g., in patients who refuse or are considered poor candidates for surgery, are needed.

▶ The neuroradiologic detection of disease has been significantly expanded by the introduction of MRI. One of the salient aspects of this increased diagnostic sensitivity is the detection of asymptomatic lesions such as cavernous angiomas and intracanalicular acoustic tumors. As a consequence, it has become increasingly important that the natural history of such lesions be determined to help physicians and patients make correct decisions about management. In the case of an acoustic neuroma, the key questions are: What is the growth rate of the tumor and how rapidly is it likely to result in hearing loss? Although Dr. Telian has constructed a reasonable decision tree, he rightfully concludes that we need better data regarding the growth rate of small acoustic tumors to help us decide whether to treat such lesions when they are asymptomatic or simply follow them.—R.H. Wilkins, M.D.

Translabyrinthine Removal of Large Acoustic Neuromas
Briggs RJS, Luxford WM, Atkins JS Jr, Hitselberger WE (House Ear Clinic and House Ear Inst, Los Angeles; Florida Otolaryngology Group, Orlando)
Neurosurgery 34:785–791, 1994   122-96-26-3

Objective.—For patients with large acoustic neuromas, preservation of hearing generally is not a realistic surgical goal and, therefore, should not influence the choice of surgical approach. Many surgeons consider tumors measuring 4 cm or greater to be too large to remove by the translabyrinthine approach, given the limited visualization and operating room within the cerebellopontine angle. However, this approach permits early identification of the distal facial nerve and tumor removal without the need for cerebellar retraction or resection. An experience with the translabyrinthine approach to large acoustic neuromas in 167 patients was described.

Patients.—The tumors all measured at least 4 cm; the mean patient age was 43 years. Seventy-seven percent of the patients had hearing loss as their initial symptom, and approximately half had loss of the corneal reflex or facial paresthesia. On preoperative audiometry, only 20% met the "30 dB/70%" rule for good hearing. The mean duration of surgery was 4 hours, and the average blood loss was 540 mL.

Outcomes.—None of the patients died. The surgeon judged that the tumor had been totally removed in 96% of the cases. In 92%, the facial nerve was anatomically intact, and three fourths of the patients had grade IV or better facial motion at follow-up. Forty-two percent had grade I or II motion. Vascular complications occurred in 5% of the patients, CSF leak in 10%, and meningitis in 7%. Eight percent of the patients with previously normal cerebellar function had postoperative ataxia, sometimes requiring inpatient rehabilitation.

Conclusions.—For patients with large acoustic neuromas for whom there is little chance of preservation of hearing, translabyrinthine surgery may offer an effective surgical approach. Most patients achieve anatomical and functional preservation of the facial nerve. Morbidity is minimal and mortality is nil in this experience.

▶ These authors are very experienced in translabyrinthine acoustic neuroma removal, which is attested to by the mean duration of surgery for these large tumors being only 4 hours. The point is well made that large acoustic neuromas can be removed by the translabyrinthine route, with a high rate of preservation of the facial nerve, because such an approach permits identification of the distal aspect of the facial nerve early in the operation. Hearing is sacrificed by the translabyrinthine approach, but it is unlikely that hearing can be preserved in the removal of such large tumors by any other approach. The main adjustment necessary for a neurosurgeon who is used to the retrosigmoid approach to acoustic neuromas (assuming that a neurotologist provides the translabyrinthine exposure) is becoming comfortable with the relatively small size of the bony opening, which permits very little visualization of anything other than the tumor if the tumor is large. This feeling of claustrophobia is overcome with experience, and the neurosurgeon eventually becomes appreciative of the advantages of the translabyrinthine approach, which include a direct view of the tumor without a significant degree of cerebellar retraction.

I was somewhat surprised by the relatively high incidence of CSF leakage (10%) and meningitis (7%) reported by the authors. With careful and complete filling of the entire dural opening with strips of fat, and the use of a tight compressive head dressing and postoperative lumbar CSF drainage, these 2 related postoperative problems can usually be prevented.—R.H. Wilkins, M.D.

Technical Modifications to the Middle Fossa Craniotomy Approach in Removal of Acoustic Neuromas
Brackmann DE, House JR III, Histelberger WE (House Ear Clinic, Los Angeles, Calif; Jackson Ear Clinic, Miss; St Vincent Med Ctr, Los Angeles)
Am J Otol 15:614–619, 1994   122-96-26–4

Rationale.—Using the retrosigmoid approach to remove an acoustic neuroma (AN), the fundus of the internal auditory canal (IAC) is often dissected blindly, which poses a risk of not removing all the tumor tissue. Such a problem can be avoided by middle fossa craniotomy; however, exposure of the posterior fossa is limited. This approach has been increasingly used with the advent of contrast-enhanced MRI to reveal small tumors.

Technical Aspects.—A larger incision of the skin is used, and it is curved posteriorly rather than being vertical. A bone flap measuring 5 × 5 cm is developed just above the zygomatic root. Bone is drilled away in an arc of approximately 270 degrees around the porus of the IAC. Drilling anteriorly and posteriorly at the medial aspect of the IAC provides good exposure without violating the superior semicircular canal or cochlea. An attempt is made to preserve the facial nerve while removing all of the tumor under ×25 or ×40 magnification. The vestibular nerves are not cut if they are not involved by tumor. Gelfoam soaked in papaverine is placed on the cochlear nerve in the IAC and at the modiolus after the tumor has been resected.

Results.—Of 24 consecutive patients in whom these modifications of middle fossa craniotomy were used, 71% retained hearing that was almost as good as, equal to, or better than their preoperative hearing. Three other patients (12%) retained some hearing. Five of the 24 patients, 2 of whom had neurofibromatosis, had some facial weakness when last seen. One patient required drainage of a postoperative epidural hematoma.

▶ These authors, who have had an extensive experience using the middle fossa approach to small vestibular schwannomas, discuss the technical modifications they have developed to increase their ability to preserve hearing.— R.H. Wilkins, M.D.

Postoperative Headache in Acoustic Neuroma
Vijayan N (Univ of California, Sacramento)
Headache 35:98–100, 1995   122-96-26–5

Objective.—A questionnaire was sent to members of the Acoustic Neuroma Association to gather data on the incidence and nature of headache after surgery for acoustic neuroma. Although disabling postoperative headache is reported to be a major problem, there has been little information on this type of headache, its cause, and treatment.

Methods.—The questionnaire was mailed to 440 members of the association and returned by 280, including 89 men and 190 women. The information obtained included patient age, the location and severity of headache before and after surgery, clinical characteristics of the headache, methods of treatment, and prognosis.

Results.—The age of the responding patients ranged from 25 to 80 years. One hundred twenty eight of the 190 women and 70 of the 89 men were aged 40–69 years. Headache was reported by 118 patients (42%) before surgery, and 96 continued to complain of headache afterward. In 113 patients headache developed for the first time after surgery, for a total of 209 patients (75%) with postoperative headache. In general, preoperative headache tended to be frontal and temporal, whereas postoperative headache was often occipital and cervical, near the site of surgery. Postoperative headache was considerably more severe and frequently described as aching, with pressure and throbbing. Only 24% of patients experienced complete relief of headache, and improvement tended to be gradual over many years. Most patients took over-the-counter remedies, particularly anti-inflammatory agents; many were not offered specific therapy.

Conclusions.—Headache affects up to 75% of patients after surgical removal of acoustic neuroma. The cause of this problem appears to be trauma to the muscles and scalp at the site of surgery. Because most headaches were of the tension type, followed by those with neuralgic elements and vasodilatory components, potentially effective treatments included tricyclic antidepressants, muscle relaxants, and behavior modification therapy, perhaps combined with anti-inflammatory agents. Patients should be examined for spinal fluid leak or nerve entrapment, both of which can be cured with appropriate therapy.

Determinants and Impact of Headache After Acoustic Neuroma Surgery
Pedrosa CA, Ahern DK, McKenna MJ, Ojemann RG, Acquadro MA (Harvard Med School, Boston)
Am J Otol 15:793–797, 1994   122-96-26–6

Purpose.—Only recently has attention been focused on the problem of postoperative headache after surgical removal of an acoustic neuroma. Past studies have reported that the incidence of headache differs with the surgical procedure used. To determine the prevalence, duration, and impact of this form of headache and to evaluate the differences in headache patterns relative to surgical approach, 155 patients recovering from resection of an acoustic neuroma were surveyed by telephone.

Findings.—Complaints of postoperative headache after resection of acoustic neuroma were reported by 73% of the patients undergoing suboccipital resection and 53% of the patients undergoing translabyrinthine resection. Only 9% of the respondents reported having troublesome or frequent headaches preoperatively. Patients undergoing the suboccipital approach reported a greater average pain intensity. Patients described their headache most often as being similar to that caused by tension, with episodic acute exacerbations. Sixty percent of the 89 patients having recurrent headaches reported that the pain interfered with their usual activites; in most patients, pain was successfully managed with various combinations of medication, relaxation therapy, and/or physical therapy, and it generally resolved over time.

Discussion.—Several underlying mechanisms may account for headache development: injury or irritation to the dura, compromised C1 sensory rootlets, or some combination thereof in conjunction with psychosocial stress factors and behavioral dispositions for reporting pain. Recent literature suggests that headache in general is probably the result of multiple influencing factors rather than a single mechanism. The authors have been able to treat successfully most cases of postacoustic neuroma surgery headache via aggressive application of reassurance, tricyclic antidepressants, nonsteroidal anti-inflammatory drugs, trigger-point injections, adjunctive stress management techniques, and physical therapy. Further study is needed to better define the natural history and healing process of this headache, as well as to determine the optimal surgical technique for acoustic neuroma resection.

▶ The authors of these 2 papers (Abstracts 122-96-26–5 and 122-96-26–6) have performed a useful service in focusing attention on a frequent—and frequently overlooked—aspect of the surgical treatment of vestibular schwannoma: postoperative headache. There are many treatment considerations in patients who have undergone the removal of such a tumor, for example, eye protection, correction of facial weakness, adaptation to hearing loss, improvement of imbalance, etc. Postoperative headache should be addressed as well.—R.H. Wilkins, M.D.

The Long-Term Growth Rate of Residual Acoustic Neurinomas
Kameyama S, Tanaka R, Honda Y, Hasegawa A, Yamazaki H, Kawaguchi T (Niigata Univ, Japan)
Acta Neurochir (Wien) 129:127–130, 1994   122-96-26–7

Introduction.—Complete removal of acoustic neuroma (AN), even with current microsurgical techniques, often risks injury to the cochlear and facial nerves. Therefore, intracapsular removal is often performed. The natural progression of residual AN after intracapsular removal has not

TABLE 1.—Summary of Follow-Up CT Findings of 19 Residual ANs

Tumour volume	No. of Cases	Follow-up interval (median)*
Regrowth	10	5–17(13)
Regression	3	5–12 (6)
Unchanged	6	5–17(10)
	19	5–17(10)

* Years.
(Courtesy of Kameyama S, Tanaka R, Honda Y, et al: *Acta Neurochir (Wien)* 129:127–130, 1994.)

been well documented. Follow-up CT images were obtained in patients who underwent intracapsular removal of AN to determine the long-term growth rate of residual AN.

Methods.—Nineteen patients who underwent intracapsular removal of AN between 1963 and 1985 underwent follow-up with at least 2 CT scans 5–17 years after surgery. Five different CT scanners were used.

Results.—Regrowth occurred in 10 of 19 patients, 3 had regression, and 6 had no change (Table 1). Of the 10 residual tumors that grew, 5 exhibited rapid growth and 5 exhibited slow growth. The CT scans identified cystic formations in the tumors that grew quickly, whereas the tumors that grew slowly were solid (Table 2). All 5 patients with cystic tumors required follow-up surgery. Patients with solid tumors had no brain stem dysfunction or involvement with any other cranial nerves during follow-up.

Discussion.—Several factors influence the growth rate of AN, which differs before and after surgery. Preoperative growth rate is affected by age, the size of the tumor, von Recklinghausen's disease, cellularity, vascularity, atypia, necrosis, and fibrosis. However, postoperative regrowth is generally affected only by cellularity or vascularity, or both. Because a neuroma larger than 2 cm is capable of angiogenesis, surgery should

TABLE 2.—Summary of 10 Patients With a Regrowing AN

Case no.	Sex	Age at operation (yrs)	Pre-operative postoperative facial palsy	Interval of follow-up CT scan (yrs)	CT finding of the last scan	Tumour doubling time (yrs)
1	M	57	+++	5	cyst formation	4.5
2	F	41	+++	9	cyst formation	5.0
3	M	46	−−	6	cyst formation	4.8
4	F	34	−−	5	cyst formation	1.0
				0.5	cyst formation	0.15
5	M	62	+++	5	cyst formation	2.5
6	F	38	−+	13	solid	11.5
7	M	57	−−	14	solid	34.0
8	M	37	−−	17	solid	15.3
9	M	52	+++	13	solid	9.0
10	F	41	−−	15	solid	19.5

Note: +, palsy; ++, paralysis; −, intact.
(Courtesy of Kameyama S, Tanaka R, Honda Y, et al: *Acta Neurochir (Wien)* 129:127–130, 1994.)

reduce the residual AN as much as possible. Similarly, because cyst formation was always associated with rapid growth and the need for repeated surgery, as much of the tumor capsule as possible should be removed. Patients with cystic residual AN should have follow-up CT scans every 6 months.

▶ The authors have followed a series of 19 patients who had subtotal resection of an AN with CT scans to assess the growth rate of the residual tumor. During a median of 10 years, approximately half the tumors remained unchanged or regressed and half enlarged. For the tumors that recurred, cyst formation was associated with a more rapid tumor doubling time (.15–5 years) than that of tumors that enlarged without cyst formation (9–34 years). For the surgeon who has resected the majority of an AN (including most of its capsule), little is to be gained by injuring the facial nerve or destroying its anatomical continuity to completely remove an AN that is strongly adherent to the facial nerve.—R.H. Wilkins, M.D.

27 Other Intracranial Tumors

General

Surgical Implications of Magnetic Resonance-Enhanced Dura
Ahmadi J, Hinton DR, Segall HD, Couldwell WT (Univ of Southern Calif, Los Angeles)
Neurosurgery 35:370–377, 1994   122-96-27-1

Objective.—A "thickened-enhanced dura" is sometimes noted adjacent to an intracranial neoplasm on MRI. There is debate as to whether this finding represents inflammation or dural invasion; the distinction has important surgical implications, because the surgeon must decide whether to resect the "enhanced dura" to prevent or reduce the likelihood of local recurrence. The tissue changes responsible for dural enhancement and the clinical implications thereof were investigated in a prospective surgical, histopathologic, and MRI study.

Methods.—The subjects were 73 patients who had possible abnormal dural enhancement resulting from a variety of causes. Diagnoses included meningiomas in 29 patients, craniofacial tumors with possible intracranial extension in 21, gliomas and brain metastases in close proximity to the dura mater in 9, and a variety of non-neoplastic lesions in 14. Each patient underwent contrast-enhanced MRI within 5 days before operation, and some had repeat MRI within 3 days afterward. Specimens of resected or biopsied dura from all 59 patients with neoplasia and from selected patients with nonneoplastic processes were subjected to histopathologic examination.

Results.—Histopathologic examination confirmed dural invasion in 18 of 29 meningiomas, 15 of 21 craniofacial neoplasms, 3 of 5 gliomas, and 3 of 4 brain metastases. In each case, the dural invasion was focal and directly continuous with the tumor. On MRI, the invaded dura showed either a break in the continuity of dural enhancement or no discernible enhancement; the association between patterns of dural enhancement and tumor invasion was significant. Thickening and enhancement of the dura on MRI corresponded to reactive changes. There were some false negative findings of dural invasion, involving 4 intracranial neoplasms and 1 extracranial neoplasm. After surgery, postoperative enhancement was noted as early as 24 hours; the histologic findings in these cases showed vasodilation and reactive changes.

Conclusions.—The MRI finding of dural enhancement is a nonspecific one that may be noted in many pathologic conditions. A dural inflammatory reaction appears as a fairly uniform "enhanced dura" adjacent to a tumor; dural invasion usually appears as a discontinuous dural enhancement. There are some false negative findings, underscoring the limitations of contrast-enhanced MRI in predicting dural invasion.

▶ When the MRI appearance of dural enhancement adjacent to a neoplasm was first noted, this dural "tail" was thought to represent tumor invasion of the dura. Since then, exemplified by this report, this sign has been found to be a nonspecific phenomenon.—R.H. Wilkins, M.D.

Electrocardiographic Changes in Patients With Brain Tumors
Koepp M, Kern A, Schmidt D (Universitätsklinikum Rudolf Virchow, Berlin; Freie Universität, Berlin)
Arch Neurol 52:152–155, 1995   122-96-27–2

Objective.—In retrospective study of 85 patients who had brain tumors, the incidence of ECG changes was determined, and abnormal ECG results were correlated with the site of the cerebral lesion. A previous study reported ECG abnormalities in 56% of patients who had intracerebral tumors.

Patients and Methods.—The 85 patients were part of a group of 169 consecutive patients with brain tumors who underwent surgery between January 1985 and June 1989. Fifty-seven were excluded from this analysis because of preexisting conditions or use of drugs that might influence findings; an additional 27 patients were not included because neuroimaging showed multiple lesions or suggested raised intracranial pressure. Each tumor was assigned to 1 of 14 anatomical regions and classified as limbic system (25), frontal (23), temporoparieto-occipital (27), or brain stem/cerebellum (10) tumors.

Results.—The average patient age was 47.7 years. Thirty-four (40%) had an abnormal ECG. A prolonged QT interval was present in 10, including 8 of the patients who had limbic system tumors. Eight of the 10 cases of sinus bradycardia/sinus tachycardia also occurred in the limbic system tumor group. Eight patients had abnormal U waves, 7 had arrhythmias, 6 had displaced ST segments, and 4 had abnormal T waves. Among patients who had limbic system lesions, those who had epilepsy (85%) were more likely to have ECG abnormalities than those who did not have epilepsy (58%). For the group as a whole, however, abnormal ECG activity was present in 33% of patients who had epilepsy vs. 45% of those who did not have epilepsy.

Conclusion.—The ECG changes in otherwise healthy patients who had brain tumors and no evidence of increased intracranial pressure occurred most often when tumors were located within the limbic system (72%) rather than at extralimbic locations (27%), suggesting that the limbic system is directly involved in the regulation of cardiac function. The presence of ECG changes was not related to surgical or postoperative outcome.

▶ It is well known that patients with a ruptured intracranial aneurysm frequently will have ECG abnormalities that may, at times, suggest myocardial infarction. Koepp and associates remind us that ECG changes also may occur in otherwise healthy patients with brain tumors, emphasizing the close associations between the brain and heart (1, 2), as reflected in the development of a field of study entitled *neurocardiology* (3).—R.H. Wilkins, M.D.

References

1. Loewy AD, Spyer KM: *Central Regulation of Autonomic Functions.* Oxford, Oxford University Press, 1990.
2. Talman WT: Cardiovascular regulation and lesions of the central nervous system. *Ann Neurol* 18:1–13, 1985.
3. Skinner JE: Neurocardiology: Brain mechanisms underlying fatal cardiac arrhythmias. *Neurol Clin* 11:325–351, 1993.

Microvessel Count and Cerebrospinal Fluid Basic Fibroblast Growth Factor in Children With Brain Tumours

Li VW, Folkerth RD, Watanabe H, Yu C, Rupnick M, Barnes P, Scott RM, Black PM, Sallan SE, Folkman J (Dana-Farber Cancer Inst, Boston; Children's Hosp, Boston; Harvard Medical School, Boston; et al)
Lancet 344:82–86, 1994   122-96-27–3

Background.—Angiogenesis is necessary for solid tumor growth. Brain tumors are known to produce basic fibroblast growth factor (bFGF), a potent angiogenic molecule. Therefore, CSF from 26 children with brain tumors and 18 controls was examined for biologically active bFGF.

Methods.—The CSF samples were tested for bFGF by immunoassay. The ability of samples to stimulate proliferation was assessed on cultured capillary endothelial cells. The density of microvessels was assessed in a blinded manner by immunohistochemical staining of tumor sections.

Results.—Basic fibroblast growth factor was not detected in any of the control CSF samples. However, bFGF was detected in 62% of the CSF samples from patients with brain tumors (table). The CSF samples containing bFGF stimulated proliferation of capillary endothelial cells. This proliferative response was blocked by antibodies to bFGF. The presence of bFGF was significantly correlated with the in vitro mitogenic activity of CSF samples and the density of microvessels in histologic tumor sections. A high tumor microvessel count was associated with both recurrence and mortality.

Conclusions.—These results suggest that bFGF is an angiogenic mediator found in the CSF of patients with brain tumors. Therefore, bFGF has the potential to serve as a clinical marker for neural neoplasia and as a

Summary of Results

Assay	Result	p	n
bFGF concentration (immunoassay)	bFGF is elevated in the CSF of 62% of brain tumour patients and is not present in the CSF of controls.	≤ 0.0001	44
	bFGF ≥ 30 pg/mL is associated with tumour recurrence.	0.1	17
Endothelial cell stimulation (DNA synthesis) in vitro	CSF from patients with brain tumours has higher biological activity than CSF from control donors.	≤ 0.0001	24
	bFGF level in CSF correlates with biological activity in vitro (Spearman $\gamma = 0.87$) in newly diagnosed patients.	≤ 0.0001	16
Neutralising antibody studies (anti-bFGF 3H3)	Endothelial proliferative activity in vitro in brain tumour CSF is inhibited by 55% to 82%.	≤ 0.001	6
Tumour microvessel density (Factor VIII or CD34 stain)	Microvessel density (per 200 × field) correlates with bFGF level in CSF (Spearman $\gamma = 0.64$)	≤ 0.005	17
	Microvessel density (per 200 × field) correlates with stimulation of endothelial cells by CSF in vitro (Spearman $\gamma = 0.59$)	≤ 0.02	16
	Microvessel density of ≥ 68 (per 200 × field) is associated with tumour recurrence.	0.005	17
	Microvessel density of ≥ 68 (per 200 × field) is associated with mortality.	0.02	17

(Courtesy of Li VW, Folkerth RD, Watanabe H, et al: *Lancet* 344:822–86, 1994.)

therapeutic target. It is also possible that evaluation of the presence of bFGF in CSF and of microvessel quantity in histologic sections may provide prognostic information for the management of patients with brain tumors.

▶ Dr Folkman has had an interest in tumor angiogenesis for many years, both from the standpoint of understanding how tumors invade tissues and grow, and as a potential target for treatment. This article presents the results of a well-designed study of one growth factor with angiogenic properties in relation to brain tumors in childhood.—R.H. Wilkins, M.D.

Brain Tumors in Children: Long-Term Survival After Radiation Treatment

Jenkin D, Greenberg M, Hoffman H, Hendrick B, Humphreys R, Vatter A (Toronto-Bayview Regional Cancer Ctr, Canada; Hosp for Sick Children, Univ of Toronto; et al)
Int J Radiat Oncol Biol Phys 31:445–451, 1995   122-96-27–4

Introduction.—Many studies of treatment for brain tumors in children do not report the results beyond 10 years after diagnosis. Most long-term survival data in these patients come from registries. A 33-year review was conducted to determine the long-term survival of children with brain

TABLE 1.—Survival Rates at 5, 10, 20, and 30 Years For All Patients and For Individual Tumor Types

Tumor type	N	5	10	20	30
			% Survival years		
All	912	51	44	37	26
Astrocytoma					
low grade	112	64	57	46	
high grade	92	34	28	19	
Medulloblastoma	187	55	47	41	
Brain stem	132	24	20	17	
Ependymoma	85	44	29	29	
Basal ganglia	66	50	41	41	
Germ cell	48	66	63	54	
Optic glioma	37	100	85	68	
Glioma (clinical)	32	74	67	59	

(Courtesy of Jenkin D, Greenberg M, Hoffman H, et al: *Int J Radiat Oncol Biol Phys* 31:445–451, 1995.)

tumors, focusing on the causes of death among patients who survived for longer than 5 years after radiation treatment.

Methods.—The analysis included 929 children with primary brain tumors treated from 1958 to 1991. The institutions at which the children were treated had the only radiation resources in the Toronto metropolitan area for the years considered. There were 912 evaluable patients; complete radiation treatment data were available for 90%. Three hundred seventy-seven children lived for more than 5 years.

Results.—Overall survival was 44% at 10 years and 37% at 20 years (Table 1); relapse-free survival was 44% and 42%, respectively. Among 5-year survivors, 83% of subsequent deaths resulted from inadequate

TABLE 2.—Causes of Death More Than 5 Years From Diagnosis for All Patients and for Individual Tumor Types

				5-year survivors						
				Cause of death					% Survival (yrs)	
Tumor type	N	Later deaths	Disease	Toxicity	SMT	Trauma	Other	Unknown	10	20
All	377	83	67	2	10	2	1	1	78	67
Astrocytoma	63	15	14	—	1	—	—	—	76	72
—low grade*										
—high grade	30	12	8	1	3	—	—	—	68	49
Medulloblastoma	91	16	13	—	2	1	—	—	80	74
Brain stem†	25	5	3	1	—	—	1	—	87	71
Ependymoma	25	8	8	—	—	—	—	—	67	67
Basal ganglia†	23	5	4	—	1	—	—	—	81	60
Germ cell	24	3	3	—	—	—	—	—	82	—
Optic glioma	29	7	7	—	—	—	—	—	85	68
Glioma (clinical)‡	22	6	4	—	1	—	—	1	86	71

Note: Ten- and 20-year survival rates are given for 5-year survivors measured from the fifth year from diagnosis.
* Excludes astrocytomas of the brain stem or basal ganglia and optic glioma.
† With or without a histologic diagnosis.
‡ No histology. Any site other than brain stem or basal ganglia and optic glioma.
Abbreviation: SMT, second malignant tumor.
(Courtesy of Jenkin D, Greenberg M, Hoffman H, et al: *Int J Radiat Oncol Biol Phys* 31:445–451, 1995.)

TABLE 3.—The Cause of Death in Patients Who Died Before and After 5 Years From Diagnosis

Cause of death	Before 5 years Number of deaths (%)	After 5 years Number of deaths (%)
"Disease"	419 (97)	67 (81)
Toxicity	1 (0.2)	2 (2)
Second malignant tumor	1 (0.2)	10 (12)
Trauma	1 (0.2)	2 (2)
Other	3 (1)	1 (1)
Unknown	7 (2)	1 (1)
Total	432	83

(Courtesy of Jenkin D, Greenberg M, Hoffman H, et al: *Int J Radiat Oncol Biol Phys* 31:445–451, 1995.)

control or relapse of the original tumor or postoperative complications (Table 2). Ten-year survival after relapse was 9% for patients whose first relapse occurred within 1 year after diagnosis, compared with 17% when relapse occurred within 1–2 years, and 31% when relapse occurred after 3 or more years. At 30 years after diagnosis, the cumulative actuarial incidence of second malignancies was 18%. Incidence of death from these malignancies was 13% (Table 3).

Conclusions.—Children with primary brain tumors commonly die more than 5 years after diagnosis. Most of these deaths result from progressive disease in patients with slowly evolving low-grade tumors. Beyond 15 years after diagnosis, death is more likely to result from a second malignancy than from the original tumor. There is no overall survival advantage for children treated since 1975 (i.e., the modern neurosurgery era).

▶ The authors have conducted a thorough analysis of long-term survival of a large and fairly homogeneous population of children whose treatment for a brain tumor included radiation therapy. It is evident that a significant percentage of children treated for a brain tumor live for many years and that these individuals will require prolonged management of their original tumor, as well as management of complications of treatment and second malignant tumors.—R.H. Wilkins, M.D.

Gliomas

Lightning Injury and Glioma
Cherington M, Yarnell PR, Todd HM (St Anthony Hosp, Denver, Colo; Fort Lauderdale, Fla)
Injury 25:687–688, 1994   122-96-27–5

Introduction.—A patient who had been struck by lightning died of a glioma about 1 year later.

Case Report.—Woman, 64, was struck by lightning while horseback riding. She lost consciousness and was revived by CPR. The results of CT and MRI scans were normal. One year later, she had nausea and complained of unusual smells. Magnetic resonance imaging revealed a 3- to 4-cm mass lesion centered at the right basal ganglia. Histopathologic analysis of samples obtained by stereotactic biopsy revealed a glioblastoma multiforme. She died 1 month after diagnosis.

Discussion.—Delayed neurologic complications can occur after high-voltage electric trauma, (e.g., lightning). Complications include parkinsonism, seizure, myelopathy, motor neuron disease, post-traumatic syndrome, and progressive cerebellar syndrome. It is not known how these complications develop. The development of a glioma in a patient who had lightning encephalopathy might be a tragic coincidence. However, there might be a connection between cancer and exposure to a high-voltage electric current.

▶ As an isolated incident, the case reported in this article does not prove a cause-and-effect relationship between lightning injury and glioma; however, the article does add to the expanding body of knowledge about the possible oncogenetic properties of electromagnetic fields.—R.H. Wilkins, M.D.

MR Imaging in Cerebral Gliomas: Tissue Component Analysis in Correlation with Histopathology of Whole-Brain Specimen

Tovi M, Hartman M, Lilja A, Ericsson A (Univ Hosp, Uppsala, Sweden)
Acta Radiol 35:495–505, 1994   122-96-27-6

Introduction.—There are interpretive difficulties in correlating MR images and histopathologic findings in primary brain tumors. A comparative analysis was done between MR examinations and histopathologic whole brain specimens in 5 patients with malignant glial brain tumors.

Methods.—The mean patient age was 50.2 years. Histopathology and in vitro MRI was performed for all 5 brain specimens. A comparative analysis was possible between findings of the intravital MR, postmortem MR, and histopathologic whole-brain specimens in cases 4 and 5.

Case Report.—Woman, 28, had a grade III–IV astrocytoma, 5 cm in diameter, in the medial aspects of the temporal lobe that was diagnosed 2 years before her death. Palisading and micronecrosis were found in the most hypercellular region only in this patient. Hemorrhagic and necrotic features were more pronounced in the ventrally located tumor part.

Results.—Identification of the heterogeneous components of the hypercellular core was possible during in vivo MRI only in T2-weighted imaging (T2WI). However, in vitro MRI identified these tumor parts by T1-, T2-, and proton density-weighted imaging. In all except case 2, distant tumor spread of benign-appearing cells was found in areas depicted as normal on T2WI, outside the margins of the peritumoral edema. A sample from the white matter in the temporal lobe in case 4 showed the largest presence of antigenic sites to albumin. Samples of gray and nonedematous white matter, depicted as nonedematous on MRI and histopathologic examination, showed a larger water content in gray than in white matter. Non-edematous white matter from cases 3 and 4 showed no presence of antigenic sites to albumin.

Conclusion.—Magnetic resonance imaging is capable of reflecting underlying heterogeneous histopathologic composition in malignant glioma lesions. However, malignant gliomas cannot be properly delineated using MRI.

▶ Peter Burger and others have correlated the features of malignant cerebral gliomas seen on axial CT slices with those of comparable postmortem whole-brain slices from the same patients, as studied histologically (1, 2). This study is similar, but the pathologic correlations are with MRI. Although data were collected from only 5 patients, the authors have made useful observations. They concluded that the most homogeneous hypercellular area in malignant gliomas, giving the highest tumor grade, is not visualized on MRI as an isolated entity, either during life or after death. Heterogeneous signal patterns from accompanying tumor features, such as hemorrhage and necrosis, can override the signal pattern produced by homogeneous hypercellularity alone. In agreement with the conclusions of previous pathologic and clinical studies by others, tumor cells infiltrate the brain in areas beyond the limits of abnormality noted on CT or MRI.—R.H. Wilkins, M.D.

References

1. Burger PC, Dubois PJ, Schold SC Jr, et al: Computerized tomographic and pathologic studies of the untreated, quiescent, and recurrent glioblastoma multiforme. *J Neurosurg* 58:159–169, 1983.
2. Burger PC, Heinz ER, Shibata T, et al: Topographic anatomy and CT correlations in the untreated glioblastoma multiforme. *J Neurosurg* 68:698–704, 1988.

Tectal Plate Gliomas: II. CT Scans and MR Imaging of Tectal Gliomas
Bognar L, Turjman F, Villanyi E, Mottolese C, Guyotat J, Fischer C, Jouvet A, Lapras Cl (Hosp Pierre Wertheimer of Lyon, France)
Acta Neurochir (Wien) 127:48–54, 1994   122-96-27-7

Objective.—The neuroradiologic findings were reviewed in 12 patients, seen in a 15-year period, who had gliomas of the tectal plate. Seven lesions were low-grade astrocytomas, and 2 were high-grade astrocytomas. There were single cases of oligodendroglioma, oligoastrocytoma, and ependymoma.

Findings.—Hydrocephalus was demonstrated by CT scanning in all cases, and abnormalities of the quadrigeminal plate were seen in 7 patients. Three lesions exhibited tectal calcifications. In 5 cases the tumor was partially enhanced. Three of the gliomas had a cystic component. All 9 MR studies demonstrated a distorted tectum. On T1-weighted sequences, the lesions appeared isointense or hypointense with the corpus callosum. All 5 postcontrast images showed enhancement, and the tectum was consistently increased in intensity on T2-weighted images. Six lesions were exophytic, whereas 2 infiltrated the tegmentum.

Conclusions.—An intrinsic tectal tumor is likely to be a low-grade astrocytoma that may be followed by MRI. An exophytic tectal tumor must be distinguished from a tumor of the pineal region.

▶ This is the second in a three-part series (1, 2) concerning tectal plate gliomas, from the Department of Neurosurgery of Hospital Pierre Werthe-imer of Lyon, France. The authors have also published information about other aspects of these tumors in other journals—for example, in *Neurosurgery* (3).—R.H. Wilkins, M.D.

References

1. Bognar L, Fischer C, Turjman F, et al: Tectal plate gliomas: Part III. Apparent lack of auditory consequences of unilateral inferior collicular lesion due to localized glioma surgery. *Acta Neurochir (Wien)* 127:161–165, 1994.
2. Lapras C, Bognar L, Turjman F, et al: Tectal plate gliomas: Part I. Microsurgery of the tectal plate gliomas. *Acta Neurochir (Wien)* 126:76–83, 1994.
3. Fischer C, Bognar L, Turjman F, et al: Auditory early- and middle-latency evoked potentials in patients with quadrigeminal plate tumors. *Neurosurgery* 35:45–51, 1994.

Low-Grade Glial Neoplasms and Intractable Partial Epilepsy: Efficacy of Surgical Treatment

Britton JW, Cascino GD, Sharbrough FW, Kelly PJ (Mayo Clinic, Rochester, Minn)
Epilepsia 35:1130–1135, 1994   122-96-27-8

Introduction.—In 10% to 30% of patients undergoing surgery for medically refractory seizures, the cause of partial epilepsy is primary brain tumors. Most of these tumors are low-grade glial neoplasms. They are best identified by MRI, and their detection has a direct impact on the diagnostic and operative approach. Resection of the tumor may significantly reduce the seizure tendency of such patients. The long-term efficacy of epilepsy surgery for patients with refractory partial seizures associated with low-grade intracerebral neoplasms was assessed retrospectively.

Methods.—The patients underwent surgery over a 6-year period. All had partial seizures that were refractory to medical treatment and a mass lesion detected on neuroimaging studies. The mean patient age at surgery was 27 years, and the mean time from the onset of seizures to detection of the tumor was 9 years. Thirty-four patients underwent surgical extirpation of the lesion with resection of the epileptogenic cortex; 17 had lesionec-tomy. The patients were followed up for a mean of 4 years after surgery.

Results.—At follow-up, two thirds of the patients were free of seizures. Eighty-eight percent had at least an 80% reduction in frequency of sei-zures, and 31% were able to stop taking antiepileptic drugs. Of 31 eligible patients, 25 were able to obtain a driver's license after successful surgery. The outcomes were best for patients who had complete tumor resection and no interictal epileptiform activity on postoperative EEG. For selected patients with intractable tumor-associated epilepsy, surgery yielded long-term improvements in seizure control and quality of life.

Conclusions.—For patients with intractable seizures related to low-grade intracerebral tumors, excision of the tumor may have beneficial long-term effects on seizure tendency. These benefits may accrue even in patients with a long history of medically refractory seizures. For patients with intractable tumor-associated partial epilepsy, surgery remains an important treatment alternative.

▶ These authors studied a series of 51 consecutive patients who were surgically treated for intractable partial epilepsy related to low-grade intracerebral neoplasms. They document the value of this approach in terms of reduction or cessation of seizures, successful discontinuation of antiepileptic medication, and return to driving.—R.H. Wilkins, M.D.

Low-Grade Gliomas of the Cerebral Hemispheres in Children: An Analysis of 71 Cases
Pollack IF, Claassen D, Al-Shboul Q, Janosky JE, Deutsch M (Univ of Pittsburgh School of Medicine, Pa; Children's Hosp of Pittsburgh, Pa)
J Neurosurg 82:536–547, 1995   122-96-27–9

Objective.—Experience with low-grade cerebral hemispheric gliomas was reviewed in 71 children with astrocytomas, oligoastrocytomas, or oligodendrogliomas seen between 1956 and 1991.

Patients and Management.—Twenty-three of the 71 patients were younger than 5 years of age when given a diagnosis. The most common feature seen was seizure. Nearly half of the children had focal abnormalities, but only 6 children had severe neurologic deficits. Recent patients had CT or MRI preoperatively. Resection was considered complete in 21 cases and nearly complete in 12 others. Thirty-eight children had subtotal resection.

Outcome.—Only 7 patients died during a median follow-up of over 8 years. Five deaths resulted from progressive disease, and 1 resulted from perioperative complications. Thirteen patients have had confirmed progression of disease. Of 70 patients who survived the perioperative period, 79% were living without disease at 10 years and 76% at 20 years. The only factor that on multivariate analysis correlated independently with progression-free survival was the extent of resection. Radiotherapy did not significantly improve overall survival. Fifteen children had significant cognitive problems related to treatment, and 10 had intermittent seizures. Three patients given radiotherapy had anaplastic changes develop near the site of the original tumor, and irradiated children also were at increased risk of late cognitive and endocrine dysfunction.

Recommendations.—Low-grade hemispheric gliomas in children generally have an excellent long-term prognosis, especially when totally resected. Radiotherapy presently is deferred if aggressive resection is possible, even if a small amount of tumor is left in place. Occasional patients, younger than 6 years of age, who have progressive disease despite extensive resection should receive chemotherapy. Older patients generally should receive focal conventional radiotherapy. In selected patients, residual or progressive disease may be removed a second time.

▶ This study emphasizes that children who are treated for a low-grade hemispheric glioma are expected to live for many years. Treatment must be tailored not only to the best control of tumor growth but also to the avoidance of long-term complications of treatment.—R.H. Wilkins, M.D.

Treatment of Malignant Gliomas Using Ganciclovir-Hypersensitive, Ribonucleotide Reductase-Deficient Herpes Simplex Viral Mutant
Mineta T, Rabkin SD, Martuza RL (Georgetown Univ Med Ctr, Washington, DC)
Cancer Res 54:3963–3966, 1994   122-96-27–10

Introduction.—Despite therapeutic advances, the prognosis for patients with malignant brain tumors has not improved dramatically; the 5-year survival for glioblastoma multiforme is still no better than 5.5%. This situation has prompted the use of genetically engineered viruses in novel treatment approaches. In a previous study, attenuated mutants of herpes simplex virus (HSV) were shown to have therapeutic potential for malignant brain tumors. A ribonucleotide reductase-deficient (RR⁻) HSV mutant was tested as an experimental treatment for these tumors.

Methods.—The study used the HSV-RR⁻ mutant hrR3. This mutant contains an *Escherichia coli* lacZ gene insertion in the *ICP6* gene that encodes the large subunit of RR. In vitro experiments were performed to assess the cytopathic effect of hrR3, 0.1 plaque-forming unit/cell, on the human glioblastoma cell line U-87MG. In vivo studies were also done, in which athymnic BALB/c-*nu/nu* mice with U-87MG tumors were randomized to receive intraneoplastic treatment with either hrR3, 5 × 10⁶ plaque-forming units, or medium alone.

Results.—In the in vitro studies, just 0.2% of U-87 cells were alive 67 hours after infection with hrR3. Hypersentivity of hrR3 to ganciclovir was documented on drug sensitivity assays. In the mouse studies, animals treated with hrR3 showed significant inhibition of tumor growth (Fig 27–1). The treated tumors showed expression of the *lacZ* gene in hrR3, as visualized by 5-bromo-4-chrolo-3-indolyl-β-D-galactopyranoside histochemistry.

Conclusions.—The HSV-RR⁻ mutant hrR3 destroys human glioblastoma cells both in vitro and in vivo. Understanding of the mechanism of HSV tumor therapy requires further characterization of viral spread with HSV mutants containing *lacZ*. Clinical application of this therapy will require examination of different attenuated HSV strains and mutants affecting neurovirulence.

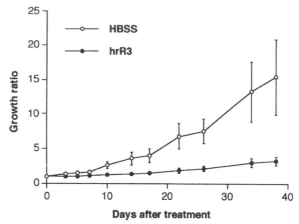

Fig 27–1.—Subconfluent U-87MG tumor growth in BALB/c-*nu/nu* mice. Mice harboring subconfluent U-87MG tumors (> 6 mm in diameter, 3 weeks post implantation) were treated with either 5×10^6 hrR3 on days 0 and 10 or control medium (n = 5/group). The mean tumor growth rate was significantly inhibited in hrR3-treated tumors compared with control tumors treated with medium alone. (Courtesy of Mineta T, Rabkin SD, Martuza RL: *Cancer Res* 54:3963–3966, 1994.)

▶ As indicated by this report, Dr. Martuza and his colleagues are continuing their important investigations into the treatment of glioblastoma multiforme with genetically engineered viruses. This approach, several variations of which are currently being studied by divers investigative teams, has real potential for curing patients with this fatal disease.—R.H. Wilkins, M.D.

Radiation Necrosis or Glioma Recurrence: Is Computer-Assisted Stereotactic Biopsy Useful?
Forsyth PA, Kelly PJ, Cascino TL, Scheithauer BW, Shaw EG, Dinapoli RP, Atkinson EJ (Mayo Clinic and Mayo Found, Rochester, Minn)
J Neurosurg 82:436–444, 1995   122-96-27–11

Objective.—Stereotactic biopsy was performed in 51 patients with supratentorial glioma who had received external beam irradiation but had clinical or radiographic evidence of progressive disease develop, in an attempt to distinguish between recurrent tumor and radiation necrosis.

Patients.—Forty of the original tumors (78%) were low-grade (Kernohan grade 1 or 2) lesions. Diffuse or fibrillary astrocytoma was present in 41% of patients, oligoastrocytoma in 33%, and oligodendroglioma in 26%. Radical subtotal resection was performed in 7 patients, subtotal resection in 20, and biopsy only in 24. All patients then received external beam radiotherapy, the median total dose being 59.5 Gy. The median time from initial surgery to stereotactic biopsy was 28 months.

Results.—The tumor types found at the time of biopsy were similar to those present initially, but only 37% of tumors remained low-grade. Thirty patients had biopsy findings of recurrent tumor only, 3 had changes of radiation necrosis, and 17 had both recurrent tumor and radiation necrosis. One patient had a radiation-related chondroblastic osteosarcoma. Seventy-three percent of patients had died of progressive disease at last follow-up. Eight of the 14 surviving patients were severely disabled. All patients with radiation necrosis alone survived. Those with recurrent tumor only had a median survival of 0.8 year compared with 1.9 years for those having both recurrent tumor and radionecrosis. High-grade tumor was an adverse prognostic factor.

Conclusion.—Stereotactic biopsy is a useful means of evaluating patients with glioma who may have progressive disease after initial surgical treatment.

▶ Patients who receive radiation therapy for a brain tumor will often have clinical and radiologic evidence of worsening develop after an initial period of improvement or stability. In these individuals, the cause of the decline is usually either further growth and/or increasing malignancy of the tumor or radiation necrosis. Despite the fact that a stereotactic biopsy provides only a small sample of the affected tissue, the value of this approach as a guide to prognosis and further treatment is shown in this study by Dr. Forsyth and his colleagues.—R.H. Wilkins, M.D.

Prognostic Significance of Flow Cytometry Deoxyribonucleic Acid Analysis of Human Astrocytomas
Coons SW, Johnson PC, Pearl DK (Barrow Neurological Inst, Phoenix, Ariz; Ohio State Univ, Columbus)
Neurosurgery 35:119–126, 1994   122-96-27–12

Background.—The value of assessing gross DNA content abnormalities by flow cytometry (FCM) ploidy analysis in predicting the survival of patients with astrocytomas has been equivocal. The FCM analysis of one series with ploidy and cell cycle analysis was reported.

Methods.—The DNA ploidy and proliferative activity were determined by FCM in 230 astrocytomas. Relationships among survival, ploidy, proliferation, histologic features, and clinical variables were tested.

Findings.—Multivariate analysis confirmed that S-phase fraction, ploidy, age at diagnosis, extent of surgery, and sex were independently significant prognostic indicators. Three patient groups with significantly different survival rates were identified according to S-phase fraction ranges of less than 3%, 3% to 5.9%, and 6% or more.

Conclusions.—The strong association between S-phase fraction and survival confirms the importance of quantitative proliferation assays in predicting tumor behavior. It also shows that specific reference ranges can be defined for clinical application. The weaker relationship between ploidy and survival casts doubt on the value of determining ploidy with FCM.

▶ In his discussion of this paper, David Hinton made several points (1). First, in their analysis of a large number of specimens, Coons et al. have provided convincing evidence that flow cytometry is an independent prognostic indicator for nonpilocytic primary astrocytic tumors. Second, they demonstrated that the S-phase fraction has value as a prognostic indicator in both low-grade and high-grade astrocytoma. Third, the authors found no association between aneuploidy and survival, but they did find an increased percentage of near-diploid cells to be correlated with worse prognosis. Finally, analysis of flow cytometry requires an experienced laboratory; other measures of proliferative activity, such as Ki-67 immunoreactivity, are more practical in routine practice.—R.H. Wilkins, M.D.

Reference

1. Hinton, DR: Comment. *Neurosurgery* 35:126, 1994.

Treatment Options and Prognosis for Multicentric Juvenile Pilocytic Astrocytoma
Mamelak AN, Prados MD, Obana WG, Cogen PH, Edwards MSB (Neuro-Oncology Service of the Brain Tumor Research Ctr, San Francisco; Univ of Calif, San Francisco)
J Neurosurg 81:24–30, 1994   122-96-27–13

Background.—Juvenile pilocytic astrocytoma (JPA) is a relatively benign variant of astrocytoma that rarely spreads in the craniospinal axis. Even subtotal resection, with adjuvant radiotherapy, has yielded 20-year survival rates as high as 80%. Nevertheless, the lesion frequently recurs, and it occasionally behaves agressively.

Series.—The risk of multicentric spread was examined in a series of 90 patients who, in 1986–1992, received a primary diagnosis of JPA. Thirty-three tumors were in or near the hypothalamic region, including the optic chiasm and third ventricle. Many of the others involved the cerebellum.

Course and Management.—Eleven of the 90 patients (12%) had multicentric disease develop. Their median age at the time the primary tumor was found was 16 months. All but one of these patients had a primary tumor in the hypothalamic region. Two patients had multicentric disease when initially diagnosed. Five of the 11 patients with multicentric spread had had subtotal resection of the primary tumor, and 5 had biopsies. Six of the 8 children aged 5 years or younger and 1 adult patient received chemotherapy. In 8 of the 11 patients, disease progressed within 2 years of initial diagnosis. Five patients had disease at more than one site in the craniospinal axis. Multicentric disease stabilized or regressed in 7 patients after a median follow-up of 31 months.

Implications.—All patients with JPA involving the hypothalamic region should undergo MRI of the craniospinal axis each year, especially for the first 5 years after diagnosis. A solitary metastatic nodule that is acessible may be grossly removed, and either chemotherapy or radiotherapy should be administered.

▶ The authors call attention to the fact that some JPAs (11 of 90 in their series) develop multicentric spread. The incidence of this phenomenon is greater than previously recognized.—R.H. Wilkins, M.D.

Survival After Stereotactic Biopsy and Irradiation of Cerebral Nonana-plastic, Nonpilocytic Astrocytoma
Lunsford LD, Somaza S, Kondziolka D, Flickinger JC (Univ of Pittsburgh, Pa; Presbyterian-Univ Hosp, Pittsburgh, Pa)
J Neurosurg 82:523–529, 1995   122-96-27–14

Background.—Nonanaplastic, nonpilocytic astrocytomas are found in young adults, peaking in the third decade of life. They make up about 15% of operatively diagnosed brain tumors. Early detection and treatment may promote survival, but there is no agreement on the efficacy of cytoreductive surgery or radiotherapy.

Series.—The results of stereotactic biopsy and radiotherapy were examined in 35 consecutive adults seen between 1982 and 1992 with nonanaplastic, nonpilocytic astrocytomas, whose median age at the time of presentation was 32 years.

Management.—All patients underwent stereotactic biopsy and received fractionated external-beam radiotherapy. The treatment volume was based on the CT or MR findings and included a margin of 2–3 cm. The median total dose was 56 Gy in 31 fractions, delivered over 5½ weeks. Two patients also received intracavitary irradiation with radiophosphorus.

Results.—After an average follow-up of approximately 4 years, 60% of surviving patients had a Karnofsky Performance Scale rating of 90 or 100, and 4 patients had a rating less than 70. Nearly 70% of patients remained able to work at full capacity. Six patients (17%) had delayed transformation to a malignant glial neoplasm and died as a result. Three patients died of unrelated causes. Only 3 patients required delayed cytoreductive surgery. The median survival time after the onset of symptoms was 148 months, and after biopsy, 118 months.

Conclusions.—All patients who are clinically suspected of having an astrocytoma should definitively be given a diagnosis. Those without significant mass effect need not undergo cytoreductive surgery.

▶ The treatment of nonanaplastic, nonpilocytic astrocytomas has generated considerable controversy. This study does not settle the issue of which form of therapy is best, but it does analyze the outcome of 35 patients managed in one way.

Astrocytomas of this sort grow slowly without treatment, so any form of treatment must be evaluated over many years. Ideally, the results of any treatment should be compared with those of no treatment in identical populations of patients who are randomly assigned to either the treatment group or control group immediately after the diagnosis is established, and who are then followed for at least 20 years. Because such stringent requirements are almost impossible to fulfill, treatment decisions are usually based on uncontrolled studies, such as the one summarized in this abstract.—R.H. Wilkins, M.D.

Complete Regression of Anaplastic Astrocytoma by Intravenous Tumor Necrosis Factor-Alpha (TNFα) After Recurrence: A Case Report

Maruno M, Yoshimine T, Nakata H, Nishioka K, Kato A, Hayakawa T (Osaka Univ, Japan; Ohno Mem Hosp, Japan)
Surg Neurol 41:482–485, 1994   122-96-27–15

Case Report.—Man, 61, had a Jacksonian seizure starting in the right upper limb and was admitted with a mild right hemiparesis. A tumor was detected in the left parieto-occipital region, and stereotactic biopsy revealed an anaplastic astrocytoma. The patient was given 55 Gy as well as 130 mg of ACNU, but the hemiparesis subsequently increased and a Gerstmann syndrome developed. Magnetic resonance imaging confirmed enlargement of the lesion, and a second biopsy confirmed recurrent tumor. When symptoms continued to progress, the patient was given human tumor necrosis factor-alpha (TNF-α) intravenously starting in a daily dose of 5,000 Japan Reference Units for 5 days. A dose of 10,000 units daily, 5 days a week, was then given for 5 weeks. The enhanced lesion became markedly smaller. Intratumoral injections of TNF-α were given twice weekly for 2 weeks, followed by a second session of IV treatment, after which the tumor again regressed and the hemiparesis lessened. The total IV dose was 785,000 units. The patient was doing well when last seen and had no further recurrence on MRI. Side effects were controlled by indomethacin. The platelets decreased to 59% of baseline.

Conclusion.—Although not all patients treated with TNF-α have done this well, it is clear that some malignant gliomas can be effectively treated in this way without major adverse effects.

▶ As pointed out by William Sweet (1), a single case report can be valuable. For example, it can lead to a better understanding of the nature of a condition or can provide a clue as to a more effective treatment of that condition. This case report documents the complete regression of an anaplastic astrocytoma in response to treatment with TNF-α.

The follow-up in this case has only been 2 years. Furthermore, it is well documented that, using the usual current treatment modalities, malignant gliomas can be cured in a small percentage of patients. However, despite these caveats, this report may provide a lead to a more effective treatment for malignant gliomas; this agent should be tested further.—R.H. Wilkins, M.D.

Reference

1. Sweet W: The difference between zero and one. *Clin Neurosurg* 23:32–51, 1976.

Cerebral Oligodendroglioma: Prognostic Factors and Life History

Celli P, Nofrone I, Palma L, Cantore G, Fortuna A (La Sapienza Univ, Rome)
Neurosurgery 35:1018–1035, 1994   122-96-27–16

Background.—Oligodendroglioma is rare in the brain, accounting for 1% to 4% of intracranial tumors and 4% to 8% of cerebral gliomas. The prognostic factors and results in patients treated for this disorder before and after the introduction of CT were examined.

Patients and Findings.—Records of 137 patients who were surgically treated for supratentorial oligodendroglioma between 1953 and 1986 were examined. Tumors were histologically rated as benign or malignant. Overall, 105 patients underwent follow-up for a minimum of 5 years to December 1991. In these patients, the mean postoperative survival was 90.2 months, median survival was 64 months, and 5- and 10-year survival rates were 52.4% and 24%, respectively. Univariate methods and multivariate analysis according to Cox's stepwise proportional hazards model were used to evaluate 16 possible prognostic factors, which were broken down into 2 or more variables. Variables that positively correlated with survival on multivariate analysis included benign histologic findings, postoperative radiation therapy, and time of operation from 1977 to 1986 in the 105 patients, as well as surgery in the period from 1977 to 1986, subtotal or total tumor resection, and radiation therapy in a subgroup of 79 patients who had surgery for benign tumors. The relevance of admission clinical status to the survival of patients not receiving radiation therapy and to the prognostic response of those who did ultimately emerged as the most interesting factor.

In 40 patients with seizures and negative neurologic status (clinical syndrome A), the 10 not receiving radiation therapy survived as long as the 30 who did. Conversely, in 65 patients with intracranial hypertension or neurologic deficits, or both (clinical syndrome non-A), the 18 patients not receiving radiation therapy had shorter survival times compared with the 47 who did, all of whom had significantly better prognoses. After excluding malignant tumors, both the response to radiation therapy and the survival of nonirradiated patients remained significantly different in each syndrome. Multivariate analysis showed that patients undergoing surgery for benign tumors had different prognostic variables according to the clinical syndrome and radiation therapy. In the 47 patients with syndrome non-A, these included radiation therapy and preoperative history of less than 12 months; in the 32 with syndrome A, these included subtotal or total surgical tumor resection and second operations.

Conclusions.—These findings provide a reasonable explanation for the improved survival and the unresponsiveness to radiation therapy in patients receiving treatment since the introduction of CT from 1977 to 1986. Patients with histologically benign tumors should be classified by clinical status at admission. Treatment should then be organized and survival evaluated on that basis, as the 2 clinical syndromes appear to correspond to different periods in the tumor's life history.

▶ Celli et al. provide a careful review of a relatively large series of patients with oligodendroglioma treated at their institution. Their study includes an analysis of the benefits of postoperative radiation therapy. On the basis of this retrospective review, the authors recommend that treatment decisions for patients with benign oligodendrogliomas be based to some extent on the preoperative clinical syndrome. In patients with seizures only and nonenhancing lesions, the tumor should be resected to the extent consistent with the preservation of neurologic function, and radiation should be kept in reserve for later use. On the contrary, in patients with intracranial hypertension or neurologic deficits, or both, aggressive surgery is less beneficial and radiation therapy is recommended after the diagnosis has been established.—R.H. Wilkins, M.D.

Outcome for Children With Medulloblastoma Treated With Radiation and Cisplatin, CCNU, and Vincristine Chemotherapy
Packer RJ, Sutton LN, Elterman R, Lange B, Goldwein J, Nicholson HS, Mulne L, Boyett J, D'Angio G, Wechsler-Jentzsch K, Reaman G, Cohen BH, Bruce DA, Rorke LB, Molloy P, Ryan J, LaFond D, Evans AE, Schut L (George Washington Univ, Washington, DC; Univ of Pennsylvania, Philadelphia; Univ of Texas, Dallas; et al)
J Neurosurg 81:690–698, 1994   122-96-27–17

Introduction.—Although it remains a poorly understood disease, treatment for medulloblastoma/primitive neuroectodermal tumor (MB/PNET) has progressed, resulting in an increase in overall disease-free survival rates for children with this malignancy. Craniospinal irradiation combined with chemotherapy (CCNU and vincristine) has been shown to increase the progression-free survival in some children with MB/PNET. Children with larger primary tumors and disseminated disease at diagnosis appear to benefit more from this combination than children with localized, resected MB/PNET. The addition of cisplatin to CCNU and vincristine was found to further improve survival. To better evaluate this combination of chemotherapy, the outcomes of 63 children with MB/PNET treated during a 10-year period with the 3-drug regimen are examined.

Methods.—Children recently diagnosed with posterior fossa MB/PNET were included in the study. After surgical resection of the tumor, children received craniospinal radiation therapy (full or reduced dose) with vincristine, 1.5 mg/m^2, given weekly. Radiologic studies were conducted both preoperatively and postoperatively to assess tumor stage and extent of tumor resection. Tumor resections were graded as total or near total, partial, or biopsy. Six weeks after radiation therapy, 8 cycles of chemotherapy consisting of CCNU, 75 mg/m^2; cisplatin, 68 mg/m^2, every 6 weeks; and vincristine, 1.5 mg/m^2, every week for 3 weeks, were administered. Audiologic examination, renal function, hematologic monitoring, myelography, CSF, and MR studies were performed to assess drug toxicity and progression of disease.

Results.—Fifty-five of 63 children (87.3%) remain alive and progression-free. Estimations of progression-free survival were calculated as 90% ± 4% at 3 years and 85% ± 6% at 5 years. Overall event-free survival was 83% ± 6 % at 5 years, with 3 patients having a second malignancy (brain stem glioma, glioblastoma multiforme, and acute myelogenous leukemia). Progressive disease has developed in 8 patients. Factors such as young age at diagnosis, brain stem involvement, reduced-dose radiation, and subtotal resection did not affect progression-free survival. Progression-free survival was significantly affected by the presence of metastatic disease at diagnosis as compared with children with localized disease (5-year survival rates of 67% ± 15% and 90% ± 6%, respectively). Significant audiologic toxicity was observed in 30 of 63 (47.6%) patients, with 2 children eventually requiring a hearing aid. Significant loss of renal function has not yet occurred; however, grade 3 or 4 renal toxicity was found in 13 children. Eleven children required platelet transfusions because of thrombocytopenia. Neurotoxicity from vincristine manifested as ileus or significant weakness in 6 children. Adjustment of cisplatin therapy (either reduction or omission) was needed in 35 patients.

Discussion.—The progression-free and event-free survival rates observed in these children receiving the three-drug regimen (CCNU, cisplatin, and vincristine) are consistent with those previously reported in the literature and have further characterized the role of chemotherapy in the treatment of MB/PNET. The subgroup of patients who would benefit the most from this treatment still remains to be identified; less than 35% of the children in this study had disseminated disease and/or subtotal resection. Although still effective, treatment was less beneficial in children who had disseminated disease at the time of diagnosis. Additionally, the risk of the development of secondary malignancies with this three-drug regimen as compared with radiotherapy alone needs to be assessed.

▶ Over the past 2 decades, cooperative studies such as this have led to increasingly better survival rates for children treated for medulloblastoma. They have also documented the negative effects of such treatment as well, such as the hearing loss reported in this article. Despite the progress made, much remains to be done with regard to increasing the effectiveness of treatment while decreasing its adverse effects.—R.H. Wilkins, M.D.

Multivariate Analysis of Prognostic Factors in Adult Patients With Medulloblastoma: Retrospective Study of 156 Patients

Carrie C, Lasset C, Arapetite C, Haie-Meder C, Hoffstetter S, Demaille M-C, Kerr C, Wagner J-P, Lagrange J-L, Maire J-P, Seng S-H, Man YOCTK, Murraciole X, Pinto N (Centre Léon Bérard, Lyon, France; Institut Curie, Paris; Institut Gustave Roussy, Villejuif, France; et al)
Cancer 74:2352–2360, 1994   122-96-27–18

Introduction.—Medulloblastoma occurs relatively frequently in children but is rare in adults. Its rarity in the adult population means that data are sparse. Therefore, adult patients are often treated with pediatric protocols. In a retrospective, multicenter study of adult medulloblastoma, prognostic factors and the impact of postoperative chemotherapy and radiation therapy were examined.

Methods.—Clinical data regarding 156 adult patients with histologically proven medulloblastoma treated at 13 French centers between 1975 and 1991 were examined. Data on demographics, preoperative and postoperative clinical status, histologic findings, the completeness of resection, postoperative treatment, and post-treatment clinical status were reviewed. Associations between these factors and event-free survival rates were analyzed.

Results.—In the whole study population, the 5- and 10-year overall survival rates were 70% and 51%, respectively, and the 5- and 10-year event-free survival rates were 61% and 48%, respectively. Postoperative performance status of at least 3, the classic histologic subtype, and fourth ventricular floor involvement significantly predicted shorter event-free survival, whereas the desmoplastic histologic subtype predicted longer event-free survival. Combined radiation therapy and chemotherapy did not significantly prolong event-free survival compared with radiation therapy alone, and the whole brain radiation dose did not affect survival.

Discussion.—The outcome of medulloblastoma is similar in adults and children. The same prognostic features—histologic subtype, radiation dose, and fourth ventricular floor involvement—are valid in both populations. However, chemotherapy has greater toxicity and less benefit in adults than in children. Further study should test the efficacy of lowering the total brain irradiation dose to 30 Gy.

▶ Carrie et al. have analyzed information about 156 adult patients with medulloblastoma and have concluded that the prognostic factors and treatment outcomes in adults are generally similar to those of children with medulloblastoma. However, in the adults, no benefit of concomitant chemotherapy was demonstrated, and complete tumor resection resulted only in severely reduced postoperative performance status.—R.H. Wilkins, M.D.

Meningiomas

Meningiomas: Genetics, Malignancy, and the Role of Radiation in Induction and Treatment
Wilson CB (Univ of California, San Francisco)
J Neurosurg 81:666–675, 1994   122-96-27–19

Objective.—The author of this study reviews his own surgical experience with meningiomas and analyzes available published information on the molecular genetics, pathology, and cell kinetics of these tumors. The role of radiation, both as treatment for meningiomas and as a cause of the lesion in patients treated with radiation for other malignancies of the head, was also examined.

Molecular Genetics.—Initial development of a meningioma appears to follow the loss of genetic material from the long arm of chromosome 22. The gene has been mapped to a region between the myoglobin locus and the *c-sis* proto-oncogene. Progression may occur as a consequence of sequential deletions or modifications of other genes, with the acquisition of increasingly aggressive characteristics, a model supported by the finding of a more aggressive form in cases of recurrence.

Pathology.—There are 3 classic types of meningiomas, namely syncytial, fibroblastic, and transitional, as well as a number of histologic variants or subtypes. One third of meningiomas occur in childhood, one third have distant metastases, and one third are associated with a hemangiopericytic type, with 30% to 40% of these showing a papillary pattern. The Helsinki group has proposed a useful microscopic classification by cytologic features. The first 5 of these 6 features are graded on a scale of 0–3, yielding a total score for the tumor and 4 possible tumor grades: benign, atypical, anaplastic, and sarcomatous.

Cell Kinetics.—Determination of the mitotic labeling index, expressed as a percentage, is of powerful predictive value. The labeling index is the portion of the cells in a tumor that incorporates a thymidine analogue into nuclear DNA during brief exposure. A higher labeling index indicates a reduced time to tumor recurrence, and the formula has agreed well with clinical experience. This information can serve as a guide to determine the optimal frequency of follow-up scans.

Malignant and Radiation-Induced Meningiomas.—Whereas benign meningiomas are commonly found in women, malignant forms affect the sexes equally. Approximately 12% of the tumors prove to be malignant, and recurrent meningiomas have a higher rate of malignancy. Both CT and MRI findings aid in diagnosis. Gross or total resection is the primary treatment, and most patients require reoperation. Surgery alone is inadequate, however, and postoperative radiotherapy is more effective than chemotherapy. Radiation-induced tumors occur years after irradiation of the primary condition. Children, particularly girls, are more susceptible to tumor induction.

Discussion.—The method proposed by Simpson in 1957 for grading operations for meningiomas focuses on the importance of excision of involved dura. Wide removal of dura adjacent to the tumor reduces the risk of recurrence, and aggressive resection is generally recommended. Progression-free survival has been markedly improved by new irradiation techniques. Doses greater than 52 Gy prevent the regrowth of subtotally removed benign tumors and of all malignant meningiomas.

▶ Dr. Wilson was instrumental in establishing the Brain Tumor Research Center at the University of California, San Francisco, and for many years directed its productive efforts. This review, given as the Richard C. Schneider Lecture at the 60th Annual Meeting of the American Association of Neurological Surgeons in San Francisco, April 15, 1992, is a thoughtful analysis of certain aspects of meningiomas (molecular genetics, pathology, cell kinetics, malignant transformation, radiation induction, the role of the dura mater in meningioma recurrence, and the value of radiation therapy of subtotally removed meningiomas). Because of the difficulty in summarizing the considerable amount of worthwhile information contained in this analysis, the reader is referred to the full paper in the *Journal of Neurosurgery.*— R.H. Wilkins, M.D.

Necrosis in a Meningioma Following Systemic Chemotherapy
Bernstein M, Villamil A, Davidson G, Erlichman C (The Toronto Hosp; Univ of Toronto)
J Neurosurg 81:284–287, 1994   122-96-27–20

Introduction.—The effect of chemotherapy on meningiomas is not well known. Systemic chemotherapy for a rectal carcinoma was associated with necrosis in a meningioma in 1 patient.

Case Report.—Man, 54, was seen for resection of an adenocarcinoma of the rectum. During the workup, a CT scan was obtained of a firm swelling at the vertex of the head, which had been growing slowly for at least 10 years. Results of neurologic examination were normal. The CT scan revealed a large bilateral meningioma of the falx with bone thickening. It was decided that rectal cancer therapy should proceed, with elective review of the meningioma at follow-up. Two weeks after initiation of chemotherapy, the patient had headaches and somnolence with rapid onset. Papilledema and a left hemiparesis were detected upon examination. Both CT and MRI revealed a new area of low density in the meningioma. Surgical removal of the tumor was performed. Pathologic examination of the tumor revealed a typical syncytial meningioma with large areas of necrosis.

Purpose.—The purpose of this report is to indicate that systemic chemotherapy may be capable of producing necrosis in meningiomas. Therefore, systemic chemotherapy should be investigated as a treatment option in meningiomas that are refractory to surgery or radiotherapy.

▶ This serendipitous observation should stimulate investigation of the possible therapeutic efficacy of chemotherapy (intravenous 5-fluorouracil, intravenous folinic acid, and oral levamisole) in the treatment of meningiomas.— R.H. Wilkins, M.D.

Miscellaneous Tumors

Stereotactic Radiosurgery for the Definitive, Noninvasive Treatment of Brain Metastases
Alexander E III, Moriarty TM, Davis RB, Wen PY, Fine HA, Black PM, Kooy HM, Loeffler JS (Harvard Med School, Boston; Harvard School of Public Health, Boston)
J Natl Cancer Inst 87:34–40, 1995   122-96-27–21

Introduction.—Patients with cancer commonly experience brain metastases. Untreated, these metastases typically are fatal within 1 month.

Surgical resection or whole brain radiotherapy can significantly increase survival. Stereotactic radiosurgery is a minimally invasive treatment option that delivers a high-energy, focal dose of radiation. Its effectiveness in treating brain metastasis was retrospectively evaluated.

Methods.—The records of all patients with brain metastasis treated with radiosurgery over 7 years were reviewed. All patients had a Karnofsky performance score above 70, had no clinical evidence of emergent neurologic deterioration, and were treated with prior whole brain radiotherapy. Follow-up consisted of neurologic examination and contrast-enhanced CT or MRI 6–10 weeks after treatment, and then every 3 months. Survival and local tumor control were analyzed. Patient and treatment characteristics were analyzed to determine an association with survival or local tumor control.

Results.—Survival ranged from .5 to 88 months, with a median of 9.4 months. There was local failure in 11% of the tumors at a median time of 8.4 months after treatment. Reduced survival was associated with systemic disease at the time of radiosurgery, age above 60 years, male sex, and 3 or more brain lesions, with age and systemic disease contributing independently. Local tumor control failure was associated with infratentorial tumors, tumors larger than 3 cm^3 in volume, and previously treated lesions, with infratentorial and recurrent lesions contributing independently. Karnofsky performance scores changed by a median of 15% at 6 months, and 10% at 1 year. There was low perioperative morbidity and mortality, with a 2% 30-day mortality.

Discussion.—Radiosurgery may be a treatment option with outcomes comparable with those of craniotomy in patients with brain metastasis. Radiosurgery may be particularly suitable for patients with inoperable lesions or multiple metastases, but it is unsuitable for treating large tumors causing acute neurologic deterioration, especially when they are located infratentorially.

▶ The authors document the outcomes of 248 consecutive patients with 421 brain metastases that were treated with whole brain radiotherapy (median dose of 3,000 centigray in 10 daily fractions) followed, at an average of 6.3 months, by stereotactic radiosurgery using a linear accelerator. The authors conclude, on the basis of their own data as well as published information, that such treatment provides rates of local tumor control that are equivalent to those from surgical series, and that it is also effective in treating patients with surgically inaccessible lesions, those with multiple lesions, and those with tumor types that are resistant to conventional treatment.—R.H. Wilkins, M.D.

Estrogen Receptor Gene Expression in Craniopharyngiomas: An In Situ Hybridization Study

Thapar K, Stefaneanu L, Kovacs K, Scheithauer BW, Lloyd RV, Muller PJ, Laws ER Jr (Univ of Toronto; Mayo Clinic and Found, Rochester, Minn; Univ of Virginia, Charlottesville)
Neurosurgery 35:1012–1017, 1994   122-96-27–22

Background.—Although craniopharyngiomas are generally histologically benign epithelial neoplasms of the sellar region, they may lead to a wide range of clinical effects and can be extremely resistant to treatment. To improve currently available therapeutic approaches, a further understanding of the subcellular mechanisms guiding the genesis and progression of these neoplasms is needed. Therefore, the presence and cellular distribution of estrogen receptor (ER) messenger RNA was investigated in 23 surgically removed craniopharyngiomas to further elucidate their biological aspects.

Methods and Findings.—Nineteen adamantinomatous and 4 papillary variants were investigated via in situ hybridization. Immunohistochemical techniques were also used to study the expression of both ER and progesterone receptor proteins. All craniopharyngiomas uniformly expressed the ER gene. An intense ER messenger RNA hybridization signal was also noted in all cases, one of which was localized exclusively to the epithelial tumor cells. Hybridization signals were not observed in connective tissue and vascular elements. As demonstrated via immunohistochemistry, the ER protein was focally but conclusively identified in only 2 tumors, in spite of the relative abundance of ER message in all 23 instances. The reason for this discrepancy was not determined. The definitive presence of progesterone receptor protein was found in only one instance and was limited to occasional nuclei.

Conclusions.—A possible hormonal component may play a role in the genesis or progression, or both, of craniopharyngiomas. If so, therapeutic hormonal manipulation may lead to a potential treatment response in patients with these neoplasms.

▶ In recent years, it has been recognized that estrogens have the capacity to modulate the growth of some neoplasms. With regard to intracranial tumors, interest has been focused on meningiomas. The findings of this study are unexpected because the occurrence and growth rate of craniopharyngiomas have not been recognized as being influenced by female sex hormones.—R.H. Wilkins, M.D.

Craniopharyngiomas: A Clinicopathological Analysis of Factors Predictive of Recurrence and Functional Outcome
Weiner HL, Wisoff JH, Rosenberg ME, Kupersmith MJ, Cohen H, Zagzag D, Shiminski-Maher T, Flamm ES, Epstein FJ, Miller DC (New York Univ; Univ of Pennsylvania, Philadelphia)
Neurosurgery 35:1001–1011, 1994   122-96-27–23

Objective.—Although craniopharyngiomas are relatively rare, the consequences of these tumors include serious endocrine dysfunction and visual impairment. A retrospective study was conducted to delineate the clinical behavior of adamantinomatous and squamous papillary tumors and to determine whether brain invasion is predictive of recurrence.

Methods.—Specimens from 30 adults, aged 26–70 years, and 26 children, aged 1–19 years, were evaluated pathologically. Patients received either gross total resection or subtotal resection. Some patients had postoperative radiation therapy.

Results.—Adamantinomatous tumors were found in 66% of the adults and 96% of the children. Squamous papillary tumors were found in 28% of the adults and none of the children. Calcification was found in 95% of adamantinomatous tumors and 13% of squamous papillary tumors. There was brain invasion in 37% of adamantinomatous tumors and 13% of squamous papillary tumors. Gross total resection was performed in 27% of the adults and 77% of the children. Gross total resection was achieved in 54% of adamantinomatous and mixed tumors and 63% of squamous papillary tumors. The mean follow-up was 49 months. There were significantly fewer recurrences with totally resected tumors. After subtotal resection, with or without radiation, the recurrence rate was 58%. After gross total resection, the recurrence rate was 17%. The mean time to recurrence was 34 months. Of subtotally resected tumors, 2 of 3 squamous papillary and 11 of 21 adamantinomatous and mixed craniopharyngiomas recurred. For totally resected tumors, zero squamous papillary tumors and 5 adamantinomatous and mixed tumors recurred. There were no significant differences in Karnofsky performance status, visual outcome, or endocrine outcome. Ten patients died, 7 of their tumors.

Conclusion.—Subtotally resected tumors tended to recur. Recurrence rate is associated with the extent of resection rather than histologic type. Brain invasion is not associated with recurrence rate. Gross total resection yields a lower rate of recurrence and does not affect functional outcome.

▶ In 1973, Kahn and associates brought to our attention the 2 histologic variants of craniopharyngioma, emphasizing their clinical differences (1). During the past 2 decades, a number of clinical assessments have focused on the outcome of treatment of these 2 tumor types, particularly in relation to the completeness of surgical resection and the inclusion of postoperative radiotherapy. This study by Weiner and associates adds to this body of information.—R.H. Wilkins, M.D.

Reference

1. Kahn EA, Gosch HH, Seeger JF, et al: Forty-five years experience with the craniopharyngioma. *Surg Neurol* 1:5–12, 1973.

Surgical Resection of Third Ventricle Colloid Cysts: Preliminary Results Comparing Transcallosal Microsurgery With Endoscopy
Lewis AI, Crone KR, Taha J, van Loveren HR, Yeh H-S, Tew JM Jr (Univ of Cincinnati, Ohio; Mayfield Neurological Inst, Cincinnati, Ohio)
J Neurosurg 81:174–178, 1994   122-96-27-24

Background.—The best surgical option for third ventricle colloid cysts has not been established. The use of a steerable fiberscope and microsurgery through a transcallosal approach were compared.

Methods and Findings.—The steerable fiberscope was used to remove colloid cysts in 7 patients, and microsurgery through a transcallosal approach was used in 8. The operating times for microsurgery averaged 206 minutes and for endoscopy, 127 minutes. The average combined days spent in the intensive care unit and on the ward were 9.5 after microsurgery and 4 after endoscopy. Five patients undergoing microsurgery and 1 patient undergoing endoscopy had postoperative complications, which were transient and were mainly associated with short-term memory loss. Preoperative symptoms resolved in all patients, and none has had cyst recurrence. After surgery, 1 patient needed a ventriculoperitoneal shunt after microsurgery, but all patients were shunt-independent after endoscopy. Patients returned to work a mean of 59 days after discharge after microsurgery and 26 days after endoscopy.

Conclusions.—Compared with transcallosal microsurgery for colloid cyst removal, a steerable endoscope reduces operating time and number of days spent in the hospital. Patients undergoing the steerable endoscope technique were also able to return to work sooner.

▶ Lewis and his colleagues make the case for endoscopic resection of colloid cysts of the third ventricle.—R.H. Wilkins, M.D.

Hypothalamic Hamartomas: With Special Reference to Gelastic Epilepsy and Surgery

Valdueza JM, Cristante L, Dammann O, Bentele K, Vortmeyer A, Saeger W, Padberg B, Freitag J, Herrmann H-D (Univ Hosp Hamburg-Eppendorf, Hamburg, Germany)
Neurosurgery 34:949–958, 1994   122-96-27–25

Background.—The hypothalamic hamartoma is a non-neoplastic malformation consisting of hyperplastic neuronal tissue that resembles gray matter. It most often arises in the area of the tuber cinereum and mamillary bodies, and extends into the interpeduncular cistern. Most patients exhibit precocious puberty, gelastic ("laughing") epilepsy, other types of seizures, and behavioral abnormalities.

Review of Six Cases.—Six patients seen at a university hospital in a 10-year period had hypothalamic hamartomas diagnosed by MRI. The 4 females and 2 males ranged from 4½ to 30 years of age. None had clinically evident neurofibromatosis. Four of the patients had gelastic seizures as well as other forms of seizures, and 2 had precocious puberty. Two were visually impaired. All the lesions consisted of irregularly grouped multipolar ganglionoid cells and small bundles of myelinated fibers. Three of the patients did well after resection of the hamartoma.

Recommendations.—Magnetic resonance imaging is the best means of detecting hypothalamic hamartomas. Young patients having a small hamartoma that produces symptoms should be considered for surgical resection. Surgery also may be helpful when a larger hamartoma produces severe epileptic activity and behavioral abnormalities that are difficult to control.

▶ The authors provide a useful review of hypothalamic hamartomas.—R.H. Wilkins, M.D.

Pathology With Clinical Correlations of Primary Central Nervous System Non-Hodgkin's Lymphoma
Miller DC, Hochberg FH, Harris NL, Gruber ML, Louis DN, Cohen H (New York Univ Med Ctr, NY; Massachusetts General Hosp, Boston, Harvard Medical School, Boston; et al)
Cancer 74:1383–1397, 1994   122-96-27–26

Background.—The occurrence of non-Hodgkin's lymphoma of the CNS (NHL-CNS), an enigmatic disease of uncertain origin, appears to be increasing. The pathologic features, clinical data, and natural history of this tumor in one series of patients were reported.

Methods.—Neurologic specimens and autopsy tissues were available for 99 of 104 patients. Immunostaining and clinical data were obtained from the relevant physician offices and hospital charts.

Findings.—Between 1958 and 1989, NHL-CNS tripled in frequency. It currently represents 6.6% of all primary brain neoplasms. Eighty-nine percent of the 99 tumors classified histologically were of high grade. Intermediate-grade lymphomas, which were once the second most common subtype, have not been encountered since 1983. Architecture was diffuse in all tumors. Seventy-seven percent were large-cell subtypes. Two patients had intravascular lymphoma. All 41 tumors assessed were B-cell types, with one exception. Thirty-two of 40 had monotypic surface immunoglobulin. One T-cell lymphoma was identified. Of 64 tumor recurrences, 29 were at the initially defined site. Twelve were in the leptomininges, 29 in other neuroaxis sites, and 8 in systemic sites. Systemic metastases have not been seen since 1984. The 68 patients who survived after diagnostic surgery and for whom follow-up data were available had a median survival of 19 months. This survival rate was 9 months for patients with high-grade tumors and 30.5 months for those with intermediate-grade tumors. This difference was nonsignificant. Another 7 patients had focal tumorlike lymphoid infiltrates consisting of benign-appearing lymphocytes associated with good long-term survival. The differential histologic diagnosis of NHL-CNS was difficult in some cases. The spectrum of this differential was broader than is generally reported.

Conclusions.—The frequency of NHL-CNS has increased, even in this series of nonimmunocompromised patients. This increase is accompanied by the disappearance of intermediate-grade histologic types, which suggests a fundamental shift in the biology of the neoplasms. The introduction of chemotherapy regimens seems to have changed the natural history so that systemic metastases no longer occur outside the CNS. There are now some long-term survivors of this once fatal disease.

▶ The authors have studied a large series of NHL-CNS and have documented significant changes that have occurred since 1958.—R.H. Wilkins, M.D.

Preirradiation Methotrexate Chemotherapy of Primary Central Nervous System Lymphoma: Long-Term Outcome

Glass J, Gruber ML, Cher L, Hochberg FH (Temple Univ Cancer Ctr, Philadelphia, Pa; Univ of Calif, Los Angeles; Harvard Medical School, Boston)
J Neurosurg 81:188–195, 1994   122-96-27–27

Background.—The frequency of primary CNS lymphoma continues to increase. The disease has a poor outlook if not treated, and whole brain irradiation has increased survival only modestly. More consistent responses have been achieved in patients given methotrexate intravenously before cranial radiotherapy. Twelve of 13 such patients achieved a partial or complete radiographic response.

Study Plan.—Twenty-five patients, including the original 13, have received methotexate therapy in a dose of 3.5 g per m^2 of body surface area with leucovorin rescue. As many as 6 cycles of treatment were given every 10-21 days, and whole brain radiotherapy was begun within 3 weeks of the end of chemotherapy or sooner if disease was progressing. The minimum dose was 3,000 cGy, delivered in daily fractions of 180 cGy. Steroid doses were tapered as allowed by the clinical response.

Results.—Only 4 of 17 evaluable patients responded to preliminary steroid treatment. Fourteen patients completely responded to methotrexate therapy, and 6 others had major partial responses. Two patients had a lesser response, and 3 continued to progress during chemotherapy. Ten patients who responded completely received whole brain radiotherapy immediately afterward, and all maintained their responses. Thirteen of 22 patients had recurrences after 3 to 52 months of follow-up; the median interval was 32 months. Two patients were successfully retreated. The overall median survival time was 33 months; for patients who responded to treatment, median survival was 42.5 months. Two patients died without evidence of disease. Toxicity included individual cases of pulmonary embolism, transient encephalopathy, and acute renal failure.

Conclusion.—Administration of methotrexate before whole brain irradiation can prolong survival in patients treated for primary CNS lymphoma without undue toxicity.

► The authors make a strong case for the inclusion of methotrexate chemotherapy in the treatment protocol for primary lymphoma of the CNS.—R.H. Wilkins, M.D.

28 Pseudotumor Cerebri

Optic Nerve Sheath Decompression for the Treatment of Visual Failure in Chronic Raised Intracranial Pressure
Acheson JF, Green WT, Sanders MD (Natl Hosp for Neurology and Neuro-surgery, London; St Thomas's Hosp, London)
J Neurol Neurosurg Psychiatry 57:1426–1429, 1994   122-96-28–1

Background.—At least 50% of patients with benign intracranial hyper-tension have visual loss over time. Moreover, pronounced field and acuity deficits occur in as many as 10% of these patients. The results of optic nerve sheath decompression performed on patients with chronic elevated intracranial pressure and visual failure are examined. The relation between optic nerve sheath decompression, visual outcome, and other CSF diver-sion procedures is also discussed.

Patients and Findings.—The records of all patients undergoing optic nerve decompression during a 15-year period were evaluated. All patients had chronic raised intracranial pressure complicated by visual failure, and none had responded to maximal medical treatment. Follow-up informa-tion of at least 12 months' duration was available for 20 eyes in 14 patients. Eleven patients had benign intracranial hypertension (idiopathic intracranial hypertension), whereas the remaining 3 were given a diagnosis of dural venous sinus occlusive disease. Unilateral and bilateral surgery was performed in 8 and 6 patients, respectively. Improved or stabilized visual acuity and fields were noted in 17 of 20 eyes. The other 3 eyes deteriorated. In 8 patients undergoing unilateral surgery, the untreated eye remained stable in 7 and deteriorated in 1. Optic nerve sheath decompres-sion was necessary in 4 patients, even though previous shunting or sub-temporal decompression had been performed. Shunting or subtemporal decompression was required after optic nerve sheath decompression in 5 patients because of persistent headache in 3 and uncontrolled visual failure in 2. No vision was lost as a direct result of surgery.

Conclusions.—Optic nerve sheath decompression is a safe treatment alternative for managing chronic elevated intracranial pressure compli-cated by visual loss. Vision can be saved after shunt failure and may be maintained without the need for a shunt in some instances. However, shunts may still be necessary after optic nerve sheath decompression, particularly in patients with recurring headaches.

▶ This paper emphasizes two facts: First, optic nerve sheath decompression has value in preserving or improving vision in some patients with the chronic intracranial hypertension associated with pseudotumor cerebri or venous sinus thrombosis. Second, no single treatment approach is 100% successful in ameliorating the symptoms and signs of these two conditions, so it is not unusual for a patient to require several different treatment approaches during the course of the disorder.—R.H. Wilkins, M.D.

29 Intracranial Aneurysms and Intracranial Hemorrhage

Perimesencephalic and Nonperimesencephalic Subarachnoid Haemorrhages With Negative Angiograms
Canhão P, Ferro JM, Pinto AN, Melo TP, Campos JG (Hosp ST, Maria, Lisbon, Portugal)
Acta Neurochir (Wien) 132:14–19, 1995   122-96-29-1

Background.—Ten years ago, perimesencephalic (PM) hemorrhage was identified as a distinct, benign, nonaneurysmal subarachnoid hemorrhage. However, only one retrospective series outside The Netherlands has been reported. The clinical course and long-term follow-up in a consecutive series of patients hospitalized with PM subarachnoid hemorrhage were reported.

Methods.—Seventy-one patients with subarachnoid hemorrhage and negative cerebral angiography admitted between January 1985 and April 1992 were included. The patients were categorized as PM and non-PM bleeding based on the distribution of blood on a CT scan obtained within 72 hours of onset.

Findings.—There were 36 PM and 35 non-PM hemorrhage cases. The 2 patient groups were similar in sex and age distribution. The PM group typically had a normal examination on admission. Only one patient with PM bleeding had a complication—transient neurologic signs during angiography. There was no mortality or morbidity during follow-up. Three patients in the group with non-PM hemorrhage had rebleeding, 4 had hydrocephalus, and 2 had delayed cerebral ischemia. The mean length of follow-up in the groups with PM and non-PM were 27.6 months and 30.8 months, respectively. A fatal rebleed occurred in the latter group after discharge. In both groups, 22% to 25% had headaches and depression.

Conclusions.—Perimesencephalic hemorrhage is a distinct entity within the larger group of subarachnoid hemorrhage. Patients with PM bleeding have negative angiograms, good short-term and long-term prognoses, and no need for repeated angiographic investigation.

▶ These authors add to the literature on PM subarachnoid hemorrhage with this report of a series of 36 patients who were followed for an average of 27.6 months. They also report 35 control patients who had other forms of subarachnoid hemorrhage with negative cerebral angiography. Although the authors emphasize the "benign" nature of PM hemorrhage, with no fatal rebleeding or mortality occurring during the follow-up in their patients, the following facts are worth noting: Of the 33 patients with PM hemorrhage who were followed, 11 had only a partial subjective recovery, 8 had headaches, 8 had symptoms of depression, 3 had neck pain, and 2 had postural vertigo; four patients retired from work. The outlook for patients with subarachnoid hemorrhage and negative cerebral angiography (especially those with PM hemorrhage) is better than the outlook for patients with a ruptured aneurysm, but the condition is not entirely benign.—R.H. Wilkins, M.D.

Blinded Prospective Evaluation of Sensitivity of MR Angiography to Known Intracranial Aneurysms: Importance of Aneurysm Size
Huston J III, Nichols DA, Luetmer PH, Goodwin JT, Meyer FB, Wiebers DO, Weaver AL (Mayo Clinic and Found, Rochester, Minn)
AJNR 15:1607–1614, 1994   122-96-29–2

Introduction.—Traditionally, conventional angiography has been used to diagnose and assess intracranial aneurysms. However, studies have shown that MR angiography, a noninvasive technique, can retrospectively diagnose aneurysms of at least 3 mm. In a blinded, prospective study, the accuracy was evaluated of transaxial T1- and T2-weighted standard MR and time-of-flight and phase-contrast (PC) MR angiography in detecting intracranial aneurysms.

Methods.—Sixteen patients with 27 conventional angiography-proven intracranial aneurysms and 19 control patients underwent standard sagittal T1-weighted and transaxial T2-weighted MR head imaging, 3-dimensional (3-D) time-of-flight imaging, and 3-D PC imaging. The images were interpreted by 3 blinded, experienced neuroradiologists. Aneurysms were diagnosed if detected by at least 2 examiners.

Results.—Time-of-flight MR angiography had the best overall sensitivity, detecting 55% of the aneurysms and 87.5% of the 16 aneurysms measuring at least 5 mm. The overall sensitivity of PC MR angiography was 44% and increased to 75% with aneurysms of at least 5 mm. The T2-weighted MR images had the best sensitivity for aneurysms smaller than 5 mm. Time-of-flight MR angiography demonstrated false positive diagnoses of subacute thrombus, which did not occur with PC MR angiography.

Discussion.—Although retrospective examinations of MR angiographic images have allowed identification of aneurysms as small as 3 mm, these data show that 5 mm is the critical size for prospective examination. Time-of-flight MR angiography is superior to PC MR angiography in detecting intracranial aneurysms. However, neither was sensitive enough to be recommended for routine screening.

▶ Magnetic resonance angiography is still being refined, but it has not yet reached the accuracy of standard angiography in the identification of intracranial aneurysms.—R.H. Wilkins, M.D.

Three-Dimensional Computed Tomographic Angiography in the Preoperative Evaluation of Cerebrovascular Lesions
Harbaugh RE, Schlusselberg DS, Jeffery R, Hayden S, Cromwell LD, Pluta D, English RA (Dartmouth-Hitchcock Med Ctr, Lebanon, NH)
Neurosurgery 36:320–327, 1995   122-96-29–3

Background.—Three-dimensional CT angiography (3D-CTA) was initially used as a screening tool for patients with suspected cerebrovascular disease. However, 3D-CTA has proved to be most useful in planning operations for patients with unusual or large intracranial aneurysms and vascular malformations.

Patients—During a 1-year period, 49 patients with intracranial aneurysms and 12 patients with cerebral arteriovenous malformations underwent catheter angiography and 3D-CTA and subsequent operation. The images obtained with 3D-CTA provided important information regarding the size and configuration of the lesion, the presence and extent of intra-aneurysmal thrombus, the relationship of the vascular lesion to normal cerebral vessels, aneurysm wall thickness, and the presence and orientation of an aneurysm neck (Fig 29–1). Although 3D-CTA did not change the decision to operate or the operative approach used for any of the patients, for those with large or unusual lesions, the anatomical detail obtained from 3D-CTA provided information not readily available from other neuroradiologic studies. This information allowed the surgeon to better envision various approaches to the lesion and in some cases modify the planning and decision-making.

Conclusions.—Intra-arterial angiography remains the "gold standard" in the preoperative evaluation of cerebrovascular lesions, but as experience with 3D-CTA accumulates, this imaging modality may well take its place.

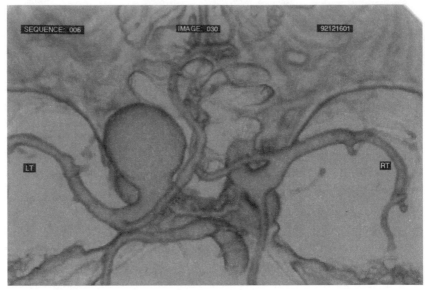

Fig 29–1.—Three-dimensional CT angiographic image demonstrating the large aneurysm with surrounding cranial base and cerebrovascular structures. (Courtesy of Harbaugh RE, Schlusselberg DS, Jeffery R, et al: *Neurosurgery* 36:320–327, 1995.)

Three-Dimensional Computed Tomographic Angiography of Cerebral Aneurysms

Tampieri D, Leblanc R, Oleszek J, Pokrupa R, Melançon D (Montreal Neurological Hosp and Inst, Quebec, Canada; McGill Univ, Montreal, Quebec, Canada)

Neurosurgery 36:749–755, 1995   122-96-29–4

Objective.—The value of high-definition, reformatted, 3-dimensional CT angiography was examined in 18 patients in whom intra-arterial digital subtraction angiography had demonstrated a cerebral aneurysm after subarachnoid hemorrhage or CT or MRI had shown a large or giant aneurysm.

Method.—In 15 cases 3-dimensional CT angiography was performed in the axial plane centering on the circle of Willis. A bolus injection of 80 mL of iohexol was administered. Three patients were examined in the coronal plane to avoid clip-related artifacts.

Results.—No complications occurred. All aneurysms larger than 3 mm in diameter and 3 of the 6 smaller aneurysms were demonstrated. The fundus, sac, and neck of the aneurysms all were well visualized, and it was possible to distinguish the filling part of the aneurysm from the thrombosed portion. The relationships of the aneurysm to the vessel of origin, associated vessels, and surrounding bony structures also were well demonstrated. The relationship of a previously coated aneurysm to the acrylic was visualized. It was possible to visualize the reformatted images in any plane and orientation.

Conclusion.—Three-dimensional CT angiography is an effective means of evaluating complex aneurysms of the circle of Willis.

▶ The authors of these 2 papers (Abstracts 122-96-29–3 and 122-96-29–4) provide a sample of what can now be shown by three-dimensional CT angiography. Vascular relationships can be visualized in greater detail than with two-dimensional angiography, which has the potential of adding valuable information for the preoperative assessment of complex vascular lesions.—R.H. Wilkins, M.D.

Three-Dimensional Display of the Orifice of Intracranial Aneurysms: A New Potential Application for Magnetic Resonance Angiography
Bontozoglou N, Spanos H, Lasjaunias P, Zarifis G (Athens Med, Greece; Centre Hospitalier Universitaire de Bicêtre, Paris)
Neuroradiology 36:346–349, 1994   122-96-29–5

Background.—Selective intra-arterial angiography is the method of choice for detecting intracranial aneurysms, with CT and MRI providing useful complementary information preoperatively. However, the endovascular approach to intracranial aneurysms requires different pretherapeutic data. Endoluminal assessment of the aneurysmal orifice is key in determining the feasibility of filling the aneurysmal sac or blocking the orifice. The value of MR angiography in the three-dimensional display of the orifice of intracranial aneurysms was investigated.

Methods.—Twelve patients with 17 intracranial aneurysms were studied. Fifteen aneurysms had been shown previously by digital subtraction angiography.

Findings.—In 10 patients, the overall image quality of three-dimensional display MR angiography was excellent. The orifice was clearly seen in 13 aneurysms (76%) (Fig 29–2). Unique information about the size, shape, and orientation of the orifice was provided by MR angiography. In 2 aneurysms (12%) the orifice was not demonstrated. In another 12%, MR angiography did not detect the aneurysms.

Conclusions.—These preliminary findings indicate that MR angiography is potentially useful in demonstrating the orifice of intracranial aneurysms. The anatomical and technical reliability of three-dimensional display MR angiography is currently being investigated.

▶ Although MR angiography (MRA) is not as sensitive as digital subtraction angiography in detecting intracranial aneurysms, three-dimensional MRA does permit in many instances a spectacular display of the aneurysm orifice, as is shown in the 4 case examples in the original of this report.—R.H. Wilkins, M.D.

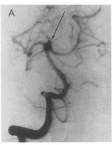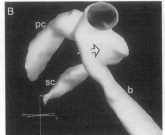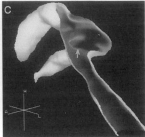

Fig 29–2.—Aneurysm at the tip of the basilar artery demonstrated in 2 planes. A, anteroposterior digital subtraction angiography. An aneurysm 1 cm in diameter is seen (*long arrow*). B and C, lateral projection from 3-dimensional display MR angiography. *Open arrow* represents aneurysm; *b*, basilar artery; *pc*, posterior cerebral artery; *sc*, superior cerebellar artery; *white arrow*, orifice of right superior cerebellar artery; *white arrowhead*, artificial object representing background noise. (Courtesy of Bontozoglou N, Spanos H, Lasjaunias P, et al: *Neuroradiology* 36:346–349, 1994.)

Cranial Base Approaches to Intracranial Aneurysms in the Subarachnoid Space

Sekhar LN, Kalia KK, Yonas H, Wright DC, Ching H (George Washington Univ, Washington, DC; Univ of Pittsburgh, Pa)
Neurosurgery 35:472–483, 1994   122-96-29–6

Background.—The exposure and treatment of cerebral aneurysms can be improved by cranial base approaches developed primarily for use in surgery for tumors or for developmental malformations. A critical analysis of the experience of these surgeons was provided.

Methods.—The surgical approaches to and clinical outcomes of surgical treatment of intracranial aneurysms in 38 patients over 9 years were summarized and presented.

Results.—The 38 patients had aneurysms involving the anterior communicating artery complex, proximal internal carotid artery, basilar artery, or vertebral artery. The cranial base approaches taken to surgically treat these aneurysms included orbital osteotomy, orbitozygomatic osteotomy, petrous apicectomy, presigmoid petrosectomy, and extreme lateral transcondylar methods (table). Author-developed modifications of these approaches are described in detail. In the more recent cases, the technique of three-dimensional CT angiography was used to plan the approach to the aneurysm. One partial ptosis and 2 CSF leaks occurred in 3 separate patients as postoperative complications that resolved with treatment. Long-term outcomes have largely been very positive with most patients returning to independent living with minimal disability.

Conclusions.—Excellent exposure with minimal brain retraction results from selectively applied cranial base approaches to intracranial aneurysms.

▶ In this paper, Sekhar and colleagues show how developments in one area of medicine can be applied to advantage in another. Within a single specialty,

Cranial Base Approaches Used in Aneurysm Surgery, 1984–1993*

Aneurysm	Number of Patients ($n=38$)	Approaches Used
Anterior communicating artery	7	Subfrontal-transorbital
Carotid-hypophyseal	10	Frontotemporal-transorbital
Carotid-ophthalmic	2	Frontotemporal-transorbital
Basilar apex	6	1) Transcavernous-transclinoidal
		2) Orbitozygomatic-transsylvian
		3) Subtemporal, transzygomatic, transpetrous apex
Basilar superior cerebellar artery	4	1) Orbitozygomatic-transsylvian
		2) Retrolabyrinthine petrosal
Distal superior cerebellar artery	1	Retrolabyrinthine petrosal
Basilar anterior inferior cerebellar artery	2	1) Retrolabyrinthine petrosal
		2) Transcochlear petrosal
Vertebrobasilar junction	1	Subtemporal-infratemporal
Vertebral artery	5	Extreme lateral, transcondylar, transjugular

* Most of the aneurysms were large or giant.
(Courtesy of Sekhar LN, Kalia KN, Yonas H, et al: *Neurosurgery* 35:472–483, 1994.)

this is relatively easy to accomplish. It is harder to accomplish between medical specialties because of the increasing lack of communication and cross-fertilization resulting from specialization itself.—R.H. Wilkins, M.D.

Hunterian Proximal Arterial Occlusion for Giant Aneurysms of the Carotid Circulation

Drake CG, Peerless SJ, Ferguson GG (Univ of Western Ontario, London, Canada; Mercy Neuroscience Inst, Miami, Fla)
J Neurosurg 81:656–665, 1994   122-96-29-7

Background.—At one center, Hunterian proximal arterial occlusion has been performed on all major intracranial arteries, mostly for giant aneurysms considered otherwise inoperable, but sometimes as a safer alternative to attempted clipping of the neck of an aneurysm.

Methods and Findings.—From 1961, 723 patients with giant aneurysms were treated. Three hundred thirty-five patients had giant aneurysms of the anterior circulation. Hunterian proximal artery occlusion was used in 160 of these patients. Aneurysms arose from the internal carotid arteries in 133, from the middle cerebral arteries in 20, and from the anterior cerebral arteries in 7. Outcomes were satisfactory in 90% of the patients. The use of preoperative cerebral blood flow studies and test occlusion with an intracarotid balloon to identify patients who needed preliminary extra-cranial-to-intracranial bypass greatly improved the safety of internal carotid artery occlusion. The leptomeningeal collateral flow of the anterior cerebral artery prevented infarction, even without cross flow. Aneurysm obliteration by thrombosis was complete or nearly complete in all but 4 patients finishing treatment. In the 16 patients with poor outcomes, hemodynamic ischemic infarction was known to occur after only 2 of the carotid occlusions.

Conclusions.—Clinical outcomes were good in 84% of these patients with anterior aneurysms, including those in poor condition before surgery. Considering the poor outcomes expected when giant aneurysms are untreated, these outcomes seem reasonable.

▶ The authors report what undoubtedly is the most extensive experience ever accumulated with proximal arterial occlusion for the treatment of giant aneurysms of the carotid circulation. This encyclopedic information will be of value to any neurosurgeon contemplating such treatment.—R.H. Wilkins, M.D.

Intraarterial Papaverine Infusion for Cerebral Vasopasm After Subarachnoid Hemorrhage
Clouston JE, Numaguchi Y, Zoarski GH, Aldrich F, Simard JM, Zitnay KM (Univ of Maryland, Baltimore)
AJNR 16:27–38, 1995   122-96-29–8

Objective.—The techniques and efficacy of intracranial intra-arterial papaverine infusion for symptomatic vasospasm after subarachnoid hemorrhage caused by aneurysm rupture were evaluated.

Methods.—Intracranial intra-arterial infusion was administered on 19 occasions in 14 patients between 6 hours and 2 days after spasm became clinically apparent. Of the 60 vascular territories treated, infusion was made into the supraclinoid internal carotid artery 20 times, the cavernous internal carotid artery once, the selective A1 anterior cerebral artery 8 times, the selective M1 middle cerebral artery 7 times, and the basilar artery 3 times. Papaverine doses ranged from 150 to 600 mg and exceeded 400 mg on 8 occasions. The follow-up ranged from 2 to 12 months.

Outcome.—Angiographic improvement occurred in 18 (95%) of the 19 treatment sessions, being excellent in 3 sessions, moderate in 8, and mild in 7. The best angiographic results were observed more frequently with superselective infusion. Clinically, 7 (50%) patients showed dramatic acute improvement within 24 hours of papaverine therapy, and none of those patients showed clinical evidence of recurrent vasospasm. Four patients had repeat treatment, but only 1 patient showed dramatic acute recovery after a second treatment. There was no correlation between clinical results and angiographic response. Likewise, there was no correlation between clinical outcome and elapsed time from subarachnoid hemorrhage or surgery, Fisher grade related to admission CT scans, duration of new neurologic symptoms, dose or site of infusion of papaverine, or distribution of angiographic spasm. There were no episodes of systemic hypotension during or after treatment. Three patients had procedural complications, including permanent monocular blindness resulting from papaverine being infused near the ophthalmic artery, internal carotid artery dissection during catheter placement, and brief generalized tonic-clonic seizures.

Conclusion.—Intra-arterial infusion of papaverine effectively dilates spastic arteries in most patients who have symptomatic vasospasm after subarachnoid hemorrhage. The clinical results are encouraging, with no recurrence of neurologic deterioration being observed in patients who respond well to papaverine. Superselective infusion appears to be indicated in some patients for adequate papaverine delivery.

▶ Although infusion of papaverine will result in angiographic improvement in most patients who are treated for cerebral vasospasm, clinical improvement does not occur as often, and the two phenomena do not necessarily coincide. The exact pathophysiology of symptomatic intracranial arterial spasm is still not well understood, and its successful prevention and treatment remain elusive.—R.H. Wilkins, M.D.

Surgical Treatment of Extracranial Internal Carotid Artery Dissecting Aneurysms
Schievink WI, Piepgras DG, McCaffrey TV, Mokri B (Mayo Clinic and Found, Rochester, Minn)
Neurosurgery 35:809–816, 1994   122-96-29–9

Introduction.—The extracranial internal carotid artery (ICA) is a rare site of aneurysms. Operations for such aneurysms typically comprise less than 1% of the operations performed on the ICA. When the aneurysm does occur, it usually results from dissection from an intramural clot that extends outward toward the adventitia, resulting in aneurysmal dilatation. Traumatic dissection can result in transient cerebral or retinal ischemia, whereas spontaneous dissection rarely becomes symptomatic. In the acute phase, the aneurysm may enlarge for a few weeks and then remain unchanged, shrink, or resolve; this occurs most often in spontaneous aneurysms. In the chronic phase, enlargement or rupture of the aneurysm is rare, but there is a chance for distal thromboembolization, primarily in dissecting aneurysms. Experience with surgical treatment of extracranial ICA dissecting aneurysms at one center was reviewed.

Methods.—During a 13-year period, 22 of 200 patients evaluated had surgical treatment of ICA aneurysms caused by dissection. Follow-up was by clinical examination, letter, or phone contact. The average follow-up was 6.6 years. The patients were 7 women and 15 men (average age, 39 years). There were 11 patients with traumatic ICA lesions and 11 with spontaneous lesions; the aneurysm was located on the distal segment in all patients. Although risk factors of atherosclerotic heart disease were rare in this group, 5 were hypertensive, 9 were smokers, and 1 had chronic obstructive lung disease.

Results.—Five patients had cervical ligation, 13 patients had the aneurysm resected and the artery reconstructed, and 4 had cervical-to-intracranial ICA bypass. There were 2 postoperative strokes. Although facial and lower cranial nerve palsies were seen after high cervical exposure, the palsies were transient, and no long-term neurologic problems were noted in follow-up.

Conclusions.—The need for surgery on the ICA dissecting aneurysm is rare; however, the limited experience evaluated had acceptable morbidity. No generalization regarding the optimal surgical method can be made because the use of surgery in these patients is limited.

▶ These authors have a special interest in this subject and speak with authority about the management of these unusual lesions.—R.H. Wilkins, M.D.

Hemorrhagic Dilation of the Fourth Ventricle: An Ominous Predictor
Shapiro SA, Campbell RL, Scully T (Univ Med Ctr, Indianapolis, Ind)
J Neurosurg 80:805–809, 1994   122-96-29–10

Introduction.—Studies of CT-documented intracranial hemorrhage have suggested that a large amount of hemorrhage is a poor prognostic factor for patients with intraparenchymal hemorrhage and subarachnoid hemorrhage (SAH). However, few studies have addressed the presence of blood in the fourth ventricle and its effects on the surrounding ependyma and brain stem.

Patients.—A total of 50 patients who had CT-documented fourth intra-ventricular hemorrhage (fourth IVH) treated over a 5-year period were reviewed. The cause was intraparenchymal hemorrhage with secondary fourth IVH in 19 patients, spontaneous SAH in 18, spontaneous IVH in 7, and trauma in 6. The ventricle was dilated in 56% of the patients, all of whom sustained brain death, even with aggressive therapy. Of the 44% without dilation, 41% died and 59% survived in a functioning state. The difference in survival between the dilated and nondilated groups was significant.

Findings.—Diffuse clot—involving the lateral and third ventricles as well as the fourth ventricle—was present in 89% of the patients in the dilated group and 59% of those in the nondilated group. Mortality was increased among patients with diffuse clot in the group receiving no dilation. The Glasgow Coma Scale (GCS) score was 3 or 4 in 86% of patients with a fourth IVH associated with dilation; the GCS scores were higher in patients without dilation. On logistic regression multivariate analysis, fourth IVH with hemorrhagic dilation was the most significant outcome predictor, followed by GCS score and diffuse IVH.

Conclusions.—In patients with CT–documented fourth IVH, hemor-rhagic ventricular dilation is an ominous prognostic sign. Outcome is not improved by ventriculostomy; the situation calls for more aggressive tech-niques, such as intraventricular thrombolysis. Rapid infarction in these patients likely results from pressure on the brain stem impairing perforator perfusion.

▶ It has long been recognized that a hematoma filling the fourth ventricle is associated with a poor prognosis. Shapiro et al. assessed the situation in an organized way and verified that this is the case whether the intraventricular hematoma has resulted from hypertensive intraparenchymal hemorrhage, spontaneous subarachnoid hemorrhage, spontaneous IVH, anticoagulation, or trauma. They also point out that in contrast to a hematoma that only fills the fourth ventricle, one that distends it (regardless of etiology) dramatically increases the risk of mortality and is the strongest outcome predictor for IVH. Furthermore, ventriculostomy alone has no impact on the survival of patients with hemorrhagic dilation of the fourth ventricle, a circumstance that has led the authors to recommend a more aggressive approach to treatment, such as intraventricular thrombolysis with urokinase or tissue plasminogen activator.—R.H. Wilkins, M.D.

30 Vascular Malformations and Fistulas

The Influence of Hemodynamic and Anatomic Factors on Hemorrhage From Cerebral Arteriovenous Malformations
Kader A, Young WL, Pile-Spellman J, Mast H, Sciacca RR, Mohr JP, Stein BM, the Columbia University AVM Study Project (Columbia Univ, New York)
Neurosurgery 34:801–808, 1994   122-96-30–1

Purpose.—Hemorrhage from cerebral arteriovenous malformations (AVMs) is a major cause of their morbidity and mortality. However, the physiologic and anatomical conditions that lead to such hemorrhage are unknown. A variety of clinical and physiologic variables in a large group of patients with AVMs were studied in an attempt to identify conditions predisposing to spontaneous intracranial hemorrhage (ICH).

Methods.—The retrospective/prospective analysis included 449 patients with AVMs, most treated surgically. Fifty-eight percent were initially seen with hemorrhage, 24% with seizures, 13% with headache, and 3% with neurologic deficits. Patients with and without hemorrhage were compared for such variables as AVM size, type of venous drainage, transcranial Doppler (TCD) velocities, feeding mean arterial pressure (FMAP), and draining vein pressure. The latter 3 variables were measured before treatment.

Findings.—The mean patient age was 33 years, with no difference between groups. Hemorrhage was the initial event in 90% of the patients with lesions under 2.5 cm as compared with about half of those with larger AVMs. Hemorrhage occurred in half of the patients with deep venous drainage vs. one third of those with superficial drainage. Deep drainage predicted hemorrhage even in patients with medium to large supratentorial AVMs. There was no difference between groups in draining vein pressure. Although FMAP was greater in the hemorrhage group—44 vs. 34 mm Hg—it was not strongly related to the size of the lesion. Transcranial Doppler velocity was related to the size of the lesion but less so to the propensity for hemorrhage.

Multiple logistic regression analysis was performed in the patients with medium to large AVMs with superficial venous drainage, i.e., the subset with the lowest identified risk of ICH. The findings showed a strong influence of FMAP, but not TCD velocities, on the incidence of ICH.

Conclusions.—The risk of ICH from AVMs appears to be elevated in patients with a smaller nidus size and the presence of deep venous drainage. Elevated FMAP seems to play an important role in the pathophysiology of hemorrhage from AVMs rather than being just a consequence of lesion size. The presence of a lower feeding artery pressure may have important protective effects against hemorrhage.

▶ The basic associations found by these authors, such as the increased risk of AVM hemorrhage with smaller nidus size, have been noted by other investigators in the past. What marks this study is the large cohort of patients studied and the comprehensive manner in which they have been investigated.—R.H. Wilkins, M.D.

Vascular Malformations and Intractable Epilepsy: Outcome After Surgical Treatment
Dodick DW, Cascino GD, Meyer FB (Mayo Clinic, Rochester, Minn)
Mayo Clin Proc 69:741–745, 1994   122-96-30–2

Background.—Authorities disagree on the value of surgical treatment in reducing seizure activity in patients with vascular malformations and intractable epilepsy. One recent experience was reviewed.

Methods.—Twenty consecutive patients who had surgery for medically refractory partial epilepsy at the Mayo Clinic were studied. All had cerebral vascular malformations. Eighteen patients had remote hemorrhage associated with the vascular lesion. On MRI, 36 vascular malformations were seen in 20 patients. In all patients, surgery included a complete resection of the vascular malformation.

Findings.—Fifteen patients were free of seizures after surgery, and 3 had at least a 90% reduction in the number of seizures. Unfavorable outcomes were seen in only 2 patients. Outcome was unaffected by age at onset of a seizure and the duration of a seizure. The site of the vascular malformation was less important than the exact correlation between the site of onset of seizure and the corresponding vascular malformation.

Conclusions.—In patients with intractable partial epilepsy and cerebral vascular malformations, in the absence of dual pathologic conditions, lesionectomy can yield a seizure-free outcome. The possibility of coexisting ipsilateral atrophy of the hippocampal formation should be pursued, and the surgical strategy should be modified appropriately.

▶ Of the cerebral vascular malformations reported in this article, 32 were cavernous angiomas and only 4 were arteriovenous malformations. Twenty of the 36 lesions were in the temporal lobe. The favorable outcome in regard to cessation or reduction of seizures reflects this bias toward cavernous angiomas of the temporal lobe.—R.H. Wilkins, M.D.

Linear Accelerator Radiosurgery for Arteriovenous Malformations: The Relationship of Size to Outcome

Friedman WA, Bova FJ, Mendenhall WM (Univ of Florida, Gainesville)
J Neurosurg 82:180–189, 1995   122-96-30–3

Purpose.—An earlier study of LINAC radiosurgery in patients who had intracranial arteriovenous malformations (AVMs) reported that AVM size does not significantly affect the cure rate, even though larger AVMs must be treated with smaller radiation doses to avoid radiation-induced complications. The relationship between AVM size and outcome was conducted.

Patients.—Between 1988 and 1993, 80 male and 78 female patients aged 13 to 70 years who had AVMs were treated radiosurgically. Twenty-two patients had undergone prior attempts at AVM excision, and 14 had had at least 1 embolization procedure. The lesions were graded using the Spetzler-Martin classification. The mean lesion volume was 9 cc, and the range was 0.5–45.3 cc. The mean radiation dose was 1,560 cGy. There were 8 possible outcomes, 3 of which were selected as definitive end points for success or failure: angiographic cure (success), retreatment (failure), and death resulting from AVM hemorrhage or radiosurgical complications (failure). The mean follow-up was 33 months.

Results.—Using traditional reporting standards, there was angiographic cure in 81% of AVMs 1–4 cc in volume, 89% of AVMs 4–10 cc in volume, and 69% of AVMs greater than 10 cc in volume (Table 1). The overall angiographic cure rate was 80%. Fifty-six patients reached 1 of the end-

TABLE 1.—Outcome Categories and Volume Size of Arteriovenous Malformations (AVMs) of 85 Patients Who Received Linear Accelerator Radiosurgery

Outcome	Size Category			
	A	B	C	D
angiographic cure		21	16	11
angiographic failure (> 24 < 36 mos)		3	2	2
re-treated (> 36 mos)		2		3
deceased*		2	1	2
MR-documented cure (angiogram pending or refused)			3	1
MR-documented failure (< 36 mos)			1	4
refused follow-up review	1	1		4
lost to follow-up review	1	2	1	1
total	2	31	24	28

A, < 1 cc; *B* 1–4 cc; *C*, 4–10 cc; *D* > 10 cc.
* One patient died secondary to fatal hemorrhage from AVM; the others died of intercurrent disease.
(Courtesy of Friedman WA, Bova FJ, Mendenhall WM: *J Neurosurg* 82:180–189, 1995.)

TABLE 2.—Summary of End Point Outcome by Lesion
Volume Size Category

Outcome	Category			
	A	B	C	D
angiographic cure	0	21	16	11
re-treatment	0	2	0	3
fatal hemorrhage	0	0	0	1
percentage success	0	91	100	79

There is a statistically significant ($P > 0.04$) difference between outcomes in category C and category D. A, < 1 cc; B, 1–4 cc; C, 4–10 cc; D, > 10 cc.
(Courtesy of Friedman WA, Bova FJ, Mendenhall WM: *J Neurosurg* 82:180–189, 1995.)

points. Successful end points were seen in 91% of AVMs 1–4 cc in volume, 100% of AVMs 4–10 cc in volume, and 79% of AVMs greater than 10 cc in volume (Table 2).

Conclusions.—Arteriovenous malformations greater than 10 cc in volume can be safely and effectively treated with LINAC radiosurgery.

► Experts in the use of radiosurgery and stereotactic radiotherapy continue to "push the envelope," trying to achieve the maximum benefits of these valuable techniques while avoiding or minimizing the complications. The accurate collection and analysis of data, such as those reported in this article by William Friedman and colleagues, are essential to this process.—R.H. Wilkins, M.D.

Hereditary Hemorrhagic Telangiectasia (Rendu-Osler-Weber Disease) Presenting With Polymicrobial Brain Abscess: Case Report
Hall WA (Univ of Minnesota, Minn)
J Neurosurg 81:294–296, 1994   122-96-30–4

Introduction.—Central nervous system manifestations of hereditary hemorrhagic telangiectasis are rare but include brain abscess and cerebral and spinal vascular malformations. Brain abscesses may develop as a result of a right-to-left pulmonary shunt with reduced arterial oxygen saturation.

Case Report.—Man, 26, had weakness of the right arm for 1 week before having a generalized seizure. A CT study showed an enhancing mass in the left frontal region surrounded by edema. The patient reported having had frequent exertional dyspnea and recurrent epistasis since childhood. A severe expressive aphasia was present as well as right-sided hemiparesis and hyperactive reflexes on the right. Small telangiectasias were present in the oral mucosa, and the digits of the hands and feet were clubbed. The hemoglobin level was 7.2 g/dL. The blood PO_2 was 57 mm Hg. Magnetic resonance imaging showed that the frontal lesion projected to the cortical surface. Pus containing various organisms was aspirated, and the patient was given penicillin G and chloramphenicol intravenously on the basis of results of sensitivity testing. Thoracic CT showed arteriovenous fistulas in both lungs, and echocardiography showed a large right-to-left shunt. Five of the fistulas were embolized, after which the PO_2 increased to 93 mm Hg. Small arteriovenous malformations in the colonic mucosa were coagulated by laser. Both the aphasia and the hemiparesis improved gradually. The abscess had completely resolved at 6 months.

Discussion.—Brain abscesses develop in 5% to 10% of patients with pulmonary arteriovenous fistulas. As this case indicates, a brain abscess of polymicrobial origin may be the initial manifestation of hemorrhagic telangiectasis. Aspiration of the abscess should be followed by obliteration of the pulmonary malformations.

▶ Hall and colleagues remind us with this case report that hereditary hemorrhagic telangiectasia can manifest as a brain abscess. They indicate that the mechanism responsible for the development of brain abscess in patients with this condition is septic embolization through the pulmonary capillary circulation into areas of cerebral microinfarction, with such areas resulting from vascular thrombosis that may be caused by polycythemia and cerebral hypoxia resulting from imperfect oxygenation. The patient whose case is discussed in this abstract had bilateral pulmonary arteriovenous fistulae; brain abscess occurs in 5% to 10% of patients with hereditary hemorrhagic telangiectasia and pulmonary arteriovenous fistulae.—R.H. Wilkins, M.D.

Angiographically Occult Vascular Malformations: A Correlative Study of Features on Magnetic Resonance Imaging and Histological Examination

Tomlinson FH, Houser OW, Scheithauer BW, Sundt TM Jr, Okazaki H, Parisi JE (Mayo Clinic and Found, Rochester, Minn)
Neurosurgery 34:792–800, 1994   122-96-30–5

Introduction.—Architecturally, cavernous vascular malformations show a compact growth pattern with no intervening brain parenchyma. Histologically, the vessels appear hyaline and collagenous, without the microscopic features of arteries or veins. The term *cavernous angioma* has traditionally been assigned to lesions showing both features. The MRI findings of 25 angiographically occult vascular malformations, including a critical analysis of the histologic findings, were described.

Patients.—Twenty-five of 106 patients undergoing surgery for cerebral vascular malformations met the inclusion criteria for the study. All had an angiographically occult lesion and had T1- and T2-weighted MRI scans and histologic sections available for review. There were 17 females and 8 males (mean age, 30 years; 28% were children). Presenting symptoms included a subacute focal neurologic deficit in 36%, seizure in 44%, and headache in 16%. The lesion was located in a supratentorial position in two thirds of the cases, and all were intraparenchymal. Surgery improved the patients' clinical condition in all cases.

Findings.—On histologic review, the vascular channels of all lesions but 1 were cavernous in nature. The specimen from the remaining case was inadequate for classification. Eighty-four percent of lesions had a partially racemose architecture, and 25% had a capillary component. Ninety-four percent had evidence of thrombosis, and 63% showed recanalization. On review of T2-weighted MRI scans, the pattern of cavernous malformation varied, the most common being a multifocal hyperintense center surrounded by a hypointense ring. The MRI findings reflected the histologic appearance. There were no thrombosed arteriovenous malformations.

Conclusions.—These findings suggest that the growth of cavernous malformations arises from intraluminal thrombosis and subsequent recanalization; thrombosed arteriovenous malformations are apparently rare. It is not always possible to distinguish resolving hematomas from cavernous lesions. Magnetic resonance imaging is the method of choice for evaluating angiographically occult vascular malformations, and treatment is by microsurgical excision. The histologic picture of such malformations is almost always cavernous, which suggests they should be designated cavernous angiomas. At least for CNS lesions, the criterion of architectural compactness is somewhat artificial and should be abandoned.

▶ The morphological pattern (and, therefore, the diagnosis) of angiographically occult vascular malformations has received the attention of several investigators in recent years. The inclusion criteria for this study were the presence of an angiographically occult lesion, the availability of MRI scans with T1- and T2-weighted imaging, and the availability of histologic sections. Twenty-five such lesions were obtained from 25 patients. One of the specimens was not adequate for classification. Histologically, all of the other 24 lesions demonstrated cavernous types of vessels, although in some there were other components as well (capillaries were observed in 6 cases, and arteries were demonstrated outside the lesion in 5). However, only 3 lesions demonstrated a purely compact or cavernous pattern of vessel distribution. In one lesion there was a purely racemose pattern, in which parenchyma intervened between the vascular channels, and in the remaining 20 lesions, there was a mixed cavernous and racemose pattern. The authors recommend that the diagnosis of cavernous angioma be based solely on the histologic appearance of the vessels rather than on the vessel appearance plus the feature of architectural compactness. Using this terminology, all of their evaluable angiographically occult vascular malformations were cavernous angiomas.

In contrast, Robinson et al. (1) examined the histology of 34 consecutive angiographically occult vascular malformations of the brain and stressed their pathologic heterogeneity. They classified the lesions as 21 cavernous malformations, 3 arteriovenous malformations, 3 venous malformations, 2 capillary malformations, and 5 mixed malformations.

Although various factors, including chance occurrence, may explain the differences between these 2 studies, the main difference seems to be one of interpretation and emphasis. In other words, Tomlinson et al. can be viewed as "lumpers" and Robinson et al. as "splitters."—R.H. Wilkins, M.D.

Reference

1. Robinson JR Jr, Awad IA, Masaryk TJ, et al: Pathological heterogeneity of angiographically occult vascular malformations of the brain. *Neurosurgery* 33:547–555, 1993.

Cavernous Malformations of the Brain Stem: A Review of 139 Cases

Fritschi JA, Reulen H-J, Spetzler RF, Zabramski JM (Univ of Bern, Switzerland; Univ of Munich, West Germany; Barrow Neurological Inst, Phoenix, Ariz)
Acta Neurochir (Wien) 130:35–46, 1994   122-96-30–6

Introduction.—Some researchers have recommended that cavernous malformations (CMs) of the brain stem be surgically removed whenever they are accessible and symptomatic. However, because of the difficulty of the surgical approach and because little is known about the natural history of brain stem CMs, surgery is not a generally accepted recommendation. Patient and disease characteristics and outcomes were investigated in a retrospective evaluation of brain stem CMs.

Methods.—A total of 41 patients with brain stem CMs were seen in centers in Phoenix, Bern, and Munich. The clinical data from these patients, together with published data on 98 well-documented, symptomatic patients, were examined with particular attention to patient age, location and size of the lesion, bleeding, enlargement, and the type and results of treatment.

Results.—Patients ranged in age from 2 to 69 years (average age, 31.8 years). Lesions were localized in the pons in 62% (with half near the floor of the fourth ventricle, 30% infiltrating a cerebellar peduncle, and 20% located deeply), the mesencephalon in 14% (with 60% in the tectum and 40% in the tegmentum or sited ventrally), the pontomesencephalic junction in 12%, and the pontomedullary junction in 12%. Most lesions measured 10–30 mm in diameter; follow-up studies documented enlargement in 12 patients (9%). Of the 115 patients with data on hemorrhage, 88% had evidence of hemorrhage, with 55% having 1, 17% having 2, and 17% having 3 or more hemorrhages during a mean follow-up of 30.3 months. The average bleeding rate was 2.7% per year per lesion. The rebleeding rate was 21% per year per lesion. Ninety-three patients were treated surgically; 39.8% achieved complete recovery, 44.1% were minimally disabled, 15% were moderately disabled, 1 patient was severely disabled, and none died perioperatively. Of the 7 patients who had only partial resection, 2 had rebleeding within 4.1 years, and 2 had enlarging residual lesions. Of the 30 patients who did not undergo resection, 43.3% recovered to clinical grade I or II, 13.4% had moderate or severe disability, and 20% died.

Discussion.—Patients with sudden-onset symptomatology caused by a hemorrhage or with a neurologic deficit that progresses slowly may be appropriate surgical candidates. However, the surgery should only be performed by experienced neurosurgeons in properly equipped centers, as the susceptible structures require delicate handling. When the lesions are deep in the brain stem, surgery is not indicated. Asymptomatic lesions should be regularly monitored.

▶ Magnetic resonance imaging has greatly facilitated the diagnosis of CMs of the brain stem. These authors have used this advantage in an attempt to assess the natural history of these lesions. There undoubtedly was bias in patient inclusion in this series; so the recorded outcomes may not be an accurate reflection of natural history; however, the authors do present information that should be useful to neurosurgeons and neurologists, who must decide whether to recommend the surgical resection of such a lesion.—R.H. Wilkins, M.D.

Intracranial Dural Arteriovenous Fistulae: Angiographic Predictors of Intracranial Hemorrhage and Clinical Outcome in Nonsurgical Patients
Brown RD Jr, Wiebers DO, Nichols DA (Mayo Clinic and Found, Rochester, Minn)
J Neurosurg 81:531–538, 1994   122-96-30–7

Background.—Although many researchers have described the clinical appearance of dural arteriovenous fistulae (AVFs), follow-up of only a few conservatively managed patients has been reported. No reports have been done on a cohort of untreated patients monitored over time for features predicting intracranial hemorrhage (ICH) or other clinical outcomes. The natural history of dural AVF was defined in a cohort given a diagnosis before ICH or debilitating symptoms necessitated immediate intervention.

Methods.—Fifty-four patients were examined at 1 center between 1976 and 1989. A neuroradiologist examined all available cerebral arteriograms. A total of 52 patients (96%) underwent follow-up until death, until treatment intervention, or for at least 1 year after diagnosis. The mean follow-up was 6.6 years.

Findings.—Intracranial hemorrhage associated with dural AVF occurred in 5 patients, for a crude risk of 1.6% per year. The risk of bleeding at the time of mean follow-up evaluation was 1.8% per year. Angiography indicated that several features potentially predicted ICH during follow-up. Although the small numbers of patients precluded a definitive conclusion, lesions of the petrosal sinus and straight sinus had a greater tendency to bleed. Patients with a dural AVF with a venous varix on a draining vein had a greater risk of hemorrhage, whereas none of the 20 patients without a varix hemorrhaged. Lesions draining into leptomeningeal veins bled more often, although this increased risk was not statistically significant. When initial symptoms were compared with follow-up data, pulsatile tinnitus was found to be improved in more than half of the patients, resolving in 75% of those with some improvement. Patients without a sinus or venous outflow occlusion at initial cerebral angiography were more likely to improve or remain stable. Patients with an occlusion usually did not improve.

Conclusions.—There appear to be angiographic predictors of ICH and symptomatic improvement in the absence of aggressive intervention in patients with dural AVFs. The natural history described in this paper supports the consideration of differential management for dural AVF based on angiographic features predicting an increased risk of ICH or poor symptomatic outcome.

▶ Based on their assessment of the natural history and angiographic features of intracranial dural AVFs, the authors make logical recommendations about the management of such lesions.—R.H. Wilkins, M.D.

Dural Arteriovenous Fistula of the Posterior Fossa Draining Into the Spinal Medullary Veins: An Unusual Cause of Myelopathy: Case Report
Bret P, Salzmann M, Bascoulergue Y, Guyotat J (Hôpital Neurologique et Neurochirurgical Pierre Wertheimer, Lyon, France)
Neurosurgery 35:965–969, 1994   122-96-30–8

Introduction.—A very uncommon cause of chronic myelopathy is a dural intracranial arteriovenous fistula (AVF). A patient with progressive myelopathy who had an intracranial tentorial AVF draining into the spinal veins was described. Surgical excision of the fistula relieved the symptoms of the myelopathy.

Case Report.—Man, 31, had progressive difficulties with gait during a 4-month period, with complaints of coldness, bilateral paresthesia of his legs, and dysuria. Neurologic examination revealed signs of pyramidal tract involvement. An MR image showed spinal cord swelling. A myelogram showed serpentine subarachnoid filling defects traveling medially over the anterior and posterior aspects of the cervical cord. An angiogram of the right internal carotid artery showed a tentorial AVF that drained into dilated spinal medullary veins. Further angiograms revealed no additional supply to the AVF. Via a microscopic suboccipital approach, the petrosal vein beneath the tentorium was noted to contain arterialized blood. The arterial feeder was occluded, and the petrosal vein was divided at its entry into the subarachnoid space. An angiogram was repeated a week after surgery and showed that the AVF was cured. Three months later, despite some mild spasticity, the patient had full ambulation. Some mild spinal cord swelling persisted 5 months later.

Comment.—Dural intracranial AVF should be considered in the differential diagnosis of chronic myelopathy. This is especially important in patients in whom spinal angiography does not confirm a spinal vascular deformity. It is important to consider 4-vessel cerebral angiography to determine the need for AVF treatment and to avoid an uneeded hazardous laminectomy.

▶ This is one of a few reported cases in which myelopathy has resulted from retrograde venous engorgement caused by an AVF located outside of the spinal canal. This condition must be considered in a patient who has a progressive myelopathy, in whom a focal intramedullary spinal cord abnormality is noted on MRI (especially on T2-weighted images), in whom tortuous vessels are noted on the surface of the spinal cord on MRI or CT myelography, and in whom there is no evidence of a spinal AVF.—R.H. Wilkins, M.D.

31 Cerebrovascular Occlusive Disease

Technical Issues in Carotid Artery Surgery 1995
Loftus CM, Quest DO (Univ of Iowa College of Medicine, Iowa City; Columbia Univ College of Physician and Surgeons, New York)
Neurosurgery 36:629–647, 1995   122-96-31–1

Introduction.—Important changes in the practice of extracranial cerebrovascular reconstruction have taken place in the past few years. The advances made in operative monitoring and surgical techniques during the past decade were reviewed.

Anesthesia and Monitoring.—General anesthesia is now generally preferred for carotid artery surgery because of the more controlled surgical environment it provides. Monitoring methods include measuring residual stump pressure in the isolated distal common or internal carotid artery, intraoperatively estimating regional cerebral blood flow by the intracarotid injection of xenon-133, and continuous recording of systolic and mean transcranial Doppler velocities in the ipsilateral middle cerebral artery. A Doppler probe may be used to assess postarteriotomy patency. Methods of functional assessment include intraoperative electroencephalogram monitoring and recording of somatosensory evoked potentials.

Operative Aspects.—Some surgeons who find intraoperative monitoring to be unreliable in patients with a recent reversible ischemic deficit or stroke use an indwelling arterial shunt during carotid endarterectomy. Most surgeons prefer patch grafting of the internal carotid for repair in patients with recurrent stenosis and also for primary repair if there is a risk of postoperative stenosis and thrombosis. The use of tandem sutures to secure the distal carotid intima remains controversial. Excellent results have been achieved by microsurgical endarterectomy. Consideration is given as to how to best deal with such specific operative situations as critical stenosis, intraluminal thrombi, contralateral carotid occlusion, tandem lesions of the carotid siphon, and a concurrent intracranial aneurysm.

Conclusions.—Data from cooperative studies affirm the clear advantage of surgery for both asymptomatic carotid stenosis exceeding 60% and symptomatic stenosis of more than 70% of the vessel lumen. All patients with cardiac symptoms should be aggressively investigated before carotid endarterectomy is undertaken. If surgery at both sites is indicated, staged procedures are preferred unless the extent of coronary disease makes anesthesia for endarterectomy untenable.

▶ Drs. Loftus and Quest have provided a detailed review of current technical issues concerning carotid artery surgery. I recommend this article to neurosurgeons and neurologists who have an interest in vascular disease and especially to neurosurgeons who perform carotid endarterectomy and related procedures.—R.H. Wilkins, M.D.

Carotid Artery Stenosis: A Prospective Comparison of CT Angiography and Conventional Angiography
Cumming MJ, Morrow IM (Health Sciences Centre, Winnipeg, Man, Canada)
AJR 163:517–523, 1994   122-96-31–2

Purpose.—Although catheter angiography is the definitive technique for the demonstration of carotid artery stenosis, it has some risk and is an expensive procedure. The introduction of spiral CT has led to new scanning techniques for imaging vascular structures, particularly the carotid arteries. The quality and interpretation of CT images are affected by many possible technical variations and combinations of steps. One CT angiographic technique was prospectively compared with conventional angiography in the assessment of carotid artery stenosis.

Methods.—The study sample comprised 35 patients who were referred for evaluation of carotid artery disease, for a total of 70 carotid arteries. All underwent conventional angiography, which was followed 4 to 24 hours later by CT angiography. The CT angiographic technique used 40-second spiral scans with a table speed of 2 mm/second, 2-mm beam collimation, and IV injection of iodinated contrast material at a rate of 2.5 mL/second. The CT angiograms were interpreted on the CT work-station with the use of 3-dimensional shaded-surface objects and multiplanar reformations, which took 10 to 15 minutes per artery. The paired studies were read independently without knowledge of the results of the other study. The readers classified each artery as normal; mildly stenosed, 1% to 29%; moderately stenosed, 30% to 69%; severely stenosed, 70% to 99%; or totally occluded.

Results.—The CT angiographic findings were highly correlated with those of the conventional angiograms, $r = .928$. The CT angiographic technique correctly identified all occluded arteries and never wrongly identified an artery as occluded. In 16 vessels, CT angiography overesti-

---

Fig 31–1.—A, lateral conventional angiogram shows mild irregularity of internal carotid artery. No measurable stenosis is identified. B, 3-dimensional CT angiogram, lateral projection, shows extensive calcification at carotid bifurcation that obscures lumen of artery. C and D, planar reconstructions in lateral (C) and oblique sagittal (D) projections show arterial lumen to advantage. Calcified plaques and small ulcerations, which are difficult to see on A, are on C and D. (Courtesy of Cummings MJ, Morrow IM: *AJR* 163:517–523, 1994.)

(continued)

Fig 31–1 (cont).

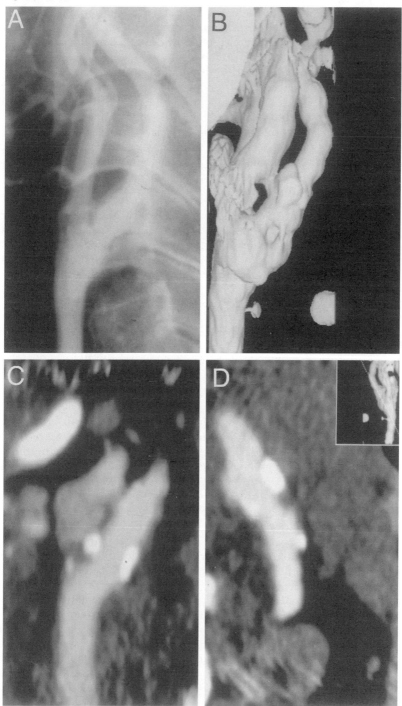

mated the degree of stenosis by more than 10%; this was most likely in vessels with calcified atherosclerotic plaques. Conventional angiography underestimated the degree of stenosis in some of these arteries. All but one artery classified as being severely stenosed on conventional angiography were correctly classified by CT angiography.

Conclusions.—In the evaluation of possible carotid artery stenosis, the results of CT and conventional angiography are highly correlated. The multiplanar capabilities of CT angiography permit differentiation of calcified plaque from contrast material, providing valuable information about plaque calcification, ulceration, and size that is unavailable with conventional angiography (Fig 31–1); this may explain some of the noted discrepancies between sonographic and angiographic findings. The described CT technique is easy to use and permits accurate measurement of stenosis at the carotid bifurcation.

▶ The development of spiral CT techniques has permitted their adaptation to carotid, vertebral, and cerebral angiography. The images provided by this less invasive and safer procedure have already advanced to the point of challenging conventional intra-arterial catheter angiography. Undoubtedly, future improvements will further enhance the value of CT angiography.—R.H. Wilkins, M.D.

Carotid Endarterectomy for Patients With Asymptomatic Internal Carotid Artery Stenosis
National Institute of Neurological Disorders and Stroke (Natl Insts of Health, Bethesda, Md)
J Neurol Sci 129:76–77, 1995   122-96-31–3

Introduction.—Interim results of the Asymptomatic Carotid Atherosclerosis Study were reported on September 28, 1994. A randomized, controlled trial of carotid endarterectomy in patients with asymptomatic carotid artery stenosis of greater than 60% reduction in diameter was done to determine whether carotid endarterectomy reduces the overall 5-year risk of fatal and nonfatal ipsilateral carotid stroke.

Methods.—Thirty-nine United States and Canadian centers were accepted after rigorous evaluation of neurologic expertise, quality of ultrasound laboratory assessment, and quality of surgical management. Participating surgeons demonstrated a perioperative complication rate of less than 3% for carotid endarterectomy in patients with asymptomatic carotid stenosis. Eligible patients were 40–79 years old, had a life expectancy of at least 5 years, had no history of TIA/stroke or previous endarterectomy on the randomized artery, and had at least 60% carotid artery stenosis near the bifurcation of the common or internal carotid artery. After randomization to surgical or medical management, all patients were started on 325 mg of aspirin daily and aggressive reduction of modifiable risk factors.

Results.—Of 1,662 patients, 828 were randomized to receive surgery and 834 were managed medically. Demographically, males outnumbered females 2:1, 95% of patients were white, and approximately 50% of patients were 60–69 years of age. Patients undergoing carotid endarterectomy had a relative risk reduction of 55% over 5 years compared with patients managed medically. Relative risk reduction in men was 69% compared with 16% in women. Additional analysis is required to determine reasons for this apparent difference.

Conclusions.—Carotid endarterectomy is beneficial for carefully selected patients with asymptomatic significant carotid stenosis who are treated at certain centers by surgeons with documented perioperative morbidity and mortality rates of less than 3%. Such treatment includes postoperative management of modifiable risk factors.

▶ In this important study, the patients were randomized to undergo treatment between December 1987 and December 1993. As a consequence of the trial reaching statistical significance in favor of endarterectomy, physicians participating in the study were notified and advised to reevaluate patients who did not receive surgery. This abstracted report is a brief clinical advisory put out by the National Institute of Neurological Disorders and Stroke. At the time it was published, the Asymptomatic Carotid Atherosclerosis Study trial group was completing follow-up, expanding the database, performing additional statistical analyses, and seeking expeditious publication of the results.—R.H. Wilkins, M.D.

Cerebral Hypoxia Detected by Near Infrared Spectroscopy
Williams IM, Picton AJ, Hardy SC, Mortimer AJ, McCollum CN (Univ Hosp of South Manchester, England)
Anaesthesia 49:762–766, 1994   122-96-31–4

Introduction.—Near-infrared cerebral spectroscopy is a recently developed technique for continuous and noninvasive monitoring of intracerebral oxygen saturation. It has potential advantages over the transcranial Doppler technique, which provides information only on blood velocity in the intracerebral vasculature and none on peripheral cortical perfusion. The detection of cerebral hypoxia with near-infrared spectroscopy was described in 3 patients undergoing carotid endarterectomy.

Methods.—During each operation, cerebral monitoring was performed with near-infrared cerebral oxygen spectroscopy, transcranial Doppler assessment of the middle cerebral artery, and jugular venous bulb sampling for measurement of oxygen saturation. The cerebral oximetry setup included a near-infrared light transmitter and 2 detectors, situated 30 and 40 mm from this source, that were housed in an adhesive plastic shield for scalp attachment. Continuous monitoring of brain oxygen saturation within the distribution of the middle cerebral artery was achieved by 2 sensors positioned over the parietal area on both cerebral hemispheres. Blood pressure and pulse oximetry were monitored as well.

Findings.—In one case, severe cerebral ischemia caused by slippage of the tracheal tube into the right main bronchus was rapidly detected by bilateral decreases in intracerebral oxygen saturation. Throughout this episode, which was confirmed by jugular bulb venous oxygen saturation, transcranial Doppler measurements of middle cerebral artery blood velocity remained stable. In the other 2 cases, decreases in intracerebral oxygen saturation were noted in association with episodes of hypotension. The oxygen saturation increased quickly once the hypotension was corrected. Pulse oximetry readings never fell below 98% oxygen saturation during these episodes.

Conclusions.—Near-infrared spectroscopy is a reliable technique of monitoring peripheral cortical perfusion during carotid artery surgery. It provides a continuous and noninvasive means of monitoring intracerebral oxygen saturation. In more than 80 patients undergoing carotid endarterectomy who were monitored with cerebral oximetry, the investigators have found that major changes in blood pressure are always associated with significant changes in intracerebral oxygen saturation.

▶ Cerebral oximetry is being used with increasing frequency as a noninvasive method of monitoring cerebral oxygen saturation. Although the accuracy of the specific measurements made by the cerebral oximeter has been questioned, the technique appears to be a reliable gauge of cerebral oxygen saturation. Williams and associates provide 3 examples of its practical value in detecting cerebral hypoxia during carotid endarterectomy.—R.H. Wilkins, M.D.

Clinical Relevance of Intraoperative Embolization Detected by Transcranial Doppler Ultrasonography During Carotid Endarterectomy: A Prospective Study of 100 Patients
Gaunt ME, Martin PJ, Smith JL, Rimmer T, Cherryman G, Ratliff DA, Bell PRF, Naylor AR (Leicester Royal Infirmary, England)
Br J Surg 81:1435–1439, 1994   122-96-31–5

Background.—Several studies have shown that transcranial Doppler ultrasonography (TCD) monitoring of the ipsilateral middle cerebral artery during carotid endarterectomy is able to detect embolization in different phases of surgery. However, these studies were not specifically designed to assess clinical outcomes. Therefore, the clinical relevance of embolization detected by TCD remains unclear.

Methods.—The clinical significance of TCD-detected microembolization was investigated by determining the quantity and nature of the emboli and correlating them with neurologic and psychometric outcome, fundoscopy, automated visual field testing, and CT brain scans. The study group was comprised of 100 consecutive patients undergoing carotid endarterectomy.

Findings.—Embolization was found in 92% of successfully monitored procedures. Most emboli were characteristic of air and unassociated with adverse clinical outcomes. However, a significant deterioration in postoperative cognitive function was associated with more than 10 particulate emboli during initial carotid dissection. Persistent particulate embolization in the immediate postoperative period was associated with both incipient carotid artery thrombosis and the development of major neurologic deficits.

Conclusions.—Embolization detected by TCD during carotid endarterectomy appears to be clinically significant. In particular, TCD can provide an early warning of incipient carotid thrombosis in the immediate postoperative period. Early intervention may decrease morbidity and mortality associated with this serious complication. Also, TCD can alert surgeons to potentially harmful embolization occurring during dissection of the carotid artery.

▶ In this study, there was evidence, by TCD, that cerebral embolization of air or particulate matter commonly occurs during carotid endarterectomy (92% of successfully monitored procedures). Fortunately, only a portion of these episodes leads to recognizable postoperative neurologic deficits. Sensitive monitoring of this sort serves a purpose in making the surgeon more aware of the risks of embolization during endarterectomy, and its routine use might make the procedure safer.—R.H. Wilkins, M.D.

Fate of the Non-Operated Carotid Artery After Contralateral Endarterectomy
Naylor AR, John T, Howlett J, Gillespie I, Allan P, Ruckley CV (The Royal Infirmary, Edinburgh, Scotland)
Br J Surg 82:44–48, 1995   122-96-31–6

Introduction.—The value of long-term follow-up with serial postoperative imaging of the nonoperated internal carotid artery (ICA) after contralateral endarterectomy has not been established. A group of 219 patients who underwent carotid endarterectomy was followed up to evaluate clinical outcome and to determine whether noninvasive surveillance is able to identify those at risk for stroke.

Patients and Methods.—The carotid endarterectomies were performed between 1975 and 1990. Demographic data, clinical features at diagnosis, concurrent diseases, and risk factors were recorded, and the results of preoperative angiography reviewed. The patients were assessed at 4 weeks, 6 months, and then annually for 10 years. Imaging was part of the follow-up after 1983, and 151 patients were studied with either IV digital subtraction angiography or duplex ultrasonography and Doppler waveform analysis.

Results.—There were 44 deaths during follow-up, including 22 resulting from myocardial infarction. The cumulative survival rate was 97% at 1 year, 82% at 5 years, and 53% at 10 years. Only 10 patients had a stroke in the nonoperated hemisphere during follow-up, giving a mean incidence of stroke of 1% per year. Cumulative freedom from stroke in the nonoperated hemisphere was 99% at 1 year, 96% at 5 years, and 86% at 10 years. Only 1 of the 10 strokes was preceded by a transient ischemic attack, and none was associated with severe (70% or greater) stenosis of the ICA. Ten patients who had an initial ICA stenosis of less than 70% were found to have significant disease progression during the surveillance period. Only 3 became symptomatic, however, and in each case the onset of symptoms preceded recognition of significant disease progression.

Conclusion.—The long-term risk of stroke in the nonoperated ICA territory was found to be very small in this series of patients. Not 1 of the high-risk patients was identified in 530 studies, and none of the observed strokes could have been prevented by the form of surveillance used. Therefore, the follow-up program is not recommended for cost-effectiveness or benefit to the patient.

▶ Among the 219 patients in this investigation who were followed after a unilateral carotid endarterectomy, the incidence of contralateral stroke was only 1% per year. It is of practical importance that none of the observed strokes could have been prevented by the postoperative surveillance used.—R.H. Wilkins, M.D.

Surgical Treatment of Recurrent Carotid Artery Stenosis
Meyer FB, Piepgras DG, Fode NC (Mayo Clinic and Found, Rochester, Minn)
J Neurosurg 80:781–787, 1994   122-96-31–7

Background.—Surgical treatment for recurrent carotid artery stenosis is frequently performed. However, because of scarring that can develop both outside and inside the vessel lumen and the friable nature of recurrent atherosclerotic plaque, this surgery is significantly more difficult than the initial endarterectomy and is associated with a significantly higher risk. In certain patients, repeat endarterectomy cannot be performed. In these instances, excision of the involved vessel and placement of an interposition graft is required. An experience with surgical repair for recurrent carotid artery stenosis was described.

Patients and Findings.—Surgical treatment for recurrent carotid artery stenosis was done in 92 vessels of 82 patients over a 21-year period. The initial surgery had been performed at the authors' facility in 55 instances and elsewhere in the remaining 37. Recurrent atherosclerosis was noted in 45 instances, myointimal hyperplasia in 20, organized thrombus without significant underlying plaque in 20, and scarring along the proximal arteriotomy site in 7. A repeat endarterectomy was done in 63 vessels, followed by a saphenous vein patch in 55, a fabric patch in 7, and a primary patch in 1. Seven patients with myointimal hyperplasia underwent enlargement of the artery lumen via an onlay patch graft without a direct endarterectomy.

Reconstruction with an interposition graft was done in 22 patients. Of these, 16 had an interposition saphenous vein graft, 4 had an interposition Dacron or bovine graft, 1 had a combination saphenous vein and Gore-Tex graft, and 1 had a direct resection and reanastomosis without an interposition graft. When performing an interposition graft, a saphenous vein can frequently be taken from the leg and dilated to adequate size. If veins cannot be harvested, a fabric graft can be used. It should be anastomosed end to end from the common carotid artery to the internal carotid artery, excluding the external carotid and superior thyroid arteries.

Five major complications, including 3 instances of intraoperative embolization during carotid artery exposure, occurred in 5 symptomatic patients. Most neurologic complications were noted in those who had intraluminal thrombus verified at surgery. Four perioperative deaths occurred. Of these, 2 patients experienced cerebral hemorrhage and 2 had myocardial infarctions. In patients whose initial surgery was performed at the authors' facility, the risk of recurrent carotid artery stenosis was 3.1% with a primary closure vs. 1.6% when a patch graft was done.

Conclusions.—Repeat endarterectomy can be accomplished in most patients with recurrent atherosclerosis. However, endarterectomy can be difficult in certain clinical situations. In these instances, the best treatment comprises excision of the diseased segment with reconstruction via an interposition graft. It is further suggested that closure of the original arteriotomy with a patch graft reduces the risk of recurrent artery stenosis.

▶ This experienced group presents a nice review of the surgical treatment of recurrent carotid artery stenosis.—R.H. Wilkins, M.D.

32 Head Trauma

Survey of Critical Care Management of Comatose, Head-Injured Patients in the United States
Ghajar J, Hariri RJ, Narayan RK, Iacono LA, Firlik K, Patterson RH (Cornell Univ Med College, New York; Baylor College of Medicine, Houston)
Crit Care Med 23:560–567, 1995   122-96-32–1

Introduction.—The use of intracranial pressure monitoring is controversial, despite evidence of its efficacy in the management of intracranial pressure in patients with severe head injuries. A nationwide telephone survey of trauma centers in the United States was conducted to ascertain neurotrauma monitoring and treatment practices.

Methods.—Of 624 trauma centers, 277 were randomly selected for telephone interviews of their neurotrauma nurses. Trauma centers from rural, suburban, and large metropolitan areas were included. A total of 261 centers (94%) participated. Of these, 219 (84%) reportedly treated patients with severe head injuries. At 6 months, 40 centers (15%) were resurveyed; the questions remained the same, but a different nurse was interviewed.

Results.—Level I, II, and III centers were represented by 49%, 32%, and 2% of respondents, respectively. There was a designated neurologic or neurosurgical ICU in 34% of the hospitals. A neurosurgeon or neurologist headed 24% of these units. Of 219 centers, 77 used intracranial pressure monitoring routinely (72% used ventriculostomy catheters) in the treatment of patients with severe head injuries, whereas 16 centers never used intracranial pressure monitoring. There was a significant correlation between the number of patients with severe head injuries and the use of intracranial pressure monitoring. Hyperventilation and diuretics were used in 83% of centers to reduce increased intracranial pressure. Cerebrospinal fluid drainage, administration of barbiturates, and administration of corticosteroids (used more than half of the time) were used in 44%, 33%, and 64% of centers, respectively. At 6-month follow-up, the frequency of intracranial pressure monitoring had significantly increased, and the types of monitoring devices used were significantly different.

Conclusion.—The care of patients with severe head injuries varies greatly. Practice guidelines are needed to improve the standard of care.

▶ This study underscores the discrepancy that frequently exists between the best-known management of a medical condition and the actual treatment that is delivered. Undoubtedly, there are many reasons for such discrepancies, but it is important that they be addressed to raise the overall level of medical care.—R.H. Wilkins, M.D.

The Effect of the 1992 California Motorcycle Helmet Use Law on Motorcycle Crash Fatalities and Injuries

Kraus JF, Peek C, McArthur DL, Williams A (Univ of California, Los Angeles; Insurance Inst for Highway Safety, Arlington, Va)
JAMA 272:1506–1511, 1994   122-96-32–2

Background.—Motorcyclists are more vulnerable to severe injuries than riders in any other type of vehicle. Despite convincing evidence that shows that motorcycle helmets reduce fatalities and nonfatal head injuries, only half of the states in the United States have motorcycle helmet laws. As of 1992 in California, all drivers and passengers are required to wear a protective helmet when riding a motorcycle or motorized bicycle on a public road or highway. With more drivers and motorcyclists than any other state, California offers the unique chance to study the effectiveness of the helmet law.

Methods.—Fatalities and injury statistics were collected from police reports and death certificates in 1991 (prelaw) and 1992 (postlaw). The statewide basis for exposure to motorcycle crash was derived from the official count of registered motorcycles. Hospital records of autopsies were obtained from 11 counties, and injury data were obtained from 28 hospitals in each of 10 of these 11 counties. Records from a total of 850 fatalities and 3,252 nonfatal injuries were examined. The number and rate of fatalities statewide were estimated, as were the number and pattern of head injuries in both nonfatal and fatal injuries.

Findings.—Statewide implementation of a helmet law resulted in a 37.5% reduction in fatalities, with an estimated prevention of between 92 and 122 fatalities. Fatality rates were reduced from 70.1 per 100,000 registered motorcycles in 1991 to 51.5 per 100,000 in 1992. There was also a significant reduction in head injuries in both fatally and nonfatally injured motorcyclists.

Comment.—The new helmet law resulted in decreases in motorcycle fatalities, fatality rate, head injuries, and head injury severity. These data reinforce the benefits of a mandatory motorcyclist helmet law. The application of this law has significantly reduced the number of crash fatalities as well as the number and severity of head injuries.

▶ This report speaks for itself. Physicians in states without a motorcycle helmet law could use the results of this study in arguing for enactment of such a law.—R.H. Wilkins, M.D.

Prevalence of MR Evidence of Diffuse Axonal Injury in Patients With Mild Head Injury and Normal Head CT Findings

Mittl RL, Grossman RI, Hiehle JF Jr, Hurst RW, Kauder DR, Gennarelli TA, Alburger GW (Univ of Pennsylvania, Philadelphia)
AJNR 15:1583–1589, 1994   122-96-32–3

Introduction.—Moderate-to-severe head injuries have been associated with diffuse axonal injury, or white matter shearing injury, changes that may well explain the decreased consciousness and cognitive dysfunction frequently observed in the absence of mass lesions. The frequency of abnormal MR findings in patients with mild head injury is not clear.

Objective.—Magnetic resonance studies were performed in a prospective series of 20 patients with mild head injury whose cranial CT findings were normal.

Methods.—Both conventional spin-echo and $T2^*$-weighted gradient-echo images were acquired using a 1.5-tesla system. Thirteen patients were examined within 48 hours of injury. Two neuroradiologists who were blinded to the patients' clinical status independently attempted to locate all foci of abnormal signal intensity in the brain.

Findings.—When interpreting T2-weighted spin-echo images, both readers found foci of high signal intensity in the white matter in 3 of the 20 patients. These lesions were in the deep white matter or at the gray-white junction, but they were not in the corpus callosum or brain stem. Gradient-echo $T2^*$-weighted images demonstrated foci of hypointensity in the white matter in 4 patients, just below the cortex. They were assumed to be small foci of hemorrhagic shear injury. In 30% of cases, the readers agreed that changes of diffuse axonal injury were present.

Conclusions.—Magnetic resonance changes consistent with diffuse axonal injury were found in 30% of mildly head-injured patients in the absence of CT abnormalities. Magnetic resonance imaging has a major role in any system of classifying head injuries.

▶ In the past, prolonged symptoms that occur after minor head injury in some patients were usually difficult to understand and were often ascribed to factors such as secondary gain from accident-related litigation. Information has gradually been accumulated from careful assessments of animals and humans with minor head injury, documenting that lesions of the brain and the vestibular system can be caused by such "minor" trauma, thereby establishing a pathologic basis for many of the symptoms that occur in this setting. Diffuse axonal injury (white-matter shearing injury) is a well-recognized pathologic change that can result from moderate or severe head injury. This study indicates that MRI abnormalities compatible with diffuse axonal injury can be demonstrated in approximately 30% of patients with a mild head injury and a normal CT scan of the brain.—R.H. Wilkins, M.D.

Inappropriate Discharge Instructions for Youth Athletes Hospitalized for Concussion

Genuardi FJ, King WD (Univ of Alabama, Birmingham)
Pediatrics 95:216–218, 1995   122-96-32–4

Background.—Concussions often are incorrectly judged to be minor injuries with no evidence of brain damage. Even when gross pathology is not found, however, microscopic changes and physiochemical abnormalities can be documented. Functional impairment also can occur. The effects of repeated concussion are now being recognized as cumulative, which should prompt efforts to prevent recurrence. The cumulative results of two apparently minor head injuries can be catastrophic. The medical care, especially discharge instructions about returning to sports participation, given young athletes hospitalized for a closed head injury were assessed.

Methods.—The records of all patients hospitalized at one center for a sports-related closed head injury during a 5-year period were reviewed. Discharge instructions were compared with the guidelines endorsed by the American Academy of Pediatrics.

Findings.—Thirty-three patients with sports-related closed head injuries were identified. Twenty-four percent had grade 1, or least severe, concussions; 30%, grade 2 concussions; and 45%, grade 3 concussions. Overall, the discharge instructions were appropriate for only 30.3% of the patients. Instructions were appropriate for all patients with grade 1 concussions, but for only 20% of those with grade 2, and for none with grade 3 concussions.

Conclusions.—All clinicians providing care for young athletes must become familiar with the guidelines for management of concussion, including instructions on when the patient may return to sports activity. Patients with grade 1 concussion, characterized by confusion without amnesia or loss of consciousness, may return to the sports event after 20 minutes of observation if no symptoms are observed at rest or on exertion. Patients with grade 2 concussion, defined as confusion with amnesia but no loss of consciousness, may return to sports participation after 1 week if there are no symptoms at rest or on exertion. Patients with grade 3 concussion, characterized by any loss of consciousness, may return to sports activity after 1 month if there have been no symptoms at rest or on exertion in the preceding 2 weeks.

▶ The neurosurgeon occasionally is called upon to make recommendations to a young athlete who is about return to participation in a sport in which the athlete has sustained a concussion. Such a sports-related concussion is not a rare event; the authors state that approximately 20% of high school football players sustain a closed head injury each season. Fortunately, there are guidelines that can be consulted. Guidelines of this sort first appeared in the early 1980s, and they were most recently summarized by the Sports Medicine Committee of the Colorado Medical Society in 1991. They are given in abbreviated form in the abstract.—R.H. Wilkins, M.D.

Neurobehavioral Effects of Phenytoin and Carbamazepine in Patients Recovering From Brain Trauma: A Comparative Study

Smith KR Jr, Goulding PM, Wilderman D, Goldfader PR, Holterman-Hommes P, Wei F (St. Louis Univ, Mo)
Arch Neurol 51:653–660, 1994   122-96-32–5

Background.—Traumatic brain injuries are a major cause of significant disability among adolescents and young adults. More than 10% of brain-injured patients have post-traumatic seizures, which can exacerbate the cognitive and behavioral sequelae of brain injury. The effects of the prophylactic anticonvulsant use of phenytoin and carbamazepine on the cognitive and emotional status of patients after brain injury were compared.

Methods.—In a double-blind, placebo-controlled trial, 40 of 64 patients who were given phenytoin and 42 of 127 who were given carbamazepine for 6 to 44 months for seizure prophylaxis after brain injury met study criteria and were assigned to continue treatment or not. A battery of neuropsychologic tests were administered twice during a 4-week baseline period, after 4 to 5 weeks of continued drug therapy or placebo, and after 4 weeks of not receiving medication.

Findings.—After the placebo phase, there were no significant differences in the performance of patients in the medication and placebo groups for either drug. Patients in the combined groups had significant improvement on several measures of motor and speed performance after cessation of drug treatment. In a multivariate analysis, additional differences between phenytoin and carbamazepine were apparent. There also seemed to be a significant practice effect on some of the measures used.

Conclusions.—Both phenytoin and carbamazepine appear to affect cognitive performance negatively, especially on tasks with significant motor and speed components. The practice effects observed may account for much of the improvement when patients stopped taking the drugs. The overall effects of the drugs were minimal and of limited clinical significance. However, there were differences among subjects that may affect selection of a particular drug for individual patients.

▶ The results of this study show that both phenytoin and carbamazepine have some negative effects on the performance of patients recovering from brain trauma. However, these effects are generally small in magnitude and are not sufficient in themselves to contraindicate the use of either of the agents when it is necessary for prevention of seizures.—R.H. Wilkins, M.D.

Treatment of Radiation-Induced Nervous System Injury With Heparin and Warfarin

Glantz MJ, Burger PC, Friedman AH, Radtke RA, Massey EW, Schold SC Jr (Brown Univ, Providence, RI; Johns Hopkins Med School, Baltimore, Md; Duke Univ, Durham, NC; et al)
Neurology 44:2020–2027, 1994   122-96-32–6

Introduction.—The most effective adjuvant treatment for CNS cancers is radiation therapy. Unfortunately, surrounding tissue can be damaged by the therapy. Damage, like subacute demyelination and myelopathy, can occur within days or months of radiation treatment. Symptoms may be severe, but resolution is generally spontaneous and complete. Delayed effects, like cerebral radiation necrosis and a gradual intellectual decline to dementia, can be progressive, resulting in disability or death, even when the cancer is stable. The similar spinal cord syndrome is termed chronic progressive myelopathy. Previous reports have described patients who responded to heparin and orally administered sodium warfarin.

Methods.—Eleven patients with documented neurologic disability linked to therapeutic irradiation underwent heparin treatment to achieve a partial thromboplastin time of about 1.5 times their control value. Orally administered sodium warfarin was then begun to achieve a prothrombin time that was 1.5 times that of control. Heparin was gradually discontinued. Anticoagulant therapy was continued for 3–6 months. Patient responses at serial clinical visits were based on the Karnofsky performance score, affected limb strength, and gait; in addition, variation in specific deficits before and after anticoagulation were assessed. Improvement in 1 category was deemed a modest response; in 2 categories, a moderate response; and in 3 categories, a marked response. If the patient was receiving either the same or a lower dose of corticosteroids, an unchanged functional status was termed stable disease. Progressive disease was defined as a deterioration in 1 or more categories in spite of stable or increased corticosteroid dosage.

Findings.—Eight of the 11 patients had cerebral necrosis. Of these 8, 5 patients had modest to marked improvement, 1 remained stable and, despite treatment, the disease progressed in 2 patients. The other 3 patients (1 with myelopathy and 2 with plexopathy) remained stable and cancer-free.

Comment.—Although no firm conclusion can be reached and numerous questions can be raised, anticoagulant therapy appears to provide a clinical benefit to a subgroup of patients with radiation-induced injury. The basic lesion of radiation necrosis, small vessel endothelial injury, may be checked with anticoagulant therapy.

▶ The treatment of delayed radiation necrosis of the brain with anticoagulant therapy began by serendipity. The first patient reported by Rizzoli and Pagnanelli (1) was a 39-year-old woman who had a metastatic follicular thyroid carcinoma resected from the right parietal lobe in May of 1979. Radiation therapy was given postoperatively. Because her neurologic status declined in 1980, she had repeat craniotomies in November 1980 and January 1981 for partial resection of what proved to be radiation necrosis. Neurologic worsening occurred again in April 1981. Because of the development of deep vein thrombosis, she was treated first with heparin and then with warfarin. Within a few days she became progressively more alert and totally oriented; there also was a dramatic improvement in the CT scan performed 3 weeks after the beginning of anticoagulant therapy. A follow-up CT scan in October 1982 showed no evidence of radiation necrosis. Subsequently, Rizzoli and Pagnanelli used this form of treatment for a patient with radiation necrosis but no venous thrombosis, again with improvement. Others have since used anticoagulation to treat delayed radiation injury to the nervous system, with benefit, as recorded in this paper.—R.H. Wilkins, M.D.

Reference

1. Rizzoli HV, Pagnanelli DM: Treatment of delayed radiation necrosis of the brain: A clinical observation. *J Neurosurg* 60:589–594, 1984.

▶ Radiation necrosis (radiation myelopathy and encephalopathy) is a feared complication of radiation treatment given either directly to the nervous system itself, or where the nervous system is inevitably included in the field of treatment for an extraneural neoplasm. Once symptoms of the necrosis have appeared, there tends to be a period of progression, followed by stabilization. Corticosteroid therapy has occasionally been shown to improve the situation, but there currently is no effective or well-accepted treatment. This study raises the possibility that anticoagulation might be of benefit. The underlying pathogenesis appears to be predominantly the result of microvascular endarteritis and infarction, with a possible additional direct effect of the irradiation on the neuronal and glial elements in the region. Intuitively, it seems unlikely that anticoagulation would be able to prevent the endarteritis obliterans; however, this study provides the basis for a scientific controlled trial.—W.G. Bradley, D.M., F.R.C.P.

33 Epilepsy

MR and Positron Emission Tomography in the Diagnosis of Surgically Correctable Temporal Lobe Epilepsy
Heinz R, Ferris N, Lee EK, Radtke R, Crain B, Hoffman JM, Hanson M, Paine S, Friedman A (Duke Univ Med Ctr, Durham, NC; Alfred Hosp, Prahran, Victoria, Australia; Univ of Calif Davis School of Medicine, Sacramento)
AJNR 15:1341–1348, 1994   122-96-33–1

Background.—Neuroimaging techniques, including MR and positron emission tomography (PET), have been used in the preoperative assessment of patients scheduled for temporal lobectomy. Accurate preoperative determination of the epileptogenic focus can lead to either a complete cure of or significant improvement in seizure activity. The association between both MR and PET abnormalities and good patient outcome in patients with temporal lobe epilepsy after lobectomy, the association of combined PET and MR findings with good outcomes after lobectomy, and MR and PET pathologic correlation were investigated.

Patients and Methods.—Twenty-seven patients who had undergone MRI and PET evaluations for temporal lobe epilepsy were included in a blinded study. All patients underwent lobectomy within 12 months of the preoperative imaging assessments. The mean patient age at surgery was 28.2 years. Follow-up was conducted for at least 12 months, with a mean of 21 months. Histologic studies were correlated with foci of increased T2 signal. In addition, 11 patients who had undergone MR studies during the same period as the study group were included as controls. These patients had pseudoseizures or conversion reaction.

Results.—Thirteen of 15 patients with mesial temporal sclerosis demonstrated increased signal or decreased volume of the hippocampus. Positive PET findings were noted in 12 of 15. Of the 24 patients with good postoperative outcomes, MR identified 83% and PET identified 71%. When both imaging techniques were combined, 95% of the patients with good outcomes were detected. In 11 study and 7 control patients, region-of-interest measurements of the hippocampus showed a significant increase in signal in patients with seizures. Increased T2 signals were related to astrocytosis in the hippocampus and adjacent white matter, as demonstrated via histologic correlative studies.

Conclusions.—Magnetic resonance significantly improved the ability to detect patients who would benefit from lobectomy. In addition, MR sensitivity was greater than that of PET.

▶ These authors demonstrate that MRI has a high sensitivity for the detection of temporal lobe abnormalities in patients who then respond to surgical treatment for the control of seizures originating from that temporal lobe. Other investigators have come to similar conclusions as a result of their own experience. What still needs to be accomplished, however, is an analysis of the MRI findings of a large series of unselected individuals studied by the same techniques, to establish the frequency of temporal lobe abnormalities in individuals who do not have a seizure disorder.—R.H. Wilkins, M.D.

Temporal Lobe Epilepsy: The Various MR Appearances of Histologically Proven Mesial Temporal Sclerosis
Meiners LC, van Gils A, Jansen GH, de Kort G, Witkamp TD, Ramos LMP, Valk J, Debets RMC, van Huffelen AC, van Veelen CWM, Mali WPTM (Univ Hosp, Utrecht, The Netherlands; Academic Hosp of the Free Univ, Amsterdam; Instituut voor Epilepsiebestrijding, Heemstede, The Netherlands)
AJNR 15:1547–1555, 1994   122-96-33–2

Patients.—Magnetic resonance signs of mesial temporal sclerosis were sought in 14 surgically treated patients with epilepsy, in all of whom mesial temporal sclerosis had been confirmed histologically. The patients, 10 women and 4 men, were 14 to 43 years of age. All of them underwent surgery when focal seizures arising from one temporal lobe had failed to respond to multiple antiepileptic drugs for 2 years or longer.

Methods.—Magnetic resonance images were acquired using a 1.5-tesla system and a head coil. Sagittal T1-weighted, axial T2-weighted, and coronal T2 images were acquired, as well as T2-weighted axial images in planes through the temporal lobes, paralleling the long axes of the hippocampi.

Findings.—All patients had foci of high signal intensity in the hippocampus, which were best visualized on T2-weighed images paralleling the hippocampal axis. The hippocampus was reduced in size in 12 patients, and 9 had a relatively small temporal lobe. Both these features were best seen in coronal images and on inversion-recovery sequences. Twelve patients exhibited ipsilateral atrophy of collateral white matter in the hippocampus on coronal T2-weighted images. Eleven patients had an enlarged temporal horn, and 10 had a reduced demarcation between gray and white matter in the temporal lobe. Seven of the latter patients had histologic abnormalities in the white matter of the temporal lobe, most often clusters of oligodendroglial cells.

Conclusion.—Multiplane MRI demonstrates abnormalities in a large majority of patients with mesial temporal sclerosis.

▶ As a variation on the MRI assessment of the temporal lobes of patients with temporal lobe epilepsy, Meiners and her associates have analyzed the MRI appearances of 14 patients who subsequently were histologically proved to have mesial temporal sclerosis.—R.H. Wilkins, M.D.

Ipsilateral Subcortical Atrophy Associated With Temporal Lobectomy
Shedlack KJ, Lee E-K, Radtke RA, Friedman AH, Crain BJ, Boyko O, Krishnan KRR (State Univ of New York, Stony Brook; Univ of California, Davis; Duke Univ Med Ctr, Durham, NC)
Psychiatry Res 54:295–304, 1994   122-96-33-3

Objective.—A retrospective study used systematic stereology applied to MRI series to determine the volume of the putamen nuclei bilaterally in 29 patients before and after unilateral temporal lobectomy. Questions of whether significant preoperative extratemporal volume differences are present with chronic complex partial seizures and whether secondary atrophy at the level of the striatum exists after surgical deafferentation by lobectomy were addressed.

Patients and Methods.—The patients, 14 males and 15 females, ranged in age from 6 to 59 years. The mean duration of seizures was 12.8 years. All underwent standard anterior unilateral temporal lobectomy for complex partial seizures unrelieved by medical treatment. Left temporal resection was performed in 14 patients, and right-sided procedures in 15. One or more postoperative MRI scans were available for 7 patients, and both preoperative and postoperative scans for 22 patients.

Results.—The mean preoperative right and left putamen volumes did not differ in patients who had preoperative scans, and the mean preoperative ipsilateral and contralateral putamen volumes were indistinguishable as well. Postoperatively, however, the ipsilateral putamen volume was significantly smaller than the contralateral putamen volume. Among patients having both preoperative and postoperative scans, the difference between contralateral and ipsilateral putamen volume before operation remained less than the difference between contralateral and ipsilateral putamen volume postoperatively. There was a significant correlation between the degree of postsurgical putamen volume asymmetry and the duration of time since resection. The 9 patients with the greatest postoperative loss of putamen volume did not differ significantly from other patients in gender, age, side of lobectomy, neuropathologic diagnosis, or postoperative seizure frequency.

Conclusions.—Patients with chronic complex partial seizures showed no preoperative volume asymmetry between the putamen nuclei but did show significant unilateral decreases in putamen volume postoperatively in association with duration of time since temporal lobectomy. Thus, in contrast to temporal structures, the putamen is not affected by significant structural loss before surgery. There may be an association between temporal lobectomy and progressive degeneration of extratemporal projections of the temporal lobe.

▶ Numerous investigators have assessed the size and morphology of the temporal lobes and their components in patients with complex partial seizure, and have correlated these findings with the outcome of temporal lobectomy. However, extratemporal subcortical nuclei and associated cortical areas have not been examined systematically by stereologic volumetric methods, and this study represents a step in that direction.—R.H. Wilkins, M.D.

Vagus Nerve Stimulation for Treatment of Partial Seizures: 3. Long-Term Follow-Up on First 67 Patients Exiting a Controlled Study
George R, Salinsky M, Kuzniecky R, Rosenfeld W, Bergen D, Tarver WB, Wernicke JF, and the First International Vagus Nerve Stimulation Study Group (Baylor College of Medicine, Houston; Oregon Health Sciences Univ, Portland; Univ of Alabama, Birmingham; et al)
Epilepsia 35:637–643, 1994   122-96-33–4

Background.—Vagus nerve stimulation (VNS) has been found to have a significant anticonvulsant effect in preclinical studies and pilot studies. After the completion of the acute phase of a multicenter, double-blinded, randomized study, a long-term follow-up was done on the first 67 patients exiting it.

Methods.—The acute phase of the study lasted for 14 weeks. At that time, 31 patients receiving high VNS and 36 receiving low VNS were assessed. Sixty-seven patients chose to continue in an open extension phase of the trial, in which all received high VNS.

Findings.—In both groups, all periods of high VNS showed a significant reduction in seizure frequency compared with baseline. For the 16–18 months of VNS, data on 26 of 31 patients randomized to receive high VNS were available. This group had a 52% decrease in the mean seizure frequency percentage compared with baseline. For those converted from low to high VNS, data on 24 of the 36 patients were available after 16 to 18 months. In this group, the mean percentage reduction in seizure frequency was 38.1% compared with baseline. There was no significant change in the safety or side effect profile in the long term. Previously reported side effects of hoarseness and voice change, coughing, and paresthesia continued to occur but were well tolerated. During the follow-up, 1 patient died of thrombotic thrombocytopenia purpura, and 5 stopped treatment because of its inefficacy.

Conclusions.—These long-term findings suggest that seizures continue to decrease between months 1–3 and months 16–18. Although these results are promising, a full analysis is needed before definitive conclusions are drawn.

▶ As indicated by the authors, it is not inherently obvious why VNS should have an anticonvulsant effect. However, the anatomical and physiologic bases for this method of treatment have been partially elucidated in animal investigations. Enough information was accumulated to justify a scientific trial in patients who were unresponsive to more standard forms of therapy. The present phase of that study documents some benefit from VNS in these otherwise treatment-resistant patients with partial seizures. Undoubtedly, the anticonvulsant effects of VNS will be investigated further in the future, to determine whether this unusual therapeutic approach will be useful from a broader clinical perspective.—R.H. Wilkins, M.D.

34 Hydrocephalus and Developmental Defects

The Role of Endoscopic Choroid Plexus Coagulation in the Management of Hydrocephalus
Pople IK, Ettles D (Frenchay Hosp, Bristol, England; Green Lane Hosp, Auckland, New Zealand)
Neurosurgery 36:698–702, 1995   122-96-34–1

Introduction.—Endoscopic coagulation of the choroid plexus has been used to treat hydrocephalus for 2 decades, during which time 156 procedures were done on 116 patients. Adequate data were available for 104 patients who underwent surgery at a median age of 5 months and were followed up for 10½ years on average.

Results.—Thirty-five percent of the 104 patients followed did not require CSF shunting. Of 80 patients first coagulated in infancy, 38% have not required a shunt. Control was achieved much more often in patients with communicating hydrocephalus than in those with obstructive hydrocephalus. The rate of progression of hydrocephalus also was an important factor. Only 2 of 16 patients with a tense anterior fontanel were controlled. The cortical sulci regularly became more prominent after successful surgery. Epilepsy developed in 48% of patients who required a shunt and in 12% of those who were controlled by choroid plexus coagulation. Infection developed in 10% of 80 evaluable patients but not since vancomycin and gentamicin were added to the irrigation solution. There were 4 major complications, but no deaths were ascribed to the procedure.

Conclusion.—Choroid plexus coagulation is an alternative to shunting in selected patients with milder forms of communicating hydrocephalus and in patients with intractable shunt failure.

▶ The authors report their experience with endoscopic choroid plexus coagulation for the management of hydrocephalus. Historically, this type of treatment was not often used after reasonably accurate and functional CSF shunts were developed. Therefore, it is of interest to see what can be achieved by this method, using modern instrumentation and technique. The best results in this series were obtained in a subset of 28 children with communicating hydrocephalus and a slow to moderate rate of increase in head circumference; 64% experienced long-term control. In the entire group, however, the results were disappointing. For example, the ventricular size was not significantly reduced by choroid plexus coagulation, and only 36 of 104 (35%) patients achieved long-term control without a shunt. Choroid plexus coagulation is still not a reasonable alternative to shunting, except perhaps for children with mild and slowly advancing communicating hydrocephalus or as a salvage procedure in patients with intractable shunt failure.—R.H, Wilkins, M.D.

Cerebrospinal Fluid Edema Associated With Shunt Obstruction
Sakamoto H, Fujitani K, Kitano S, Murata K, Hakuba A (Osaka City Univ, Japan; Children's Med Ctr of Osaka City, Japan; Shimada Municipal Hosp, Shizuoka, Japan)
J Neurosurg 81:179–183, 1994   122-96-34–2

Patients and Methods.—Four children with hydrocephalus of various origins underwent placement of a ventriculoperitoneal shunt at 1 center. Age at surgery was 10 days (patient 1), 8 months (patient 2), 17 years (patient 3), and 2 years (patient 4). The ventricular catheter was inserted from the coronal site and had inflow holes ranging from 1.8 to 2.5 cm. A shunt system with a medium-pressure valve was placed in each patient. At 1–16 months after shunt installation, all patients were seen with CSF edema along the catheter. Treatment, CT findings, and patient outcome were examined.

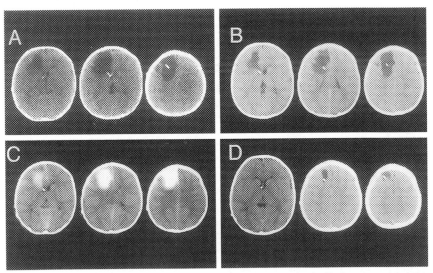

Fig 34–1.—The CT scans in 1 patient at the first examination (note the slit-like lateral ventricles) (**A**), at the second examination (**B**), after injection of contrast material into the flushing device at the second examination (**C**), and 3 years after shunt revision showing a residual small low-density lesion (**D**). (Courtesy of Sakamoto H, Fujitani K, Kitano S, et al: *J Neurosurg* 81:179–183, 1994.)

Findings.—Excessive CSF caused by shunt obstruction accumulated in the white matter along the ventricular catheter. In patients 1, 2, and 3, the ventricles remained small or slit-like without periventricular edema, despite increased intraventricular pressure. These observations indicated that the ventricles became taut after shunt installation. Patient 4 had dilated ventricles with periventricular CSF edema. In this patient, CSF edema was observed in a limited area along the ventricular catheter. After replacement of the obstructed peritoneal catheter of the shunt, a rapid resolution of edema was seen in all patients. However, patients 1, 2, and 3 still had a small lesion in the subcortical white matter along the ventricular catheter, as visualized via CT or MRI, or both, 3–5 years after shunt revision (Fig 34–1).

Conclusions.—Shunt obstruction may lead to extensive CSF edema along the ventricular catheter in children who are hydrocephalic and have ventricular tautness after instillation. This can result in irreversible, although usually asymptomatic damage to the affected area of the brain.

▶ The most striking aspect of this report is the imaging characteristics. The first 3 of the 4 reported patients had scan patterns that were almost identical (see Fig 34–1).—R.H. Wilkins, M.D.

The Detection and Management of Intracranial Hypertension After Initial Suture Release and Decompression for Craniofacial Dysostosis Syndromes
Siddiqi SN, Posnick JC, Buncic R, Humphreys RP, Hoffman HJ, Drake JM, Rutka JT (Hosp for Sick Children, Toronto, Ont, Canada; Univ of Toronto, Ont, Canada)
Neurosurgery 36:703–709, 1995   122-96-34–3

Background.—An estimated one third of children born with complex forms of craniosynostosis have clinically significant intracranial hypertension develop if not treated. The efficacy of surgical correction in reducing the risk of increased intracranial pressure (ICP) remains uncertain. There is some evidence that the ICP may be increased even after decompression and reshaping procedures.

Objective.—The prevalence of intracranial hypertension following suture release and decompression was determined in 107 patients with craniofacial dysostosis who underwent cranial vault reshaping. The most common diagnoses were Crouzon's syndrome and Apert's syndrome.

Findings.—Six patients had evidence of increased ICP months to years after initial suture release had been performed in infancy or early childhood. The mean interval was 25 months. Five patients were intermittently irritable. Three had episodic headaches and vomiting. Papilledema was apparent in 4 of the 6 patients affected, but no patient had had papilledema before initial suture release. The ventricles were normal in size in 5 patients; 1 had mild ventriculomegaly.

Course.—The patients with papilledema underwent further decompression and reshaping, with resolution of the funduscopic abnormalities. Three patients had mild ventriculomegaly a year later, but none has required ventriculoperitoneal shunting. One patient required a third operation. Four of the 6 patients probably will require further surgery for midfacial deformity.

Conclusion.—About 6% of these patients with craniofacial dysostosis had increased elevated ICP develop after initial suture release and decompression. Long-term interval assessment by a craniofacial team will minimize the risk of irreversible sequelae.

▶ The authors point out that a portion (6% in their series) of children with a craniofacial dysostosis syndrome will have significantly increased ICP after initial suture release and decompression is done early in life, probably because the cranial vault lacks adequate growth potential to accommodate the growing brain. Children who have an early operation of this sort should be followed; if evidence of increased ICP occurs, a revision craniotomy and reshaping procedure can prevent irreversible complications.—R.H. Wilkins, M.D.

Quantitative Cine-Mode Magnetic Resonance Imaging of Chiari I Malformations: An Analysis of Cerebrospinal Fluid Dynamics
Armonda RA, Citrin CM, Foley KT, Ellenbogen RG (Walter Reed Army Med Ctr, Washington, DC; Semmes-Murphy Clinic, Memphis, Tenn; Uniformed Services Univ of Health Sciences, Bethesda, Md)
Neurosurgery 35:214–224, 1994   122-96-34–4

Purpose.—Neurosurgeons are seeing more patients with Chiari I malformations who, despite having an MRI scan that demonstrates tonsillar herniation, have only vague complaints and subtle signs. All major theories regarding the cause of Chiari I malformations with an associated syrinx implicate aberrant CSF dynamics. Cine-mode MRI was used to quantify CSF flow in patients with Chiari I malformation, as well as in normal children and adults.

Methods.—The subjects were 17 patients with Chiari I malformation, including 8 who were imaged both before and after surgery, and 12 normal children and adults. All subjects underwent cine-mode MRI of the craniocervical junction, with 16 cardiac-gated velocity-encoded images arranged in a cine loop to allow measurement of the magnitude and direction of CSF velocity. A CSF velocity profile was created by plotting velocity measurements in 4 regions of interest—the foramen of Magendie, the foramen magnum, and ventral and dorsal to the spinal cord at C2—in relation to the cardiac cycle. The 8 surgical patients all underwent posterior fossa craniectomy with C1 laminectomy, lysis of arachnoid lesions, and duraplasty.

Results.—The normal subjects all showed unobstructed flow around the craniocervical junction. There was a brief period of cranial CSF flow, followed by a sustained period of caudal flow. In contrast, the patients

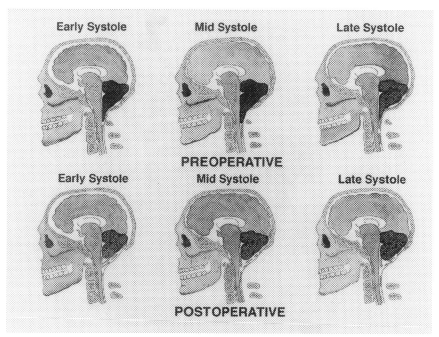

Fig 34–2.—Depiction of the changes associated with CSF flow in patients with a Chiari I malformation undergoing posterior fossa decompression with duraplasty. **Top row,** early systole with cranial CSF flow (*upward arrows*); midsystole with impaction of the foramen magnum and impaired caudal outflow (*arrow* blocked by tonsils); late systole with reversal of CSF flow and preferential cranial CSF flow (*upward arrows*). **Bottom row,** postoperative early systole with unimpaired cranial flow (*upward arrows*); midsystole with unimpaired caudal flow (*downward arrows*); sustained caudal CSF flow seen postoperatively at end systole (*downward arrows*). (Courtesy of Armonda RA, Citrin CM, Foley KT, et al: *Neurosurgery* 35:214–224, 1994.)

with Chiari I malformation with tonsillar herniation of greater than 5 mm had obstructed CSF flow, with decreased velocity and shorter periods of caudal flow. They also had preferential cranial CSF flow compared with the normal subjects. Surgery was followed by a significant increase in CSF flow velocity and in the period of caudal CSF flow in the foramen magnum, mirroring the velocity profiles of the normal subjects (Fig 34–2). The changes in CSF dynamics were associated with a more normal appearance of the foramen magnum, reduced syrinx size, and symptomatic improvement.

Conclusions.—Quantitative cine-mode MRI demonstrates the altered CSF dynamics in patients with Chiari I malformations. Although not intended as a surgical outcome study, the analysis shows significant normalization of CSF flow in patients who undergo surgical correction. This MRI method can be used in many ways to add to our knowledge of the pathophysiology of the Chiari I malformation.

▶ In recent years, these and other authors have used dynamic MRI techniques to study CSF flow at the craniocervical junction in patients with the

Chiari I malformation, with or without an associated syrinx. Such studies are helping define the pathophysiology of these related conditions. In turn, such information may lead to the development of more effective methods of surgical treatment.—R.H. Wilkins, M.D.

35 Spinal Disorders

Degenerative Diseases

Regional Variation in Tensile Properties and Biochemical Composition of the Human Lumbar Anulus Fibrosus

Skaggs DL, Weidenbaum M, Iatridis JC, Ratcliffe A, Mow VC (Columbia-Presbyterian Med Ctr, New York)

Spine 19:1310–1319, 1994   122-96-35–1

Introduction.—Many patients with spinal problems have mechanical failure of the annulus fibrosis (AF), so it is important to understand the intrinsic mechanical properties of this tissue. In previous studies, it was found that intervertebral disk tissues show both intrinsic matrix viscoelastic and biphasic viscoelastic, i.e., flow-independent and flow-dependent effects. Regional differences in the composition and ultrastructure of AF tissues suggest the presence of differing tensile properties. The relationship between structure and function in the AF of nondegenerate human lumbar intervertebral disks was examined.

Methods.—The investigators isolated single lamella specimens from the annulus from fresh human lumber spines. The tensile properites of the specimens were tested in uniaxial tension using a slow strain-rate protocol. The study compared the tensile findings and biochemical composition of lamellae from different anatomical locations.

Results.—Radial and circumferential AF specimens demonstrated significant variations in their tensile properties. Anterior specimens were stiffer than those from the posterolateral regions, whereas specimens from the outer regions were stiffer than those from the inner regions. Analysis of biochemical composition showed no significant radial or circumferential variations. There were no significant correlations between tensile modulus or strength and composition, but there were some low significant correlations between compositional parameters.

Conclusions.—Significant regional differences in the tensile properties of human lumbar AF appear to arise mainly from structural, rather than compositional, variations. These findings suggest that structural variations may play a role in the clinical frequency of posterolateral AF failure.

▶ It is well recognized that lumbar disk herniations occur preferentially in a posterolateral direction, which has been ascribed to the eccentric posterior position of the nucleus pulposus and the posterior midline reinforcement supplied by the posterior longitudinal ligament. These authors supply another reason as well, namely, that regional differences in tensile properties of the AF account for relative posterolateral weakness in this structure.— R.H. Wilkins, M.D.

Magnetic Resonance Imaging of the Lumbar Spine in People Without Back Pain

Jensen MC, Brant-Zawadzki MN, Obuchowski N, Modic MT, Malkasian D, Ross JS (Hoag Memorial Hosp, Newport Beach, Calif; Cleveland Clinic, Ohio)
N Engl J Med 331:69–73, 1994   122-96-35-2

Purpose.—Low back pain is an extremely common reason for patients to seek medical attention. There is debate as to the association between abnormalities of the lumbar spine and symptoms of low back pain, with autopsy, CT, and MRI studies showing abnormalities in a significant proportion of asymptomatic patients. It may be that well-defined morphological terms to describe disk herniation would show a better correlation with symptoms. The prevalence of MRI lumbar spine abnormalities was assessed among 98 patients without back pain.

Methods.—The subjects ranged in age from 20 to 80 years. All MRI scans were independently interpreted by 2 neuroradiologists without knowledge of the clinical findings. Twenty-seven scans of patients with back pain were randomly mixed in with the study scans to prevent bias. A standardized nomenclature was used to classify the 5 intervertebral disks in the lumbosacral spine: normal; bulge, referring to a circumferential symmetric expansion of the disk beyond the interspace; protrusion, a focal or asymmetric extension of the disk beyond the interspace; and extrusion, a more extreme extension of the disk beyond the interspace. Facet arthropathy and other nonintervertebral disk abnormalities were also recorded.

Results.—Disks at all levels were normal in 36% of the asymptomatic subjects. On averaging of the 2 readings for each subject, 52% had at least 1 bulging disk, 27% had a protrusion, and 1% had an extrusion. Abnormalities of more than 1 disk were noted in 38% of asymptomatic subjects. Bulges became more common with age, but protrusions did not. Schmorl's nodes, with disk herniation into the vertebral-body end plate was the most common nonintervertebral disk abnormality, appearing in 19% of subjects. Others included annular defects, 14%, and facet arthropathy, 8%. None of the findings were significantly different between men and women.

Conclusions.—Magnetic resonance imaging of the lumbar spine of asymptomatic subjects commonly shows bulging or protrusions of the intervertebral disks. Extrusions are not common in asymptomatic subjects. Thus, bulges and protrusions may often be a coincidental finding among patients with low back pain, or even radiculopathy.

▶ The authors confirm what others have found in previous studies using other radiologic modalities. Many asymptomatic individuals, especially older people, will have demonstrable "abnormalities" of the lumbar spine, such as bulging or protruding disks, Schmorl's nodes, and facet arthropathy. This needs to be kept in mind during the interpretation of radiologic studies of the lumbar spine in patients with low back pain.—R.H. Wilkins, M.D.

▶ Even though it is 60 years since the first surgical relief of lumbosacral radiculopathy resulting from a herniated disk was reported, we are still a long way from a complete understanding of the interplay between chronic low back pain and disk disease. It is an all too common finding in adults, particularly elderly adults, that the lumbar intervertebral disks show a variety of degenerative changes. This study elegantly demonstrates that many of these changes are present in normal control individuals who do not have low back pain. Extrusion of the disk, defined as a marked protrusion of disk material from the interspace where the base of the extrusion against the disk of origin is narrower than the diameter of the extruded material itself or where there is no connection between the material and the disk of origin, is quite rare, however. Hence, this study reaffirms the necessary skepticism that must be adopted before accepting that the patient's symptoms are caused by the observed "abnormalities" of the lumbar disks.—W.G. Bradley, D.M., F.R.C.P.

The Efficacy of Back Schools: A Review of Randomized Clinical Trials

Koes BW, van Tulder MW, van der Windt DAWM, Bouter LM (Vrije Universiteit, Amsterdam)
J Clin Epidemiol 47:851–862, 1994   122-96-35-3

Purpose.—The popularity of back schools for low back pain has increased in recent years, but the efficacy and cost-effectiveness of such programs are still under debate. The published literature on back schools was examined.

Methods.—A MEDLINE search was performed for the period 1966–1992, and references in relevant publications were further examined. Only randomized, clinical trials of low back pain that included a back school type of intervention were included in the analysis. The selected trials were scored on a predetermined set of criteria, including a score for the quality of the methodology of the trial.

Results.—Twenty-one papers reporting on 16 randomized, clinical trials were selected. Seven trials reported better results from a back school program in comparison to usual care, placebo short-waves, or a waiting-list control group. Seven trials reported negative results, and 2 trials did not report a conclusion. However, most studies had major design flaws. The 4 studies with the best methodology reported positive outcomes of the back school program. The study with the best methodological quality showed that a modified Swedish back school conducted in an occupational setting may be effective.

Conclusion.—Back school programs may be effective for patients in occupational settings in acute, recurrent, and chronic conditions.

▶ Forms of medical treatment, including surgical procedures, are often developed without proof of efficacy—a phenomenon that is compounded by the placebo effect. This study analyzes available published information on the efficacy of back schools and calls attention to the flaws in such assessments.—R.H. Wilkins, M.D.

An International Comparison of Back Surgery Rates
Cherkin DC, Deyo RA, Loeser JD, Bush T, Waddell G (Univ of Washington, Seattle; Group Health Cooperative of Puget Sound, Seattle; Western Infirmary, Glasgow, Scotland)
Spine 19:1201–1206, 1994   122-96-35–4

Background.—High geographic variation in back surgery rates have been reported in the United States. However, international comparisons have not been published.

Methods.—Back surgery rates were compared in 11 developed countries. Data were obtained from health agencies in these countries. Country-specific rates of other surgical procedures were obtained from published sources.

Results.—The U.S. back surgery rate was at least 40% greater than in any other country. It was more than 5 times higher than that in England and Scotland. Back surgery rates rose almost linearly with the per capita supply of orthopedic and neurosurgeons in the country. Countries with high rates of back surgery also had high rates of other discretionary procedures such as tonsillectomy and hysterectomy.

Conclusions.—Differences in health care systems can have a great effect on rates of back surgery. Better outcome studies are needed to establish whether Americans are being subjected to excessive surgery or whether those in other countries are suffering because of the underuse of back surgery.

▶ In this study, Cherkin and his associates document what has been assumed to be true—that the rate of back surgery (defined slightly differently in the various countries surveyed, but based on primary procedure codes indicating a spine operation) is significantly higher in the United States than in other developed countries. As the authors point out, this situation can be interpreted in various ways, and better outcome studies are needed to settle such issues as the over- or underutilization of such surgery.—R.H. Wilkins, M.D.

Outpatient Conventional Laminotomy and Disc Excision
Newman MH (private practice, Anchorage, Alaska)
Spine 20:353–355, 1995   122-96-35–5

Background.—The growing need to contain health care costs has led to an increase in outpatient surgical procedures. Certain disk procedures, such as microdiscectomy and percutaneous discectomy, have been performed on an outpatient basis, although outpatient disk excision has not yet been reported. The outcome of patients undergoing outpatient laminotomy and disk excision for herniated nucleus pulposus was thus described.

Patients and Methods.—Clinical data were collected prospectively on 75 consecutive outpatients who underwent surgery done by a single surgeon over a 7-year period. Nineteen procedures were done at a freestanding surgery center, and 56 in a hospital outpatient surgical department. The surgical procedure was essentially the same for all patients, although the amount of discectomy varied according to the pathology. Several patients received epidural steroids, placed via a small infant feeding tube. Patients were discharged approximately 2 hours postoperatively, and all had office follow-up of at least 3-months' duration.

Results.—Overall, the procedures were well tolerated. One occult spinal fluid leak attributed to instrumentation with the infant feeding tube was observed on the seventh postoperative day. This patient required reoperation to close the dural defect. After this incident, the method of instilling epidural steroids was discontinued. Another patient experienced what proved to be hysterical chest pain several days after surgery. Neither of these complications were directly related to the outpatient surgical setting. No other operative complications were noted.

Conclusions.—Outpatient laminotomy and disk excision operations are feasible and safe in select patients. Patient acceptance is high, and almost all individuals offered outpatient surgery have chosen this alternative. Furthermore, outpatient surgery is associated with a substantial cost savings when compared with inpatient procedures. There are, however, several potential drawbacks. These include the possibility of unrecognized hemorrhage, resulting in a fatal complication; urinary retention, necessitating emergency room or even inpatient catheterization; and intraoperative dural laceration, requiring transfer to an inpatient facility if surgery is performed at a free-standing center.

▶ The author documents that conventional laminotomy and diskectomy can be performed in an outpatient setting. In this series, to be considered for outpatient surgery, the patient was required to have a responsible adult living or staying with him or her for 24 hours after surgery. All patients were given detailed written and oral instructions on postoperative care, and they were instructed to stay in bed for approximately 12 hours after surgery, except to use the bathroom and eat. Patients were contacted by telephone the morning after the procedure and were then followed on a routine basis in the office.—R.H. Wilkins, M.D.

Same-Day Microsurgical Arthroscopic Lateral-Approach Laser-Assisted (SMALL) Fluoroscopic Discectomy

Savitz MH (Good Samaritan and Nyack Hosps, Rockland County, NY)
J Neurosurg 80:1039–1045, 1994   122-96-35–6

Background.—Benefits of same-day microsurgical arthroscopic lateral-approach laser-assisted (SMALL) fluoroscopic diskectomy include avoidance of general anesthesia, reduced blood loss, avoidance of spinal canal scarring, anterior fenestration of the anulus for continuing extrusion of disk material without nerve root compression, and early return to normal activity. An experience with Kambin's orthopedic instruments and frame for arthroscopic microdiskectomy was described.

Patients and Methods.—A total of 100 patients aged 18 to 73 years were included in a 2-year series. Of these, 80 patients had a single disk herniation and 20 had 2 disk herniations. All patients had been symptomatic for 6 months or more. After induction of neuroleptanalgesia, SMALL fluoroscopic diskectomy was performed in each patient within a triangular working zone (Fig 35–1). Biopsy of suspected spinal tumors was also done in 3 patients, and 1 patient underwent drainage of disk space infection. A prototype operating diskoscope was used to deliver the neodymium:-yttrium-aluminum-garnet laser beam to facilitate hemostasis.

Results.—Seventy-five ideal patients were identified, all of whom exhibited 8 specific features. These included a history of up to 6 months of unilateral sciatica symptoms that responded to bed rest, mechanical signs of nerve root irritation when erect, CT or MRI studies interpreted as having 1 protruding or prolapsed disk without extrusion, no segmental spondylosis at the level of a herniated nucleus pulposus, no motor weakness, no previous disk surgery, no obesity, and no diabetes mellitus. The remaining 25 nonideal patients failed to demonstrate 1 or more of the above criteria (table). Good outcome was judged in part by patient satisfaction, and it was not substantially different between each group. Complete success, as determined by early return to work, was noted in two thirds of the patients. However, improvement was also assessed by increased mobility and a reduction in pain medication from narcotic to analgesic agents. Repeat surgery (laminectomy) was undertaken in 3 patients, although only 1 improved.

Conclusions.—After 2 years of clinical experience, it was concluded that the use of the percutaneous endoscopic procedure under neuroleptanalgesia may become an important surgical option.

▶ As an acronym, SMALL has much to recommend it. In this report, Dr. Savitz makes the case for this smaller approach to lumbar disk surgery, and considering the mounting concern in the United States about health care costs, it may signal a trend toward using such outpatient treatment in patients who meet the criteria listed in the abstract.—R.H. Wilkins, M.D.

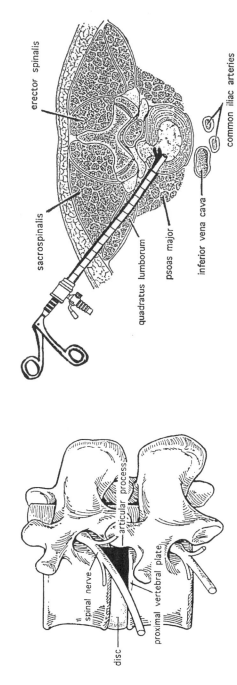

Fig 35–1.—Drawings depicting the operating area. **Left,** lateral view. The *black triangle* represents the working zone. **Right,** cross-sectional drawing of the surgical approach demonstrating the introduction of instruments into the operative area. (Courtesy of Savitz MH: *J Neurosurg* 80:1039–1045, 1994.)

Overall Results in 100 Patients Undergoing Arthroscopic Microdiskectomy

Outcome	"Ideal" Cases	"Nonideal" Cases
total cases	75	25
returned to work	50 (66%)	16 (64%)
increased mobility, reduced medication	23 (31%)	8 (32%)
reoperation, not improved	1	1
reoperation, improved	1	0

(Courtesy of Savitz MH: *J Neurosurg* 80:1039–1045, 1994.)

Report of a Controlled Clinical Trial Comparing Automated Percutaneous Lumbar Discectomy and Microdiscectomy in the Treatment of Contained Lumbar Disc Herniation
Chatterjee S, Foy PM, Findlay GF (Walton Centre for Neurology and Neurosurgery, Liverpool, England)
Spine 20:734–738, 1995   122-96-35–7

Introduction.—The typical treatment for lumbar disk herniation that fails to respond to conservative measures is an open diskectomy. Since 1985, there have been a number of studies on automated percutaneous lumbar diskectomy (APLD). The success rate is reported to range between 50% and 86%. Although there have been no reports comparing APLD with microdiskectomy, a trial comparing APLD with chemonucleolysis showed poor results from APLD. The most successful use of APLD has been in patients with small, contained herniations after 6 weeks of conservative therapy. The use of APLD was compared with that of microdiskectomy in a randomized group of patients.

Methods.—Although the original goal was to recruit 160 patients, only 71 with radiologically determined small disk herniations actually participated. The patients were randomly assigned to undergo either APLD or lumbar microdiskectomy. All had 6 weeks of prior conservative management. Postsurgical follow-up occurred at 3 weeks, and at 2 and 6 months. The assessment followed the MacNab criteria.

Results.—Automated percutaneous lumbar diskectomy was performed on 31 patients, and microdiskectomy was performed on 40. Only 29% of

TABLE 1.—Comparison of Outcome

Procedure	Excellent/Good	Fair/Bad
Microdiskectomy	32/40 (80%)	8/40 (20%)
APLD alone	9/31 (29%)	22/31 (71%)
APLD→Micro	13/20 (65%)*	7/20 (35%)
APLD alone + APLD→Micro	22/31 (71%)	9/31 (29%)

* Twenty of 22 patients with failed APLD elected to have Micro.
Abbreviations: Micro, microdiskectomy; *APLD*, automated percutaneous lumbar diskectomy.
(Courtesy of Chatterjee S, Foy PM, Findlay GF: *Spine* 20:734–738, 1995.)

TABLE 2.—Comparison of Outcome at L4–L5

Procedure	Excellent/Good	Fair/Bad
Microdiskectomy	14/17 (82%)	3/17 (18%)
APLD alone	4/12 (33%)	8/12 (67%)
APLD→Micro	5/7 (71%)	2/7 (29%)
APLD alone + APLD→Micro	9/12 (75%)	3/12 (25%)

Abbreviations: Micro, microdiskectomy; *APLD*, automated percutaneous lumbar diskectomy.
(Courtesy of Chatterjee S, Foy PM, Findlay GF: *Spine* 20:734–738, 1995.)

the APLD patients (versus 80% of the microdiskectomy group) achieved a good or excellent outcome (Table 1). The APLD results were slightly better at the L4–L5 level (Table 2) than for the L5–S1 level (Table 3). All but 3 of the microdiskectomy patients either returned to work or their prior level of activity within 3 months. Twenty-two patients with a failed APLD were offered a microdiskectomy and all but 2 accepted. Only 65% of these patients achieved an acceptable result.

Conclusions.—In this study APLD was not an effective method of treating patients with small contained lumbar disk herniations. The results of this randomized trial differ from those of unrandomized trials that have supported the procedure.

▶ In this prospective randomized study of a relatively small group of patients, the outcome after automated percutaneous lumbar diskectomy was not as good as that after microdiskectomy.—R.H. Wilkins, M.D.

TABLE 3.—Comparison of Outcome at L5–S1

Procedure	Excellent/Good	Fair/Bad
Microdiskectomy	18/23 (78%)	5/23 (22%)
APLD alone	4/19 (21%)	15/19 (79%)
APLD→Micro	9/14 (64%)	5/14 (36%)
APLD alone + APLD→Micro	13/19 (68%)	6/19 (32%)

Abbreviations: Micro, microdiskectomy; *APLD*, automated percutaneous lumbar diskectomy.
(Courtesy of Chatterjee S, Foy PM, Findlay GF: *Spine* 20:734–738, 1995.)

The Effect of Pedicle Screw/Plate Fixation on Lumbar/Lumbosacral Autogenous Bone Graft Fusions in Patients With Degenerative Disc Disease

Wood GW II, Boyd RJ, Carothers TA, Mansfield FL, Rechtine GR, Rozen MJ, Sutterlin CE III (Campbell Clinic, Memphis, Tenn; Massachusetts Gen Hosp, Boston; Bethesda North Hosp, Cincinnati, Ohio; et al)
Spine 20:819–830, 1995   122-96-35–8

Objective.—A pedicle screw/plate system, the Interpedicular Segmental Fixation (ISF) system, was used for autogenous bone graft fusion in the lumbar or lumbosacral region in 230 patients, 156 with degenerative disk disease (DDD), and 74 with spondylolisthesis. A posterior approach was used to place the plate on the spine and insert the screws into the pedicles. Pure autogenous bone graft was used in 28 of the patients with DDD.

Results.—None of the 28 patients with DDD who underwent lumbar or lumboscral fusion with autogenous bone graft had pseudarthrosis develop within 2 years of surgery. In 8 previously reported studies, the average rate of pseudarthrosis was 32%. Most of the former patients had less pain and better function after the procedure. No patient had severe pain at the time of follow-up. Six of the 22 working patients returned to work, but only 43% of all 28 patients returned to their previous social status.

Conclusion.—The ISF pedicle screw/plate system is an effective and safe means of performing lumbar or lumbosacral fusion in patients with DDD when only autogenous bone is used.

▶ There has been considerable interest in the use of pedicle screw fixation to improve the spinal stability achieved by fusion in circumstances in which instability exists or detrimental effects of segmental motion might occur. Examples of such conditions are certain types of traumatic fractures and neoplastic involvement of the spine, spondylolisthesis, and repetitive disk herniation involving the same disk. Since the early 1980s, the Food and Drug Administration has permitted the sale of pedicle screws under Investigational Device Exemptions (IDEs)(1).

This investigation was a prospective, multicenter IDE study. The patients' pain, function, complications, and fusion status were evaluated and compared with those of literature controls. Although patients with spondylolisthesis were included, the focus was on the 156 patients who had diskogenic pain resulting from DDD. Of these, pure autogenous bone grafts were used in 28 patients from 4 centers (the others had allografts). In this relatively small group of 28 patients, the pedicle screw/plate system used was shown to be a safe and efficacious method of facilitating fusion. The pseudarthrosis rate was 0%. There were no neurologic deficits or broken implants. The subjective patient evaluations of pain relief and function showed that most patients were improved in both areas.—R.H. Wilkins, M.D.

Reference

1. Wilkins RH: Introduction. *KEY Neurology and Neurosurg* 9(2):34, 1994.

Epidural Pressure Measurements: Relationship Between Epidural Pressure and Posture in Patients With Lumbar Spinal Stenosis

Takahashi K, Miyazaki T, Takino T, Matsui T, Tomita K (Ishikawa Prefectural Central Hosp, Japan; Kanazawa Univ, Japan)
Spine 20:650–653, 1995   122-96-35–9

Background.—Patients with lumbar spinal stenosis often notice that postural changes affect their symptoms. The relationship between epidural pressure and lumbar posture in patients with lumbar spinal stenosis was investigated.

Methods.—Ten patients with cauda equina symptoms at the L4–5 level were included. The catheter transducer was inserted into the epidural space through the L5–S1 interlaminar space and positioned at the L4–5 disk level. The transducer was attached to an amplifier and a recorder. Epidural pressure was continuously measured with the patient in various postures.

Findings.—In lying and sitting positions, local epidural pressure at the stenotic level was low. In standing postures, this pressure was high. Pressure was increased with extension and reduced with flexion. The highest pressure, recorded in the standing position with extension, was 116.7 mm Hg.

Conclusions.—Epidural pressure and posture are significantly associated. The pressure changes correlated with the development of cauda equina symptoms. Posture-related increases in epidural pressure may induce compression of the cauda equina. These pressure changes may explain the postural effect in eliciting symptoms.

▶ Takahashi and associates have documented what one would suspect based on the well-known effects of postural changes on the symptoms caused by lumbar spinal stenosis.—R.H. Wilkins, M.D.

Caudal Epidural Blocks for Elderly Patients With Lumbar Canal Stenosis

Ciocon JO, Galindo-Ciocon D, Amaranath L, Galindo D (Cleveland Clinic Florida, Ft Lauderdale; Veterans Affairs Med Ctr, Miami, Fla)
J Am Geriatr Soc 42:593–596, 1994   122-96-35–10

Background.—Population-based studies have shown that one fourth to one half of elderly persons have significant pain. Musculoskeletal conditions are the main source of the pain. The effectiveness of caudal epidural blocks (CEB) in alleviating pain and the duration of pain relief with CEB in elderly persons with degenerative lumbar canal stenosis (LCS) were determined.

Methods.—Thirty patients with a mean age of 76 years were enrolled in a prospective study. All had leg discomfort with or without back pain and LCS documented by MRI. None had had CEB or surgery for their leg discomfort. None had pain relief from analgesics alone. Treatment consisted of 3 doses, given at weekly intervals, of 0.5% lidocaine (Xylocaine) with 80 mg of methyprednisolone (Depo-Medrol) into the caudal epidural space through the sacral hiatus.

Findings.—On admission, LCS was moderate in 66.7% of the patients, mild in 23.3%, and severe in 10%. A mean of 2.4 lumbar vertebrae were involved. The degree of LCS was directly correlated with the level of pain before CEB. After CEB, the mean pain level changed from 3.43 to 1.5. Pain relief was significant for up to 10 months. Duration of pain relief ranged from 4 to 10 months (Fig 35–2).

Conclusions.—Caudal epidural block can significantly relieve pain in elderly patients with degenerative LCS. This treatment alternative appears to be particularly important for patients who respond poorly to drug treatment and who cannot or will not have surgery.

▶ Lumbar spondylosis with resulting stenosis of the spinal canal is a well-recognized cause of back and leg pain in older adults. The standard approach to treatment has been a decompressive laminectomy to enlarge the spinal canal and remove the pressure effect on the involved roots of the cauda equina, both centrally and laterally. It would seem unlikely, based on this mechanistic view, that one or more lumbar epidural steroid injections could result in lasting relief. Ciocon et al. present information showing that, in fact, substantial pain relief can be achieved by such injections, and that this is a worthwhile alternative to surgery, especially in elderly patients who are in poor health.—R.H. Wilkins, M.D.

▶ Lumbar canal stenosis characteristically produces neurogenic claudication, i.e., pain in the legs and other neurologic features associated with

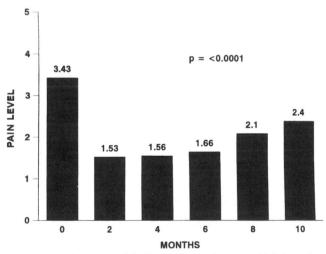

Fig 35–2.—Pain level in 30 patients with lumbar canal stenosis treated with 3 doses of caudal epidural block (CEB) and followed every 2 months up to 10 months. * $P < 0.001$ pre-CEB pain level (0-month visit) vs. each subsequent visit. (Courtesy of Ciocon JO, Galindo-Ciocon D, Amaranath L, et al: *J Am Geriatr Soc* 42:593–596, 1994.)

exercise. There typically is exacerbation by standing or extension of the lumbar spine. Chronic low back pain is, however, a less specific feature. Ideally, this syndrome is treated by surgical decompression, but many such patients are elderly and unfit for surgery. The encouraging findings of this study indicate that both the leg pain and the back pain can be significantly relieved by caudal epidural blocks combining Xylocaine and Depo-Medrol. Although there are no placebo control cases in this study, the results are sufficiently encouraging to recommend this therapy for suitable patients.— W.G. Bradley, D.M., F.R.C.P.

Spinal Cord Morphology and Pathology in Ossification of the Posterior Longitudinal Ligament
Kameyama T, Hashizume Y, Ando T, Takahashi A, Yanagi T, Mizuno J (Nagoya Univ School of Medicine, Nagoya, Japan; Nagoya Daini Red Cross Hosp, Nagoya, Japan; Aichi Med Univ, Aichi, Japan)
Brain 118:263–278, 1995   122-96-35–11

Introduction.—Ossification of the posterior longitudinal ligament (OPLL) is unusual among whites but is a significant cause of myelopathy in middle-aged and older Japanese adults. Nine autopsy cases of OPLL were examined to determine the relationship between morphology and pathology of the spinal cord.

Methods.—Cases were assessed visually, and the shape of the cross-section of the cord is classified according to the shape of the most severely affected segment. Five cases were described as having a boomerang shape (convex lateral surfaces and a concave anterior surface), and 4 as having a triangular shape (usually angular lateral surfaces and a flat anterior surface, but in one case, 1 angular lateral surface and 1 convex surface). Morphometric analysis was performed using enlarged photographs of the specimens and a computer-assisted image analyzer. Features recorded were the extent and severity of the lesions in the transverse plane, the presence or absence of the ascending degeneration of the posterior column, and the presence or absence of descending degeneration of the lateral pyramidal tracts below the level of compression.

Results.—Major pathologic changes were restricted to the gray matter in cases with a boomerang shape, whereas the white matter was relatively well preserved; this was true even when spinal cord compression was severe. There was no secondary descending degeneration of the lateral columns, and ascending degeneration of the posterior column was limited to the fasciculus cuneatus whose fibers were derived from the affected segments. Pathologic changes were more severe in cases with a triangular shape. Both gray and white matter were involved in these 4 cases, with only the anterior columns free of pathologic changes. More than a single segment exhibited severe pathologic changes, and there was both descending degeneration of the lateral pyramidal tracts and ascending degeneration of the posterior column, including the fasciculus gracilis. In most of the cases with a boomerang shape, the transverse area of the spinal cord was more than 60% of normal. Cases with a triangular shape, however, showed a reduction to less than 60% of normal in more than 1 segment. No relationship was observed between the compression ratio of the spinal cord and pathologic changes.

Conclusions.—The etiology of OPLL remains uncertain. Onset is often insidious and occurs in or after the fifth decade. Although OPLL can be asymptomatic, it is usually accompanied by cervical myelopathy. A triangular-shaped spinal cord with a transverse area of less than 60% of normal in more than 1 segment appeared to be linked with severe and irreversible pathologic changes.

▶ The authors have analyzed the pathologic changes in the spinal cord associated with OPLL in the cervical region. Their postmortem study of 9 subjects was careful and thorough. Although much has been published about the clinical and radiologic features of OPLL, there have been few investigations of its pathology.—R.H. Wilkins, M.D.

Sacral Insufficiency Fractures in the Elderly

Gotis-Graham I, McGuigan L, Diamond T, Portek I, Quinn R, Sturgess A, Tulloch R (Univ of New South Wales, Sydney, Australia; St George Hosp, New South Wales, Australia)
J Bone Joint Surg (Br) 76–B:882–886, 1994   122-96-35–12

Purpose.—The significance of sacral fractures as a cause of back pain has only recently been recognized. To emphasize the importance of these fractures as a cause of back pain and to determine the best technique for diagnosis, the records of patients with a diagnosis of sacral insufficiency fractures were examined.

Patients.—Twenty patients with sacral insufficiency fractures were identified during a 5-year period. Records were examined and data on age, gender, history of falls or minor trauma, pain duration before diagnosis, length of hospitalization, risk for osteoporosis, and other fractures were recorded. Radiographs, pelvic CT scans, and ^{99m}Tc scintigraphy were also studied. Physical examinations were performed to determine any predisposing factors. Functional outcomes (pain severity, limitations in mobility and activities, and degree of independence) were assessed within 6–9 months of the fracture.

Results.—The mean patient age was 74 years, with the group being predominately female (19 of 20). A diagnosis of sacral insufficiency fracture was made at a mean of 5 weeks after the onset of pain, with hospitalization for bedrest and analgesics required by 14 patients for a mean of 21 days. A history of low energy trauma was recorded for 9 patients. An abnormal scintigraphy was found in all 20 patients, whereas CT scanning revealed a fracture or sclerosis in 7 of 12 patients. Radiography found sclerosis in only 4 of 20 patients. Rheumatoid arthritis was seen in 6 of 20 patients. Of 18 patients who had bone mineral density measurements, 17 had severe osteopenia. Scintigraphy revealed the presence of other concurrent insufficiency fractures, including vertebral compression (15), pubic rami (10), hip (5), humerus (4), pubic body (5), and supra-acetabular ilium (3). Mild analgesics were required by 3 patients at 6-9 months follow-up, and complete resolution of pain was reported by the remaining 17 patients. Three patients had some limitations in mobility or in performance of daily activities.

Conclusion.—Bone scintigraphy was found to be the most reliable in the diagnosis of sacral insufficiency fracture, with increased uptake in the fracture area in all patients. Other techniques (e.g., plain radiography and CT scan) were less reliable. Computed tomographic scan was useful in the exclusion of other destructive processes and also in revealing the fracture line. Reduced bone density and bone formation were found in most patients. However, outcome in all patients was excellent, with most becoming pain free and fully recovered within 9 months of diagnosis. A heightened awareness of insufficiency sacral fractures as a cause of back pain may reduce the number of biopsy or MRI procedures performed in these patients. Conservative treatment with rehabilitative therapy has been shown to result in a resolution of pain and return of function and mobility in elderly patients with insufficiency sacral fractures, even in the presence of osteoporosis and other insufficiency fractures.

▶ The authors reconfirm what is known about sacral insufficiency fractures in the elderly. These are relatively easy to diagnose if the physician simply thinks of the diagnosis and confirms it with appropriate scans. Although the pain caused by such fractures can be severe, it typically resolves over the ensuing months, in a fashion similar to the resolution of spinal pain associated with insufficiency fractures in the thoracic and lumbar spine.—R.H. Wilkins, M.D.

Prevalence of Cervical Spine Subluxations and Dislocations in a Community-Based Rheumatoid Arthritis Population

Kauppi M, Hakala M (Univ of Tampere, Finland; Univ of Oulu, Finland)
Scand J Rheumatol 23:133–136, 1994   122-96-35–13

Objective.—The most common abnormalities of the cervical spine found in patients with rheumatoid arthritis (RA) are anterior atlantoaxial subluxation (AAS), vertical atlantoaxial dislocation (VD), and lateral subluxation. Posterior AAS appears to be rare. The incidence of cervical spine subluxation in patients with RA was determined in 1 Finnish community.

Methods.—Radiographs were performed on 98 patients aged 47–70 years with RA. Patients had a median duration of disease from first symptoms of 15.7 years.

Results.—Anterior atlantoaxial subluxation was diagnosed in 32 patients; a third had movement of 4 mm or more (Tables 1 and 2). Vertical atlantoaxial dislocation was found in 26 patients by the Sakaguchi-Kauppi method and in 14 patients by the McRae method. Anterior AAS and VD

TABLE 1.—Frequencies of Subluxations in the Cervical Spine Radiographs of 98 Patients With RA

	Patients	%
Anterior AAS	32	33
VD (S-K method)	26	27
VD (McRae method)	14	14
Lateral AAS	10*	14
Posterior AAS	2	2
Subaxial S	21	21
aAAS + VD (S-K)	16	16
aAAS + SAS	10	10
No AAS, VD nor SAS	47	48

* From a total of 73 patients.
Abbreviations: AAS, atlantoaxial subluxation; *VD,* vertical atlantoaxial dislocation; *S-K,* Sakaguchi-Kauppi; *aAAS,* anterior AAS; *SAS,* subaxial subluxation; *RA,* rheumatoid arthritis.
(Courtesy of Kauppi M, Hakala M: *Scand J Rheumatol* 23:133–136, 1994.)

were found in 16 patients, posterior subluxation in 2 patients, subaxial subluxation in 21 patients, and AAS plus subaxial subluxation in 10. One patient underwent surgery for subaxial staircase subluxation but still had an AAS of 4 mm. Four patients had an anterior AAS of 9 mm or more, and 6 patients had an anterior AAS of 6 to 9 mm and a vertical dislocation.

Conclusion.—The radiologic results indicate that the 11 patients with extensive AAS would be candidates for surgery, for an incidence of 10%. Severe pain, neurologic deficits, and cervical myelopathy, rather than radiographs alone, should be used as indications for surgery. In all other cases, conservative management is recommended.

▶ The authors document the common occurrence (52% in their series) of cervical subluxations in patients with rheumatoid arthritis.—R.H. Wilkins, M.D.

TABLE 2.—Severity of Anterior AAS and VD Findings in 98 Patients With RA

	Number of patients
AA diameter (mm)	
≤ 3	66
< 6	17
< 9	11
≤12	4
VD grade (S-K method)*	
I	71
II	18
III	6
IV	2

* Grading was impossible in 1 case.
Abbreviations: AA, atlantoaxial; *VD,* vertical atlantoaxial dislocation; *S-K,* Sakaguchi-Kauppi; *RA,* rheumatoid arthritis.
(Courtesy of Kauppi M, Hakala M: *Scand J Rheumatol* 23:133–136, 1994.)

Trauma

Vertebral Artery Injury After Acute Cervical Spine Trauma: Rate of Occurrence as Detected by MR Angiography and Assessment of Clinical Consequences

Friedman D, Flanders A, Thomas C, Millar W (Thomas Jefferson Univ Hosp, Philadelphia; Jefferson Med College, Philadelphia)
AJR 164:443–447, 1995   122-96-35–14

Background.—In patients with acute blunt injuries to the cervical spine, MRI examination is performed to detect such problems as cord hemorrhage and edema, disk herniation, ligamentous and osseous disruption, and epidural fluid. Vertebral artery injuries in these patients can lead to devastating intracranial neurologic complications. There have been no prospective studies of the use of MR angiography to evaluate the extracranial vertebral arteries in patients with acute trauma to the cervical spine. The frequency of vertebral artery injuries as detected by MR angiography and the clinical consequences of these injuries were evaluated.

Methods.—Magnetic resonance imaging studies were performed in 37 patients with acute, nonpenetrating cervical spine trauma. Most of these studies were done within 24 hours of the injury. In addition to routine spin-echo and gradient-echo images, the investigators performed 2-dimensional time-of-flight MR angiography of the extracranial vessels of the head and neck. Two neuroradiologists read the MR angiogram scans independently for nonvisualization, focal narrowing, or focal widening of the extracranial vessels. Angiographic correlation was obtained in 2 patients. Data on the type of spinal injury, the neurologic deficit on admission, and intracranial neurologic deficit caused by vertebral artery injury were obtained through medical record review. The specificity of MR angiography was studied through evaluation of scans from 37 control subjects, which were assessed only for the presence or absence of the vertebral arteries.

Results.—Twenty-four percent of the patients had abnormal findings on MR angiography. One vertebral artery was diagnosed as nonvisualized (i.e., occluded) or as focally narrowed in 7 patients. Bilateral vertebral artery injuries were detected in 1 patient and nonvisualization of the left common carotid and left vertebral arteries in another. Both vertebral arteries were seen on MR angiography in all control subjects—the difference in the frequency of nonvisualization was significant between the patient and control groups. In the patient with bilateral vertebral artery injuries, a massive infarction of the right cerebellar hemisphere led to death 2 days after hospital admission. Otherwise, none of the trauma patients had intracranial neurologic deficits attributable to a major arterial injury.

Conclusions.—In patients with major cervical spine trauma, vertebral artery injuries are frequently detected by MR angiography. Most of these vascular injuries remain clinically occult, but some patients may have devastating neurologic complications develop as a result of posterior fossa infarction. Thus, MR angiography for noninvasive assessment of the vertebral arteries should be a key part of the evaluation of patients with acute injury of the cervical spine.

▶ The authors demonstrate that MR angiography can add significant information to that obtained by MRI in the assessment of acute cervical spine trauma.—R.H. Wilkins, M.D.

Osteology of the Pediatric Skull: Considerations of Halo Pin Placement
Wong WB, Haynes RJ (Children's Rehabilitative Services, Phoenix, Ariz)
Spine 19:1451–1454, 1994   122-96-35-15

Background.—Halo pin placement in children is commonly associated with complications, such as loosening and dislodging, infection, and penetration. Head CT scans obtained from children were measured to identify consistently thin regions in the pediatric skull that should be avoided when pins are placed.

Methods.—Head CT scans were obtained from 48 normal children, aged 10 years and younger. The scans were divided into 4 age groups. Total skull thickness was measured in 5 areas at the level of halo insertion.

Findings.—Skull thickness tended to increase with age. Skull thickness varied greatly at each area within and between age groups. The standard pin sites were not consistently thicker. Even up to 10 years of age, the average thinnest region was only 1.9 mm.

Conclusions.—No area in the pediatric skull is safe for halo pin placement. Limited preoperative head CT scans should be acquired to determine safe areas for pin placement.

▶ Wong and Haynes have issued a warning that should be heeded by anyone applying a halo to a child's head.—R.H. Wilkins, M.D.

Prophylactic Vena Cava Filter Insertion in Patients With Traumatic Spinal Cord Injury: Preliminary Results
Wilson JT, Rogers FB, Wald SL, Shackford SR, Ricci MA (Univ of Vermont College of Medicine, Burlington)
Neurosurgery 35:234–239, 1994   122-96-35-16

Objective.—For patients with traumatic spinal cord injury (SCI), pulmonary embolism (PE) is a potentially devastating complication. These patients are at prolonged risk for venous thromboembolism because of extended perturbations in fibrinolytic activity, catecholamine effects on platelet aggregation, increased complement and acute phase reactant activity, abnormally high factor VIII concentrations, and persistent venous stasis with continuing endothelial damage. Not all patients with SCI are eligible for prophylactic measures, such as venous compression hose or low-dose heparin, which only partially reduce the risk of venous thromboembolism. The initial results with prophylactic vena cava filter insertion in patients with SCI were reported.

Experience.—The new prophylaxis protocol was prompted by the results of a 5-year retrospective study of 111 patients with SCI. Seven of these patients had 8 documented PEs, and in 3 of these 7 patients it was fatal. Three fourths of the PEs occurred after the patients had been discharged from the acute care facility. The median time to occurrence of PE was 78 days. During this period, only 4% of trauma admissions were for SCI, yet these patients accounted for 31% of all PEs in the overall population with trauma.

Under the new protocol, all patients with SCI with paraplegia or quadriplegia underwent percutaneous insertion of a vena cava filter under local anesthesia. A prospective analysis included 15 patients who underwent filter insertion. All patients were followed weekly by impedance plethysmography to detect deep venous thrombosis.

Results.—None of the 15 patients had deep venous thrombosis develop during their acute hospitalization, the median duration of which was 22 days. There were no complications of vena cava filter insertion, and no cases of PE after filter insertion. On follow-up duplex scanning of the vena cava, 30-day patency was 100% and 1-year patency was 82%, according to life-table analysis. The reduced patency rate at 1 year likely reflected trapping of thrombus.

Conclusions.—Early results suggest that prophylactic vena cava filters are safe and effective in patients with traumatic SCI. Although small, this series addresses many important aspects of venous thromboembolic disease in SCI. Vena cava filters are the only effective form of long-term prophylaxis for these patients.

► These authors have taken an aggressive approach to the prevention of PE in patients with traumatic SCI. In their relatively small series of patients (15) who were managed by the prophylactic insertion of a filter into the inferior vena cava and who were followed for a relatively short time (6–24 months), no patient had a PE, and there were no complications resulting from placement of the filter. This promising approach to the prevention of PE in patients with SCI (who are at significant risk for this frequently fatal event) should be assessed further in a larger group.—R.H. Wilkins, M.D.

Pediatric Seatbelt Injuries: Diagnosis and Treatment of Lumbar Flexion-Distraction Injuries
Greenwald TA, Mann DC (Univ of Wisconsin, Madison)
Paraplegia 32:743–751, 1994   122-96-35–17

Introduction.—Increased seatbelt use has reduced injury and deaths from motor vehicle accidents. However, motor vehicle accidents still cause more than 75% of flexion-distraction injuries of the thoracolumbar spine. While wearing a seatbelt, such an injury can occur as a result of hyperflexion of the spine about a fixed point anterior to the vertebral body axis. Six children who underwent surgery for treatment of these injuries were described.

Methods.—Six patients, including 4 boys (average age, 8 years; range, 4–15 years) were identified from reviewing charts. Additional information was obtained from interviews with patients and parents.

Results.—All 6 had been in collisions at greater than 50 mph. Only 1 had been wearing a properly fitting 3-point restraint. The others were restrained only by a lap belt or by an improperly fitting 3-point restraint. Three had purely ligamentous injuries, 2 had bony injuries (chance fractures), and 1 had combination injuries. Some also had neurologic or abdominal injuries. Spinal or abdominal injuries were initially missed in 2 patients. Preoperative kyphosis averaged 18 degrees. Within an average of 3 days after the motor vehicle accident, patients were surgically treated with open reduction and internal fixation. There were no major surgical complications. At an average follow-up of 2 years, 5 patients had excellent outcomes, with full range of motion, no back pain, and return to preinjury activity. The sixth was paraplegic from the injury.

Conclusion.—Surgery for seatbelt injuries in children is recommended in a variety of circumstances: (1) when spinal instability is apparent in a ligamentous injury or in an unstable fracture, (2) when significant kyphosis occurs and adequate reduction cannot be obtained with a cast, (3) when abdominal injury requires surgery and the patient might benefit from early mobilization and use of a cast is not appropriate, and (4) when neurologic injury is seen. Use of short-segment compression rodding using a pediatric-size rod and hook construct is advocated.

▶ The authors report their experience in treating pediatric lumbar flexion-distraction injuries that were sustained in high-speed motor vehicle accidents in which all but one of the children had been restrained only by a lap belt. Except for the child who was rendered paraplegic by the accident, the patients all achieved an excellent result, with no pain, a full range of movement, and full activity.—R.H. Wilkins, M.D.

Neoplasms

Central Neurocytomas of the Cervical Spinal Cord
Tatter SB, Borges LF, Louis DN (Harvard Medical School, Boston)
J Neurosurg 81:288–293, 1994   122-96-35–18

Introduction.—Central neurocytoma is a benign neuronal tumor that occurs supratentorially in the lateral or third ventricles. The clinical, neuroradiologic, and neuropathologic features of 2 neurocytomas arising in the spinal cord were described.

Case Reports.—Two men, 65 and 49 years, had progressive neurologic deficits referable to the cervical spinal cord. Magnetic resonance imaging revealed a homogeneous intramedullary spinal cord mass at the C3–4 level. Gliomas were initially suspected, and laminectomies were performed. In the first patient, the correct diagnosis was made after electron microscopy revealed neuronal features. Postoperatively, the patient received irradiation, and his neurologic condition remained stable 10 years after presentation. In the second patient, the initial pathologic diagnosis was probable ependymoma. Postoperatively, the patient received irradiation therapy, but neurologic deficits recurred 2 years later. A second MR image showed increased tumor size, and sagittal and axial images showed hypointense regions consistent with either flow-void areas or hemosiderin. Angiography showed faint tumor blush but no other abnormalities. The tumor was totally resected and immunostaining of the tissue revealed tumor cells that were positive for synaptophysin and neuron-specific enolase and negative for glial fibrillary acidic protein, strongly indicating a neuronal tumor. Other findings included a single mitotic figure and regions of hemosiderin deposition. The patient continues to improve in the 5 years after surgery.

Summary.—These spinal cord neoplasms should be included under the designation "central neurocytoma." Like their supratentorial counterparts, central neurocytomas of the spinal cord are vascular, although angiography does not reveal feeding vessels accessible for embolization. In the second patient, the rapid increase in tumor size and the presence of bilirubin-stained cyst cavity at the second operation are consistent with hemorrhage into the tumor, causing enlargement and clinical deterioration. Until more data are available, radiation therapy should be reserved for progressive, recurrent, or anaplastic variants similar to that in supratentorial neurocytoma.

▶ Central neurocytoma is a small-cell neuronal tumor that has been diagnosed with increased frequency in recent years. It typically is a cerebral neoplasm that grows into the lateral or third ventricle. On the basis of standard histologic analysis, it may be misdiagnosed as an oligodendroglioma. Tatter et al. document that the central neurocytoma may occur within the spinal cord.—R.H. Wilkins, M.D.

Neurinomas of the Cauda Equina: Clinical Analysis of 40 Surgical Cases
Cervoni L, Celli P, Scarpinati M, Cantore G (Univ La Sapienza, Rome)
Acta Neurochir (Wien) 127:199–202, 1994   122-96-35–19

Objective.—Cauda equina neurinomas make up 40% to 45% of all tumors in this region. Before the advent of CT, these lesions often grew quite large because of the mobility of the roots, the wide intradural space, and misinterpretation of the symptoms as the pain of lumbar disk herniation. A series of 40 patients with neurinoma of the cauda equina was reviewed.

Patients.—The patients were 30 males and 10 females with a mean age of 46 years. The average clinical history was 4 years, with all patients having pain as their first symptom. The pain was noted as low back pain with sciatica in 70% of cases; it was progressive in 73%. Pain was usually aggravated by lying down. In 75% of the patients, motor disturbances of the lower limbs developed after a mean of 12 months from the onset of pain. Sensory disturbances developed in 62%. Twenty-five percent of the patients were classified as neurologically intact, 50% as having mild sensorimotor deficits, and 25% as having severe sensorimotor deficits and sphincter disturbances with urinary retention. Only 10% of the patients had Lasègue's sign.

Diagnosis.—All patients had an elevated CSF protein level. The diagnosis was made by myelography in the 20 patients treated before 1976 and by CT myelography, sometimes with MRI, in the latter 20. Computed tomography myelography showed an isodense lesion in 85% of patients, while MRI always showed an isointense lesion.

Treatment and Outcomes.—Management was by total tumor removal, including removal of the root from which the tumor originated in 19 cases. Eighty-eight percent of the tumors were intradural, and half measured more than 50 mm. At a mean follow-up of 18 years, patients with no preoperative neurologic deficits remained the same, those with mild preoperative deficits improved, and those with severe preoperative deficits got no worse. Ten percent of the patients with nerve root resection had persistence of their preoperative deficits.

Discussion.—These findings, along with cases from the literature, suggest that it is possible but not easy to clinically differentiate neurinoma of the cauda equina from the more common lumbar disk herniation. Early-stage neurinomas cause unilateral sciatic, nonradicular pain that is ill-defined and worse in the decubitus position. In contrast, later-stage neurinomas cause bilateral, polyradicular pain with sensorimotor disturbances. As long as sacrifice of the involved nerve root does not worsen the neurologic deficit, total tumor removal appears to be the best treatment.

▶ The authors supply an up-to-date review of the topic of neurinomas of the cauda equina.—R.H. Wilkins, M.D.

Brief Report: Relief of Spinal Cord Compression From Vertebral Hemangioma by Intralesional Injection of Absolute Ethanol

Heiss JD, Doppman JL, Oldfield EH (Natl Inst of Neurological Disorders and Stroke, Bethesda, Md; Natl Insts of Health, Bethesda, MD)
N Engl J Med 331:508–511, 1994   122-96-35–20

Background.—Vertebral hemangiomas are fairly common anomalies, although neurologic symptoms are rare. Current treatments for symptomatic vertebral hemangioma are surgery, radiotherapy, and transarterial embolization, all of which are associated with some limitations. Two patients were described who had myelopathy and progressive paraparesis, caused by vertebral hemangioma, that were successfully treated via direct puncture and perfusion of the hemangioma with absolute ethanol. The technique allows the devascularization of vertebral hemangiomas as an alternative to surgery or radiation therapy.

Technique.—Two female patients, 54 and 64 years, who had histories of progressive weakness of the lower extremities for 12 months and bilateral weakness and pain in the lower extremities for 3 months, respectively, were treated using this technique. In both patients, ethanol was directly injected into the vertebral hemangioma. A transpedicular route was chosen after it was noted that a more lateral approach caused the needle to glance off the vertebral body. After patient positioning on the CT table, the CT gantry was angled to align the scan along the long axis of the pedicle. After administering 1% lidocaine for local anesthesia and IV diazepam and fentanyl for sedation and analgesia, a 17-gauge bone-biopsy needle was inserted through the skin 3 cm left of the midline. Under CT control, the needle was advanced to the cortical bone overlying the pedicle. One percent lidocaine was then used to infiltrate the periosteum, and the needle was advanced through the cortical bone and the center of the pedicle into the vertebral body. Correct positioning was verified via CT scan. A CT scan was performed while 10 mL of iopamidol was injected through the needle, which showed opacification of hemangiomatous vessels. Rapid blood flow caused the contrast medium to clear promptly from the hemangioma. Additional axial CT cuts through the adjacent spinal levels were used to exclude the possibility that the iopamidol was entering the subarachnoid space. Ten mL of absolute ethanol was then injected into the hemangioma in increments of 2 mL every 5 to 10 minutes. Occlusion of the hemangioma was verified by the prolonged retention of contrast medium in the vertebral body and by the cessation of blood flow through the biopsy needle.

Conclusions.—Injection of ethanol can be repeated, as needed, to obliterate residual hemangioma. In patient 1, a second injection was done 10 weeks after the first to eliminate residual hemangioma seen on MRI. In both patients, myelopathy was fully resolved after treatment. Further experience with percutaneous injection of ethanol should help define its role in the treatment of vertebral hemangiomas and other vertebral lesions.

▶ Heiss et al. have demonstrated in 2 patients that the percutaneous injection of absolute alcohol can be used to obliterate a symptomatic vertebral hemangioma. This technique is simpler than the standard methods of treating such lesions, and it has promise to become the preferred form of therapy.—R.H. Wilkins, M.D.

Management of the Vertebral Artery in Excision of Extradural Tumors of the Cervical Spine
Sen C, Eisenberg M, Casden AM, Sundaresan N, Catalano PJ (Mount Sinai Med Ctr, New York)
Neurosurgery 36:106–116, 1995   122-96-35–21

Objective.—In some cases, extradural tumors of the cervical spine may involve the vertebral artery on 1 or both sides. This is a major factor limiting the radical resection of such tumors; the standard anterior approach may be inadequate. The use of an anterolateral or lateral approach

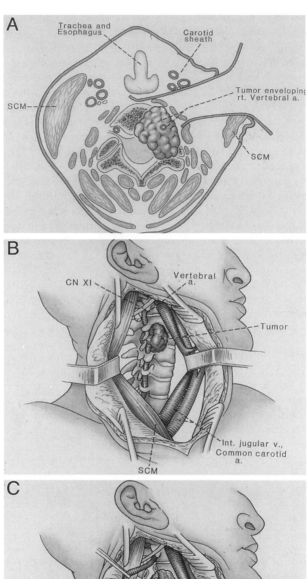

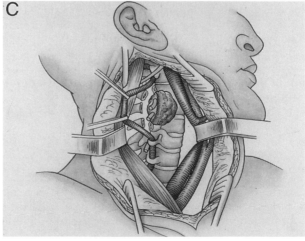

(continued)

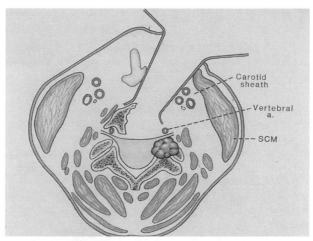

Fig 35–4.—The anterior approach, medial to the carotid sheath shown in the axial section. (Courtesy of Sen C, Eisenberg M, Casden AM, et al: *Neurosurgery* 36:106–116, 1994.)

to permit exposure and dissection of the vertebral artery, aggressive resection of the tumor, and subsequent stabilization was described.

Technique.—For patients with tumors below C2, an anterolateral approach is used to the anterior tubercles of the transverse processes of the cervical vertebrae (Fig 35–3). With careful protection of the accessory nerves, phrenic nerve, and sympathetic chain, the artery is extracted from the foramen transversarium by rongeuring the anterior bridge of bone. It is then isolated from its venous sheath through gentle coagulation and circumferential stripping. Once the vertebral artery is completely mobilized from the periosteal and venous sheath, the tumor can be dissected from the nerve roots and thecal sac. The artery is then dissected, ligated, or reconstructed as indicated. A more direct anterior approach is needed for complete vertebrectomy over to the opposite vertebral artery (Fig 35–4). After the opposite longus colli and longus capitis muscles are dissected off the vertebral body and the anterior part of the transverse process, the rest of the vertebral body is drilled away to reach the other vertebral artery. In this way, the venous sheath of the opposite artery is undisturbed. Anterior stabilization is done according to the extent of the vertebrectomy.

For tumors at C1–2 and the craniovertebral junction, a lateral approach is better than a transoral one (Fig 35–5). The incision is made behind the ear and along the posterior border of the sternocleidomastoid muscle. After the muscles in the posterior triangle are divided and detached from the transverse processes of C1 and C2, the vertebral artery is exposed from the foramen transversarium of C2 up to its dural entry. Once the foramen transversarium of C1—and of C2, if

Fig 35–3 (cont).
    Fig 35–3.—A and B, anterolateral dissection with the tumor in relation to the spine and the vertebral artery. C, vertebral artery has been dissected and laterally displaced to improve access to the tumor. (Courtesy of Sen C, Eisenberg M, Casden AM, et al: *Neurosurgery* 36:106–116, 1994.)

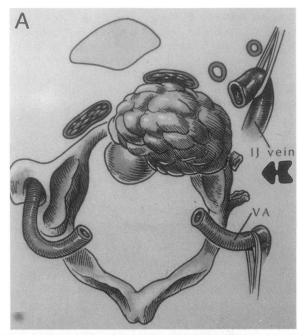

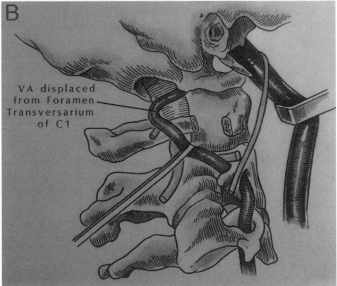

Fig 35–5.—A and **B,** lateral approach to the C1–C2 region by displacing the vertebral artery (*VA*). The *arrow* indicates the direction of the approach. (Courtesy of Sen C, Eisenberg M, Casden AM, et al: *Neurosurgery* 36:106–116, 1994.)

necessary—is opened, the vertebral artery can be displaced posteriorly to gain access to the anteriorly located tumor. The tumor is then removed piecemeal. The bone is drilled so that healthy marrow can be reached, a piece of iliac crest bone is wedged in anteriorly, and a posterior occiptiocervical stabilization is done through a posterior midline incision.

Experience.—These approaches were used in 10 patients with a variety of cervical spine tumors adjacent to or involving the vertebral arteries. Except for patients with high-grade malignancies, the goal of the procedure was to preserve the vertebral artery. Otherwise, excision of the diseased arterial segment and replacement with a vein graft were planned. The operations were done in 1 or 2 stages. Anterior and posterior stabilization were required in all patients but 1. Adjuvant therapy was used in some cases.

Discussion.—In patients with extradural tumors of the cervical spine involving the vertebral arteries, a standard anterior approach may be inadequate. Use of the described approaches to isolate the artery greatly facilitates management: The artery can then be dissected from the tumor, ligated for en bloc resection, or reconstructed. An anterolateral approach is best for tumors in the second portion of the vertebral artery, which extends from the C6 to the C2 foramen transversarium. For the third portion, from the C2 foramen to the artery's entry into the posterior fossa, a lateral approach is preferred.

▶ Sen and associates describe some techniques they have used in resecting extradural tumors of the cervical spine, especially with regard to exposing and managing the vertebral artery.—R.H. Wilkins, M.D.

Combined Microneurosurgical and Thoracoscopic Removal of Neurogenic Dumbbell Tumors
Vallières E, Findlay JM, Fraser RE (Univ of Alberta, Edmonton, Alta, Canada)
Ann Thorac Surg 59:469–472, 1995   122-96-35-22

Background.—Posterior mediastinal neurogenic dumbbell tumors are usually benign. Their removal traditionally required a 1-stage combined laminectomy and thoracotomy. A novel technique combining posterior microneurosurgical and anterior video-assisted thoracoscopic surgery (VATS) for the removal of benign dumbbell tumors was investigated.

Procedure.—In the first phase of the operation, the spinal component of the tumor is removed via a laminectomy with the aid of a neurosurgical operating microscope. The nerve root from which the tumor arises is transected. A frozen section examination of the tumor is performed before the incision is closed. A thoracotomy is done if the tumor proves to be malignant. Even if the tumor is benign, for the second phase of the operation, the patient is positioned for a full thoracotomy to enable intervention via thoracotomy if hemorrhage were to occur. The intrathoracic component of the tumor is removed by VATS.

Patients.—Over 1 year, 2 men and 2 women who had posterior mediastinal dumbbell tumors were operated on with laminectomy and thoracoscopic resection. Three patients had benign schwannomas and 1 patient had a mesenchymal hamartoma. Three patients had minimal postoperative discomfort and recovered rapidly without neurologic sequelae. The fourth patient required a limited open thoracotomy because of bleeding from an intercostal artery. This patient had near-complete neurologic recovery.

Conclusions.—Combined microneurosurgery and VATS for the removal of posterior mediastinal neurogenic dumbbell tumors is safe, and it appears to produce much less morbidity than does conventional thoracotomy.

▶ Video-assisted thoracoscopic surgery is being used with increasing frequency in the performance of thoracic sympathectomy, and its use is being investigated for the treatment of other conditions such as thoracic disc herniation. These authors add neurogenic dumbbell tumors to that list.— R.H. Wilkins, M.D.

Neurological Evaluation After Radical Resection of Sacral Neoplasms
Fujimura Y, Maruiwa H, Takahata T, Toyama Y (Keio Univ, Tokyo)
Paraplegia 32:396–406, 1994   122-96-35–23

Objective.—Eight patients who required radical resection of sacral tumors entailing severing lumbosacral nerves on both sides were evaluated functionally.

Patients.—The 6 men and 2 women had an average age of 56 years at the time of surgery. Three patients had chordoma and, in addition, there were individual instances of Ewing's sarcoma, chondrosarcoma, giant cell tumor, meningioma, and ependymoma. In 3 patients, recurrent disease had developed after they had been treated surgically. In addition to radical tumor resection, 6 patients had reconstruction of the sacrum. Fixation instrumentation was used in 3 cases.

Results.—With respect to motor function in the lower extremities, only when nerves from the L5 level and above were preserved bilaterally were patients able to walk. Patients were hypesthetic and anesthetic at spinal levels below that where the nerves were severed. Bilateral preservation of the S2 nerves and above was required to retain urinary and fecal continence and sexual function. Weak erections were possible after bilaterally severing the S2 nerves and below, but ejaculation was not.

Conclusion.—The more lumbosacral nerves that can be spared when radically resectioning a sacral tumor, the more neurologic function will be preserved.

▶ Radical resection of certain sacral neoplasms can be curative, but the patient pays a price neurologically. The authors verify that the extent of this loss of function is what one would predict based on the level of resection. They conclude that it is necessary to bilaterally preserve the L5 nerves and those above with regard to walking and to bilaterally preserve the S2 nerves and those above with regard to urinary, fecal, and sexual function.—R.H. Wilkins, M.D.

Preliminary Clinical Experience With Linear Accelerator-Based Spinal Stereotactic Radiosurgery

Hamilton AJ, Lulu BA, Fosmire H, Stea B, Cassady JR (Univ of Arizona Health Sciences Ctr, Tucson)
Neurosurgery 36:311–319, 1995   122-96-35–24

Background.—Many attempts have been made to extend radiosurgical techniques beyond the limitations of the cranium. The development, testing, and clinical application of a prototype device for extracranial stereotactic surgery were reported.

Methods and Findings.—The extracranial stereotactic radiosurgery frame (Fig 35–6) was used to deliver stereotactic radiosurgery with a modified linear accelerator to metastatic neoplasms in the cervical, thoracic, and lumbar regions in 5 patients. All neoplasms had been unresponsive to spinal cord tolerance doses delivered by standard external fractionated radiation therapy to a median dose of 45 Gy. Tumors were treated with single-fraction stereotactic radiosurgery. The spinal stereotactic frame was used for immobilization, localization, and treatment. The median number of isocenters was 1. The median single fraction dose was 10 Gy with median normalization to 80% isodose contour. One complication—esophagitis—occurred, from radiosurgery of a tumor involving the C6-T1 segments. The esophagitis resolved with medical therapy. Median follow-up was 6 months. None of the patients have had radiographic or clinical progression of the treated tumor. Two patients died of systemic metastatic disease. In the 3 survivors, CT or MRI documented regression of the treated tumor, with a reduction of thecal sac compression.

Conclusions.—This was the first clinical application of stereotactic radiosurgery in the spine. Extracranial radiosurgery may be appropriate for

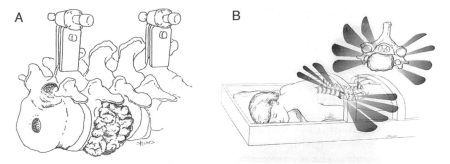

A   B

Fig 35–6.—Artist's drawing showing patient in spinal stereotactic frame. **A,** spinous process clamps that serve to immobilize the tumorous vertebral body by fixing the segment above and below the target area. **B,** the patient lying immobilized in the spinal stereotacic frame. Collimated beams of radiation could be targeted to avoid the spinal canal and treat an adjacent neoplasm radiographically. (Courtesy of Hamilton AJ, Lulu BA, Fosmire H, et al: *Neurosurgery* 36:311–319, 1995.)

the treatment of paraspinal neoplasms after external fractionated radiation therapy, even when spinal cord compression is present.

▶ The authors describe a method of performing spinal stereotactic radiosurgery. Their technique requires skeletal fixation, which is accomplished by the open surgical attachment of clamps to the spinous processes onto two vertebral segments above and below the involved vertebral segment. Because of the well-documented value of intracranial stereotactic radiosurgery, I expect that similar treatment of spinal disorders will develop as well. This report represents an important beginning.—R.H. Wilkins, M.D.

Miscellaneous

Multiplanar Magnetic Resonance Imaging of the Sacral Foramina and Presacral Space

Savolaine ER, Ebraheim NA (Med College of Ohio, Toledo)
Am J Orthop 24:139–144, 1995   122-96-35–25

Background.—Disease processes of the sacrum and presacral space are of considerable interest to neurosurgeons, orthopedic surgeons, and oncologists. Although radiologic evaluation of these complex anatomical areas can be difficult, the multiplanar capabilities of MRI can define both fracture pathology and neoplastic destruction. Alternate MRI anatomical planes were used to explore the sacral foramina and presacral space in normal volunteers and randomly selected patients.

Patients and Methods.—In 30 patients undergoing pelvic or low lumbar spine MRI scans, a coronal oblique T1-weighted scan of the sacrum was added to the protocol. The plane of the scan was oriented in the longitudinal axis of the sacrum (Fig 35–7). Imaging sections were 5 mm in thickness, and their number was determined from the sagittal plane to cover S1 through the sacrococcygeal junction. The goal was to observe the consistency of anatomical demonstration of the sacral foramina and their contents. In 3 normal volunteers, modified oblique axial MRI scans were obtained in planes parallel to individual sacral foramina to show exiting roots in profile and also the entry of nerves into presacral fat.

Results.—Pathologic involvement of the sacral foramina was noted in 12 of the 30 patients. Although lesions were seen in other conventional MRI planes, the definition of the sacral foramen margin involvement was better shown with the oblique coronal view (Fig 35–8). All 30 patients showed 4 sets of sacral foramina, and some showed 4 sets of foramina on a single frame. The exiting nerve and lateral sacral artery and vein branches were seen in all patients. The modified oblique axial planes showed individual nerves exiting into the presacral fat in all 3 volunteers. The second-order oblique sagittal plane for the sacral plexus also showed portions of the plexus in contiguous sections on volunteers. Moreover, adjacent major vessels were outlined by presacral fat.

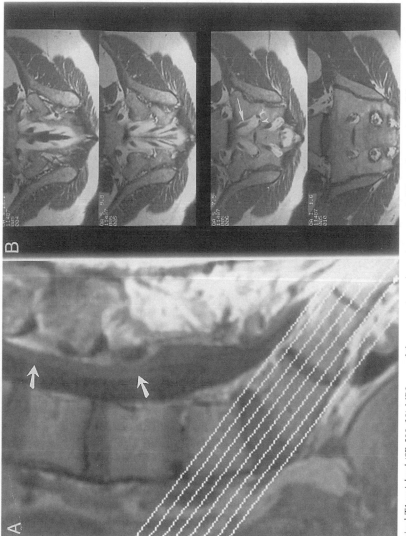

Fig 35-7.—**A,** sagittal T1-weighted (SE 500–20) MRI scan of the sacrum is used to orient coronal oblique plane sections of the sacrum (*lines*). The number of sections required to evaluate 4 pairs of sacral foramina depends on the degree of sacral curvature present in the sagittal view. Scans are obtained at 5-mm intervals, using the sagittal view as a "scout" view. In this scan of a patient with suspected pelvic or low lumbar lesions, an old meningomyelocele defect is seen incidentally. Low cord and neural placode remnant are seen (*arrows*). **B,** coronal oblique MRI sections (SE 500–20) as oriented on **A** (on a different patient) show normal thecal sac, root sleeves (*arrows*), and branches of the lateral sacral arteries and veins (*arrowheads*). Sections show normal anatomy as seen in all 30 patients. (Courtesy of Savolaine ER, Ebraheim NA: *Am J Orthop* 24:139–144, 1995.)

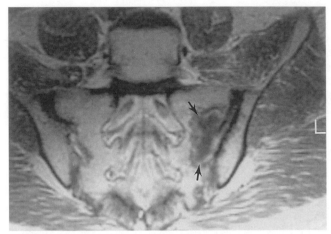

Fig 35–8.—A coronal oblique T1-weighted MRI scan (SE 500–20) demonstrates a destructive lesion in the left sacral ala which closely approaches the sacral foramina but does not produce encroachment (*arrows*). Whereas other MRI planes can show foraminal sparing, this plan provides the simplest demonstration of the foramina. At biopsy, the lesion was metastatic chondrosarcoma from the larynx. (Courtesy of Savolaine ER, Ebraheim NA: *Am J Orthop* 24:139–144, 1995.)

Conclusion.—The multiplanar capabilities of MRI can thoroughly explore the bony sacrum, sacral canal, sacral foramina, and presacral space in relation to trauma, tumor, or any other destructive or space-occupying entity.

▶ The authors demonstrate the diagnostic value of alternative MRI views of the sacrum (oblique coronal views, modified oblique axial views, and oblique sagittal views).—R.H. Wilkins, M.D.

Surgical Interruption of Intradural Draining Vein as Curative Treatment of Spinal Dural Arteriovenous Fistulas
Afshar JKB, Doppman JL, Oldfield EH (Natl Inst of Neurological Disorders and Stroke, Bethesda, Md)
J Neurosurg 82:196–200, 1995   122-96-35–26

Introduction.—Although spinal dural arteriovenous fistulas (AVFs) are amenable to curative treatment, the optimum management of this common type of spinal arteriovenous malformation has not been established. The clinical records of 19 patients were reviewed to determine whether surgical excision of the AVF or interruption of the intradural draining spinal vein are curative treatments.

Patients and Methods.—Patients eligible for the study were treated at the National Institutes of Health between 1983 and 1993 and underwent preoperative and immediate postoperative spinal arteriography. The group included 17 men and 2 women with an average age of 56 years at diagnosis. All had experienced a gradual onset and progressive deterioration of neurologic function. Sensory dysfunction was present in all patients, and most had paresis and bladder disturbance. The average duration of symptoms before diagnosis was 22 months. Eleven patients underwent complete excision of the dural AVF, and 8 were treated by intradural interruption of the vein draining the AVF. Clinical outcome was reported with a mean follow-up of 37 months.

Results.—Eight patients had neurologic improvement after surgery, and 11 showed stabilization of signs and symptoms. The 11 patients who underwent excision had no evidence of a residual lesion at immediate or delayed postoperative arteriography. Two of 8 patients who had interruption of the intradural draining vein had an AVF with both intradural and extradural venous drainage. Residual flow through the AVF into the extradural venous system occurred after intradural division of the draining vein in these 2 cases, and 1 patient required additional therapy when intrathecal venous drainage was reestablished.

Conclusion.—The goal of treatment in patients who have spinal dural AVFs is to eliminate venous congestion of the spinal cord before irreversible neurological injury occurs. Surgery is adequate treatment in most cases. Simple interruption of the intrathecal venous drainage provides lasting and curative treatment for patients with only intrathecal medullary venous drainage. Complete excision of the AVF should not be attempted in some patients because of the risk of compromise of the blood supply of the spinal cord.

▶ The group at the National Institutes of Health has had an extensive experience with arteriovenous malformations and fistulas of the spinal cord. In this article, they review their experience with the surgical management of 19 patients with spinal dural AVFs and progressive myelopathy. They emphasize the value and safety of the venous approach to treatment.

Their conclusions are threefold. In patients who had spinal dural AVFs with only intrathecal medullary venous drainage, which includes most patients with these lesions, surgical interruption of the intradural draining vein is the procedure of choice. In patients with both intra- and extradural drainage of the AVF, complete excision of the fistula or interruption of its intra- and extradural drainage is indicated. In patients in whom a common vessel supplies both the spinal cord and the dural AVF, surgical interruption of the venous drainage of the AVF is preferred because it does not risk arterial occlusion and cord infarction.—R.H. Wilkins, M.D.

Surgical Management of Spinal Tuberculosis in Adults: Hong Kong Operation Compared With Debridement Surgery for Short and Long Term Outcome of Deformity

Upadhyay SS, Sell P, Saji MJ, Sell B, Hsu LCS (Duchess of Kent Children's Hosp, Hong Kong)

Clin Orthop 302:173–182, 1994   122-96-35–27

Introduction.—In a prospective, controlled, multinational study, the Medical Research Council (MRC) reported equally good results with débridement surgery and radical resection for tuberculosis of the spine. However, previous reports have failed to address sufficiently the resulting spinal deformity: young children and adults were analyzed together, as were patients with thoracic and lumbar tuberculosis. In a 15-year longitudinal analysis of 105 patients from the MRC study, an attempt was made to overcome these deficiencies.

Methods.—Treatment was with radical resection of the tuberculous lesion followed by bone grafting in 71 patients and débridement surgery in the remaining 34. The mean age at surgery was 37 and 35 years, respectively; all patients were at least 18 years old. For the current analysis, the investigators used electronically digitalized lateral spinal radiographs to measure the kyphosis and deformity angles.

Results.—The 2 surgical groups had equally good neurologic recovery, with none of the patients reporting pain 2 years postoperatively. None had reactivated or recurrent tuberculosis. At 6 months' follow-up, there was marginal correction of deformity in the radical surgery group compared with deterioration in both kyphosis and deformity angles for the débridement group. The difference between groups from preoperative to 6-month postoperative angles was significant. At final vs. 6-month follow-up, however, the mean difference in kyphosis and deformity angles was not significant. At 6 months, 40% of radical surgery patients had a 5-degree or better improvement in deformity angle, whereas 53% of patients undergoing débridement showed deterioration. Lumbar spine lordosis was normal at final follow-up in all patients with lumbar tuberculosis treated with radical surgery compared with only 63% of those treated by débridement.

Conclusions.—These results suggest that radical resection and bone grafting yield better long-term correction of deformity than surgical débridement for patients with spinal tuberculosis. Radical surgery offers similar surgical exposure, better correction, early fusion, no kyphotic deformity of the lumbar spine, and no specific complications of bone grafting. The degree of correction noted 6 months after surgery is effectively maintained for up to 15 years.

▶ Surgeons in several parts of the world have a unique opportunity to study the most effective ways of managing spinal tuberculosis. Over the years, those in Hong Kong have led the way. In this instance, the MRC of the United Kingdom working party on tuberculosis of the spine undertook a controlled multinational prospective study to evaluate the efficacy of various treatment regimens in Korea, Zimbabwe, Hong Kong, and South Africa. As indicated in the abstract, the authors have shown that in adults, the use of radical resection and bone grafting yields better results than surgical débridement alone.—R.H. Wilkins, M.D.

The Effect of Age on the Change in Deformity After Radical Resection and Anterior Arthrodesis for Tuberculosis of the Spine

Upadhyay SS, Saji MJ, Sell P, Yau ACMC (Duchess of Kent Children's Hosp, Hong Kong; Canossa Hosp, Hong Kong)
J Bone Joint Surg (Am) 76-A:701–708, 1994   122-96-35-28

Purpose.—For children with spinal tuberculosis, radical resection of the lesion and anterior arthrodesis is a well-established operation. Progressive spinal deformity may occur for unknown reasons. One postulated cause is overgrowth of the posterior elements of the vertebral column, but this issue has not been well studied. The long-term results of radical resection for tuberculosis of the spine were examined in terms of the longitudinal pattern of the spinal deformity.

Methods.—The study included 2 groups of patients who underwent a radical operation for tuberculosis of the spine in Hong Kong. At the time of the operation, 33 patients were children aged 10 years or younger and 71 were adults at least 18 years of age. The patients were followed prospectively. The investigators used lateral spinal radiographs to measure kyphosis and deformity angles at 6 months, 1 year, 5 years, and an average of 15 years postoperatively.

Results.—The mean kyphosis and deformity angles were no different between children and adult patients at any follow-up interval. Among patients with thoracic spinal tuberculosis, correction at 6 months' follow-up was much better in children than adults, and this correction was maintained throughout follow-up. There were no such differences in deformity for patients with thoracolumbar or lumbar spinal tuberculosis.

Conclusions.—In young children with spinal tuberculosis, the performance of a short anterior spinal arthrodesis does not appear to be associated with progressive deformity during growth and development. Children and adults undergoing this type of operation show no difference in the longitudinal pattern of changes in deformity, and there is no evidence that disproportionate posterior spinal growth contributes to progressive deformity. These results suggest that prophylactic posterior spinal arthrodesis is not indicated in children undergoing a radical operation for tuberculosis of the spine.

▶ This additional study from Hong Kong shows that radical resection and bone grafting for the treatment of spinal tuberculosis provides essentially the same results as far as kyphosis and deformity angles are concerned, whether the patient is a child or an adult.—R.H. Wilkins, M.D.

36 Spinal Surgery: Technique

Trans-sternal Approach to Intraspinal Tumours in the Upper Thoracic Region

Calliauw L, Dallenga A, Caemaert J (Univ Hosp, Ghent, Belgium)

Acta Neurochir (Wien) 127:227–231, 1994   122-96-36-1

Background.—Although rare, ventrally located intraspinal tumors are difficult to manage, particularly those located in the upper thoracic area. The authors of this report advocate use of the trans-sternal approach for removal of ventrally located intradural or extradural spinal tumors.

Surgical Technique.—The patient is placed in a supine position and receives endotracheal general anesthesia; the neck is then slightly hyperextended and the head rotated to the right. A vertical incision is made in the midline of the sternum. This extends caudally to 4 cm below the xiphoid and is prolonged cranially in the cervical region along the anterior margin of the left sternocleidomastoid muscle.

After division of the platysma, the sternal portion of the sternocleidomastoid muscle is identified and separated from deeper structures. The upper portion of the manubrium is freed from the insertion of the subhyoid muscles, and the sternum is next divided with a high-speed saw. In most instances, it is not necessary to divide the innominate vein. Planes are prepared between the esophagus and trachea on one side and the carotid sheath on the other. With the recurrent laryngeal nerve protected, the superficial and deep veins are retracted downward. The prevertebral space is then prepared.

After exposing the vertebral bodies down to T4, a vertebral body located in front of the spinal tumor is removed, as are the 2 adjacent discs, thus freeing the ventral dura.

After tumor removal, a watertight closure of the dura is done. A bone graft is used to fill the gap in the vertebral bodies and is fixed with a plate and screws to the adjacent bodies. The wound is closed over vacuum drains, and the sternum parts are reattached to each other with wires. Because sternal pseudarthrosis can occur, this part of the procedure needs to be completed with care. In addition, bone wax should not be used to control bleeding for the same reason. The skin is closed after restoration of soft tissue anatomy.

Conclusions.—Because of the relative stability of the upper thoracic spine, additional posterior stabilization or a halo brace are unnecessary after surgery. After 6 weeks, fusion between the graft and the adjacent vertebral bodies occurs, and mobilization can begin. The authors' experience with the trans-sternal approach in 3 patients has yielded satisfactory results. Each patient has had a relatively benign postoperative course with no long-term morbidity.

▶ Lesions located in the ventral aspect of the upper thoracic spinal canal are difficult to expose. Calliauw et al. report their experience with one method of exposure. The neurosurgeon who has to deal with such a lesion may also want to consult papers by Lesoin et al. (1), who described a trans-sternal biclavicular approach to the upper anterior thoracic spine, and Nazzaro et al. (2), who described a "trapdoor" exposure of the cervicothoracic junction.— R.H. Wilkins, M.D.

References

1. Lesoin F, Thomas CE III, Artricque A, et al: A transsternal biclavicular approach to the upper anterior thoracic spine. *Surg Neurol* 26:253–256, 1986.
2. Nazzaro JM, Arbit E, Burt M: Trap door exposure of the cervicothoracic junction: Technical note. *J Neurosurg* 80:338–341, 1994.

A Technical Report on Video-Assisted Thoracoscopy in Thoracic Spinal Surgery: Preliminary Description
Regan JJ, Mack MJ, Picetti GD III (Texas Back Inst Research Found, Plano; Humana Med City Dallas Hosp, Tex; Presbyterian Healthcare System, Plano, Texas)
Spine 20:831–837, 1995   122-96-36–2

Objective.—Video-assisted thorascopic surgery (VATS) was performed in 12 patients undergoing surgery on the thoracic spine that otherwise would have required open thoracotomy.

Patients.—One patient had an intervertebral disk abscess drained, and 1 had a vertebral body tumor. Five diskectomies were done for disk herniation. Four patients required an anterior transthoracic procedure as part of a staged operation to correct severe scoliosis or kyphosis. One patient underwent thoracoscopic osteotomy and discectomy for previously operated Scheuermann's kyphosis before posterior corrective osteotomy and instrumentation were done.

Methods.—Exploratory thoracoscopy was performed using a 10-mm rigid 30-degree angled scope. In most cases, the procedure required 3 to 4 trocars, or more if a multilevel diskectomy was necessary. It proved helpful to have 2 working portals at the level of the disk or vertebral body being approached.

Results.—All procedures were successfully completed, and there were no deaths. Two patients had atelectasis, 1 in conjunction with pleural effusion. Intercostal paresthesias consistently resolved, and there were no neurologic sequelae. Adequate diskectomy and cord decompression were achieved in the patients with a herniated thoracic disk. Spinal deformities were satisfactorily corrected. No patient has required reoperation.

Conclusion.—Procedure-specific instrumentation will make VATS even more effective and convenient.

▶ Video-assisted thoracoscopy is becoming increasingly useful in the treatment of disorders of the thoracic spine. It has the advantages of an anterolateral approach without the disadvantages of an open thoracotomy. It is likely that this technique will be developed further, to the benefit of patients with such disorders.—R.H. Wilkins, M.D.

Removal of a Protruded Thoracic Disc Using Microsurgical Endoscopy: A New Technique
Rosenthal D, Rosenthal R, de Simone A (Univ Hosp, Frankfurt am Main, Germany; Nordwest Hosp, Frankfurt am Main, Germany)
Spine 19:1087–1091, 1994   122-96-36–3

Purpose.—Thoracic disk herniation is an unusual and difficult-to-diagnose cause of spinal cord compression. A number of surgical techniques have been proposed, all of which use thoracotomy or wide bony resection

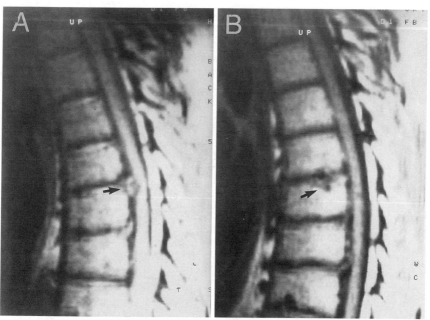

Fig 36–1.—**A,** preoperative MRI shows a herniated disk between T6 and T7 and spinal cord compression (*arrow*). **B,** postoperative MRI. The spinal cord is decompressed. The gap between T6 and T7 (*arrow*) shows where the intervertebral space was entered. The spinal cord is decompressed. (Courtesy of Rosenthal D, Rosenthal R, de Simone A: *Spine* 19:1087–1091, 1994.)

of vertebral structures to get to the ventral aspect of the spine. A microsurgical endoscopic technique was described that permits disk removal while avoiding the trauma of such approaches.

Technique.—As developed in fresh cadavers, the procedure uses a dextrolateral approach with 4 trocars inserted in triangular fashion along the middle axillary line and converging on the disk space. The parietal pleura is split, and the segmental arteries and sympathetic nerve are moved out of the way. Visualization of the spinal canal is improved by drilling off part of the posterior aspect of the vertebral body and the proximal portion of the costovertebral process. The disk and posterior longitudinal ligament are removed with the use of special forceps and rongeurs, which must be at least 33 cm long. Bone from the ribs, iliac crest, or fibula can be harvested if needed for fusion. The patient is put on chest tube drainage after surgery.

In another case, a herniated disk at T6–T7 was removed, and the spinal cord was decompressed (Figs 36–1 and 36–2). The patient was discharged 7 days after surgery and returned to work 4 weeks later.

Discussion.—This microsurgical endoscopic technique permits decompression of the spinal cord in patients with protruded thoracic disks with

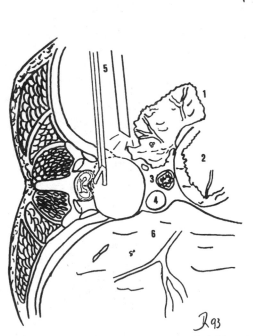

Fig 36–2.—Horizontal view at the T6 level. The patient is in the left lateral decubitus position. *1*, right lung (collapsed); *2*, heart and pericardium; *3*, esophagus; *4*, aorta; *5*, forceps and endoscope; *6*, left lung; *7*, surgeon. (Courtesy of Rosenthal D, Rosenthal R, de Simone A: *Spine* 19:1087–1091, 1994.)

a considerable reduction in surgical trauma. It may also hasten return to the patient's usual activities. The authors are exploring the application of their technique to other areas.

▶ In recent years, a number of surgical groups have reported the successful adaptation of endoscopic techniques to accomplish thoracic sympathectomy more quickly and with less surgical trauma in comparison with standard open sympathectomy techniques. This report documents a natural progression of this idea. Rosenthal et al. have developed additional techniques and instrumentation to permit the endoscopic removal of thoracic disk herniations. This probably represents the wave of the future in the surgical treatment of such lesions.—R.H. Wilkins, M.D.

In Vivo **Evaluation of Recombinant Human Osteogenic Protein (rhOP-1) Implants as a Bone Graft Substitute for Spinal Fusions**
Cook SD, Dalton JE, Tan EH, Whitecloud TS III, Rueger DC (Tulane School of Medicine, New Orleans, La; Creative BioMolecules, Inc, Hopkinton, Mass)
Spine 19:1655–1663, 1994   122-96-36–4

Objective.—A number of bone-inducing proteins have been investigated for use in place of autogenous bone. Recombinant human osteogenic protein-1 (rhOP-1) was evaluated as a bone graft substitute in a canine model of posterior spinal fusion.

Methods.—Experimental implants consisted of 800 mg of insoluble bovine bone collagen reconstituted with 2000 µg of rhOP-2. The carrier vehicle consists chiefly of type I bovine bone and does not induce cartilage or bone formation when implanted subcutaneously in rats. Implants of rhOP-1, carrier, or autogenous bone were placed for 6, 12, or 26 weeks over 1 motion segment on 1 side, after decorticating the bony surfaces of the fusion bed. New bone formation was monitored by plain radiography, CT scanning, and MRI.

Results.—The fusion segments given experimental implants achieved stable fusion within 6 weeks and were totally fused by 12 weeks. Autografted sites were fused at 26 weeks. When only the carrier was implanted, there was minimal new bone formation and no evidence of fusion. Mechanical testing showed both the experimental and autografted fusion sites to be significantly more stiff in torsion than in the other groups. The experimental fusion sites exhibited well-organized trabecular bone by 12 weeks. By 26 weeks, a cortical shell enclosed the site and a well-defined medullary cavity was present in the fusion mass.

Conclusion.—This highly purified recombinant human osteogenic protein preparation is an effective bone graft substitute with which to achieve stable posterior spinal fusion.

▶ This study represents a step in the development of agents that can enhance bone fusion and perhaps eventually can be used in place of autogenous bone to achieve spinal fusion. Such agents could also play an important role in bone replacement, for example, in cranioplasty.—R.H. Wilkins, M.D.

Interbody Lumbar Fusion Using a Carbon Fiber Cage Implant Versus Allograft Bone: An Investigational Study in the Spanish Goat
Brantigan JW, McAfee PC, Cunningham BW, Wang H, Orbegoso CM
(Creighton Univ, Omaha, Neb; Johns Hopkins Hosp, Baltimore, Md; Union Mem Hosp, Baltimore, Md)
Spine 19:1436–1444, 1994   122-96-36–5

Background.—A carbon fiber–reinforced polymer (CFRP) implant (Fig 36–3) was developed for use in posterior lumbar interbody fusion (PLIF). The cage implant provides a device designed to meet the mechanical requirements of PLIF and allows use of autologous cancellous bone for healing. The success rate of the CFRP implant using autologous bone was compared with that of standard PLIF using allografts in 27 healthy Spanish goats.

Methods.—The 27 goats were randomized to receive either the CFRP cage or a standard allografting procedure. Some animals from each group were killed and examined by autopsy, plain radiography, 3-dimensional reformatted CT and histology at 6, 12, and 24 months.

Results.—At 6 months, only 1 of the allograft specimens demonstrated fusion, whereas all 5 of the CFRP cage specimens demonstrated at least partial fusion. At 12 months, 2 of 3 allograft specimens were fused and all 3 of the cage specimens were fused. At 24 months, all of the specimens in both groups had achieved fusion.

Conclusions.—A novel CFRP cage implant was used to achieve successful PLIF in goats. Fusions done with the cage healed more quickly than those done with the standard allografting PLIF procedure. There were no

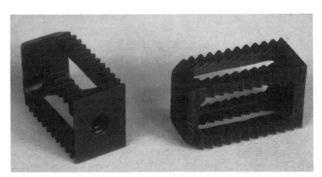

Fig 36–3.—Carbon fiber–reinforced polymer implant has struts to support weight bearing, ridges to resist retropulsion, and hollow areas to allow packing of autologous bone graft. Structure is radiolucent to allow visualization of healing with normal radiographic methods. (Courtesy of Brantigan JW, McAfee PC, Cunningham BW, et al: *Spine* 19:1436–1444, 1994.)

adverse effects of the cage implant material. A prospective controlled clinical trial is under way to determine the exact fusion and success rate of the implant in humans.

▶ These authors have developed a carbon fiber cage to facilitate PLIF. The cage is packed with cancellous bone before its insertion, in contrast to the usual freehand insertion of the bone grafts during PLIF. Whether such packing results in a better fusion in humans remains to be seen.—R.H. Wilkins, M.D.

Unintended "Incidental" Durotomy During Surgery of the Lumbar Spine: Medicolegal Implications
Goodkin R, Laska LL (Univ of Washington School of Medicine, Seattle; Veterans Administration Med Ctr, Seattle; Tennessee State Univ, Nashville)
Surg Neurol 43:4–14, 1995   122-96-36–6

Introduction.—In patients undergoing lumbar spine surgery, unintended "incidental" durotomy is a common occurrence. If recognized and primarily repaired, the occurrence should be benign. However, recent reviews have shown that unintended durotomies are frequently named in malpractice cases. The medicolegal implications of unintended durotomy were explored in a review of cases involving the lumbar spine.

Methods and Findings.—A national data set of medical malpractice cases was reviewed to identify 146 cases involving the lumbar spine from 1985 to 1992. Of these, 23 involved a dural tear; only cauda equina syndrome was more frequently named. Each case of dural tear was associated with an alleged complication or sequela, such as nerve root injury, cauda equina syndrome, pain, or CSF leak. The dural tear was recognized in 18 cases and primarily repaired in 9. Nine cases were decided in favor of the defense and 8 for the plaintiff, the rest being settled. Only 1 case involving a cauda equina syndrome was decided for the defense. Sixteen of the cases involved orthopedic surgeons, and 6 involved neurosurgeons.

Conclusions.—In some patients, unintended "incidental" durotomy appears to be associated with perioperative morbidity and long-term sequelae. Even if these incidents are recognized and repaired during surgery, there is no guarantee that the patient has not sustained a significant neurologic injury. Dural tears are frequently named in malpractice cases involving lumbar spine surgery and, therefore, cannot be considered entirely benign events. Information about this complication should be given to patients as part of the informed-consent process.

▶ Its new editor, Dr. James Ausman, has added new features to the journal *Surgical Neurology*. These include a section on medicolegal issues confronting the neurosurgeon. The first topic chosen for this section is one familiar to neurosurgeons throughout the world—unintended durotomy. (The word durotomy was chosen instead of the more descriptive and more widely used designation, dural tear, which implies carelessness.) Because of their negative connotations, surgical complications are not discussed in publications to the same extent as are the other aspects of neurosurgical practice. Articles such as the one by Goodkin and Laska can be instructive to both inexperienced and experienced neurosurgeons, if they will take the time to read them.—R.H. Wilkins, M.D.

37 Peripheral Nerve Disorders

Upper Extremity Peripheral Nerve Entrapments Among Wheelchair Athletes: Prevalence, Location, and Risk Factors
Burnham RS, Steadward RD (Univ of Alberta, Edmonton, Canada)
Arch Phys Med Rehabil 75:519–524, 1994   122-96-37–1

Background.—Soft tissue injuries of the arms and hands are some of the most common injuries of athletes with disabilities. Peripheral nerve entrapments make up a portion of these injuries. Some causes may be repetitive extrinsic hand pressure from using devices for mobility and frequent high intracarpal pressures from wrist extension posturing. There is a need to protect these nerves, but until the specific location of maximal nerve injury can be identified, placement of protective devices will be imprecise. The prevalence of peripheral nerve entrapments of the upper extremities of wheelchair athletes was determined using clinical and electrophysiologic criteria, and sites of nerve entrapment were localized. Also, demographic factors and training associated with electrodiagnostic evidence of nerve entrapment were identified.

Methods.—Clinical and electrodiagnostic assessments were performed on 52 upper extremities of 28 wheelchair athletes and 30 able-bodied control subjects. Short-segment stimulation techniques of the median nerve across the carpal tunnel and the ulnar nerve across the elbow were used.

Results.—Using clinical criteria, incidence of nerve entrapment was 23% among wheelchair athletes; this rate was 64% using electrodiagnostic methods. The most common dysfunction detected electrodiagnostically was of the median nerve at the carpal tunnel in 46% of subjects. The portion of the nerve within the proximal carpal tunnel was most often affected. The second most common entrapment detected electrodiagnostically was ulnar neuropathy at the wrist and forearm segments. The duration of the subject's disability was significantly correlated with electrophysiologic median nerve dysfunction.

Discussion.—The variation between clinical and electrodiagnostic findings presents a treatment dilemma. It would be tragic to let hand impairment continue in an individual who relies on the upper extremities to compensate for other disabilities. However, unnecessary surgery, postoperative immobilization, and possible complications would cause exceptional further disability. Strategies to minimize cumulative stress and pressure of the peripheral nerves of the upper extremities must be identified so that preventive and conservative methods of treatment can be found.

▶ The authors have added to the growing body of information on peripheral nerve entrapments in the upper extremities of wheelchair-bound athletes.— R.H. Wilkins, M.D.

Anatomical Variations of the Median Nerve in the Carpal Tunnel
Stančić MF, Eškinja N, Stošić A (Univ of Rijeka, Croatia)
Int Orthop 19:30–34, 1995   122-96-37–2

Background.—Anatomical variations in the median nerve may have an important impact on symptoms and must be considered during surgery. An anatomical study was performed to define the incidence of known variations of the median nerve and their possible clinical variations.

Methods.—The investigators looked for possible median nerve variations in 65 patients undergoing carpal tunnel release, in 10 patients with median nerve injuries, and in 25 cadaver dissections. The variations were grouped by the Lanz classification (Fig 37–1).

Findings.—Just 48 of the hands studied had the standard median nerve anatomy described in textbooks. The most common variations were thenar branch variations of subgroups 1A and 1B, referring to subligamentous and transligamentous branches, respectively. There were 17

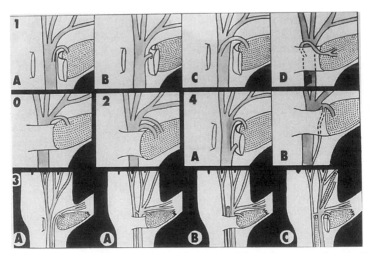

Fig 37–1.—The Lanz classification of anatomical variations of the median nerve at the wrist. **Group 1,** thenar branch variations: *1A,* subligamentous; *1B,* transligamentous; *1C,* ulnarwards; *1D,* supraligamentous. **Group 0,** extraligamentous thenar branch. **Group 2,** distal accessory thenar branch. **Group 4,** proximal accessory thenar branch: *4A,* direct in the thenar muscles; *4B,* joining another branch. **Group 3,** high division: *3A,* without an artery or muscle; *3B,* with artery; *3C,* with lumbrical muscle. (Courtesy of Stančić MF, Eškinja N, Stošić A: *Int Orthop* 19:30–34, 1995.)

hands in subgroup 1A, and 16 in subgroup 1B. Seven hands were classified as subgroup 1C or 1D, and another 7 as group 2. There was only 1 hand in subgroup 3B, and there were 4 in subgroup 4A.

Conclusions.—Anatomical variations of the median nerve may be present in about half of subjects. Knowing about these variations can help to avoid incomplete decompression in patients with carpal tunnel entrapment and injury to the thenar branch. In patients with median nerve injuries, the possibility of double thenar innervation should be borne in mind during both preoperative evaluation and follow-up.

▶ Median nerve decompression at the carpal tunnel is typically viewed as a simple procedure. However, the frequent anatomical variations of the median nerve are a trap for the unwary surgeon who inadvertently may do the following: injure the motor supply to certain thenar muscles; injure sensory components of the nerve with resulting sensory loss, neuroma formation, and pain; or fail to provide adequate nerve decompression.—R.H. Wilkins, M.D.

Endoscopic Carpal Tunnel Release: A Prospective Study of Complications and Surgical Experience
Agee JM, Peimer CA, Pyrek JD, Walsh WE (Hand Biomechanics Lab, Sacramento, Calif; State Univ of New York, Buffalo; Med Products Group, St Paul, Minn)
J Hand Surg (Am) 20A:165–171, 1995   122-96-37–3

Objective.—Complications of endoscopic carpal tunnel release were surveyed in 988 patients treated at 63 centers who underwent a total of 1,049 procedures. The participating surgeons varied widely in past experience with endoscopic release. Follow-up data were available on 883 operations.

Problems and Complications.—Problems were apparent at the time of surgery in 3.6% of cases, and 2.5% of procedures were converted to open surgery. Complications occurred in 1.8% of patients available for follow-up. Abnormal sensation was lasting and significant in 2 of 11 instances. In 0.9% of cases a second incision was added at the distal end of the ligament. The most common reason for converting to open release was aberrant anatomy. Blade entry was not visualized in 2.5% of cases, most of which were converted to either an open or an alternative endoscopic procedure. In 9% of cases it was difficult to insert the blade assembly into the carpal tunnel. An average of 2.2 passes was needed to totally divide the transverse carpal ligament. Blade height was considered too low in 2% of cases and too high in 0.6%, and more cuts were required in these cases. Mechanical malfunctions occurred in 0.9% of cases.

Conclusion.—A single-incision endoscopic technique of carpal tunnel release is feasible if done by surgeons trained in the procedure and if adequate visualization is assured.

▶ The authors review the complications in a large series of carpal tunnel releases performed with the Agee Carpal Tunnel Release System with an improved blade assembly (a revision of the system that was introduced in 1990). Considering the participating surgeons' wide variance with regard to past experience with endoscopic release, there were few complications. There were no confirmed injuries to vessels, and there were only 2 cases of persistent sensory loss. One patient experienced loss of sensibility in the distribution of the palmar cutaneous branch of the median nerve, which was known to have been injured during the initial incision before insertion of the endoscope. The second patient had sensory loss in a small area on the radial side of the ring finger; it was thought to have resulted from injury to the communicating fibers between the median and ulnar nerves.—R.H. Wilkins, M.D.

▶ Median nerve entrapment at the carpal tunnel is the most common entrapment neuropathy. Surgical release often produces gratifying results. The open procedure is relatively minor but, nevertheless, patients have restricted function of the hand for several weeks after the procedure, and even open release has a significant proportion of failures. Endoscopic ligament release is becoming more widespread in its availability. This study indicates that it can be effective in trained hands, and it can possibly have a lower frequency of failures and complications than open release.—W.G. Bradley, D.M., F.R.C.P.

Accessory Nerve Neurotization in Infants With Brachial Plexus Birth Palsy

Kawabata H, Kawai H, Masatomi T, Yasui N (Osaka Med Ctr, Japan; Hoshigaoka Koseinennkin Hosp, Osaka, Japan; Osaka Univ Med School, Japan)
Microsurgery 15:768–772, 1994   122-96-37–4

Background.—Although it is generally accepted that surgery is indicated for traumatic brachial plexus palsy in adults, its use in infants remains controversial. The surgical outcomes of 13 accessory nerve neurotizations in patients with brachial plexus birth palsy were analyzed.

Methods.—Seven boys and 6 girls with brachial plexus lesions treated with accessory nerve neurotization were followed up for an average of 5.8 years. Age at operation ranged from 3.8 to 8.7 months, with an average of 5.9 months. The accessory nerve was transferred to 3 C5 roots, 3 C6 roots, 4 posterior divisions of the middle trunk, 1 musculocutaneous nerve, and 2 suprascapular nerves.

Findings.—Sixty-seven percent of the patients acquired M4 or more in the deltoid muscle, 88% in the infraspinatus muscle, and 100% in the biceps brachii muscle. Twenty-five percent acquired M4 or more in the triceps brachii muscle and the wrist extensor muscles. Compared with previous reports of adult outcomes, these were much better. There was no functional compromise of the trapezius muscle.

Conclusions.—The results of accessory nerve neurotization in infants were satisfactory, with minimal functional compromise. Accessory nerve neurotization can safely be used in the neurosurgical reconstruction of brachial plexus palsy in infants, and it is an effective procedure.

▶ The authors report the favorable results of using the accessory nerve to reinnervate certain upper extremity muscles in infants with brachial plexus birth palsy. Patients were selected for the procedure if they demonstrated no recovery of the deltoid, biceps, triceps, or wrist extensor muscles by 3 months of age, or after 1 month of observation if the patient was older than 3 months at the first visit. The descending branch of the accessory nerve was followed as far as was practicable and was then cut for neurotization, leaving the upper portion of the accessory nerve intact. The donor and recipient nerves were coapted with 9-0 sutures, and, in some cases, fibrin glue was also used; in 1 patient interposition nerve grafting was necessary. In addition, some patients had intercostal nerve neurotizations and plex-oplexal nerve grafts. The operations were tedious, ranging from 5 hours to 13 hours and 20 minutes in length, but the results certainly justified the time and trouble. The authors demonstrated that the accessory nerve can be used as a donor nerve with minimal functional compromise, and reaffirmed that the results of nerve reconstruction are better in young children than in adults.—R.H. Wilkins, M.D.

MR Imaging of Benign Peripheral Nerve Sheath Tumors
Söderlund V, Göranson H, Bauer HCF (Karolinska Hosp, Stockholm)
Acta Radiol 35:282–286, 1994   122-96-37–5

Background.—Classifying benign neurogenic tumors is difficult in clinical practice. The MR signal pattern of benign peripheral nerve neoplasms and their stage were reported.

Methods.—Fifteen benign peripheral nerve neoplasms in 13 patients were included in the retrospective, nonblind review. One was subcutaneous; 9, intramuscular; 2, intermuscular; and 3, extracompartmental. The lesions were located on the trunk in 1 case, the upper extremity in 5, and the lower extremity in 9.

Findings.—The signal on T1-weighted spin-echo images was homogeneous and isointense when compared with adjacent muscle in 11 lesions. It was slightly hyperintense in 2 and slightly hypointense in 2. The T2-weighted spin-echo images demonstrated a hyperintense signal homogeneous in 8 and centrally inhomogeneous in 6. Postcontrast T1-weighted images of 11 lesions showed a strong signal and an inhomogeneous enhancement in the middle of the lesion, comparable to that seen in T2-weighted images. There were signal characteristics in 2 cases indicating bleeding in the tumor. In 1 lesion, both the unenhanced and contrast-enhanced T1-weighted images demonstrated a hypointense signal in the center of the tumor suggesting intramuscular myxoma. In all cases, the lesions were well delineated and had no reactive edema. The anatomical location of the tumor was assessed correctly in all cases (Fig 37–2).

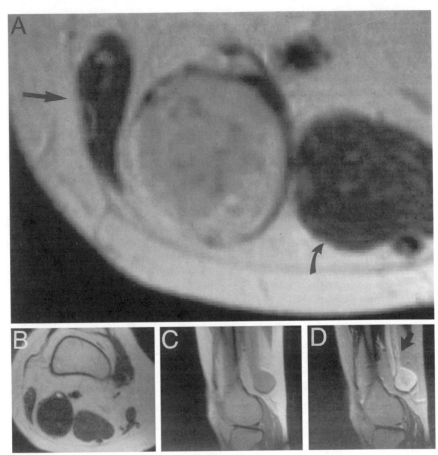

Fig 37–2.—**A**, postcontrast 4-mm image (TR/TE 440/17 ms) of an extracompartmental round neurinoma in the popliteal fossa (case 8) with a central low-intensity pattern. The neurinoma is located between the biceps femoris (*straight arrow*) and semimembranous (*curved arrow*) muscles. **B**, 5-mm axial image (TR/TE 300/17 ms). **C**, sagittal 5-mm image (TR/TE 2,000/25 ms), and **D**, 2,000/90 ms. An edematous sciatic nerve (*arrow*) is dorsal to the femoral vein. (Courtesy of Söderlund V, Göranson H, Bauer HCF: *Acta Radiol* 35:282–286, 1994.)

Conclusions.—Although MRI is not pathognomonic for neurinoma, it provides important data for preoperative assessment and for confirming clinical and cytologic evaluations. Neurinomas are usually small, have an inhomogeneous signal pattern, and do not contain necrosis.

▶ The MRI characteristics of intracranial and intraspinal tumors have been well described in many publications. In contrast, relatively little has been published about the sensitivity and specificity of MRI in detecting and differentiating peripheral nerve tumors. This study represents a step in that direction.—R.H. Wilkins, M.D.

Neural Sheath Tumors of Major Nerves

Donner TR, Voorhies RM, Kline DG (Louisiana State Univ, New Orleans)
J Neurosurg 81:362–373, 1994   122-96-37–6

Series.—In a recent 22-year period, 263 patients had surgery for 288 primary benign tumors involving major peripheral nerves. The series included 197 neurofibromas, 85 schwannomas, and 6 plexiform neurofibromas. The distribution of tumors is given in Table 1. In 15 cases, the tumor was first encountered at exploration. Complete excision was attempted in all cases. Follow-up of 229 patients averaged 15 months.

Results.—All but 2 of the 85 schwannomas were completely removed. Of the 76 patients available for follow-up, 87% had improved or stable motor function, and 85% of those with pain were improved (Table 2). One brachial plexus schwannoma recurred and was successfully reexcised. All neurofibromas in patients without von Recklinghausen's disease were totally removed using a fascicular approach. All but 10% of those who were followed up had stable or improved motor function, and pain had resolved at least partially in 88% of cases. Fifty-nine patients with von Recklinghausen's disease had 80 tumors removed, 74 fusiform lesions and 6 plexiform tumors. Of 48 patients evaluated after gross total removal of a fusiform tumor, 83% had at least stable motor function and 74% had less pain than before. Symptoms progressed, however, in all 6 patients with plexiform tumors. Several of these tumors recurred after having been incompletely removed.

Discussion.—The structure of the various forms of benign neural sheath tumor predicts how readily they can be excised (Fig 37–3). Excision of schwannomas has generally yielded good clinical results, but the best way of treating neurofibromas remains uncertain. Some consider them to be intrafascicular tumors and, as such, believe they require the division of one or more parent fascicles to achieve complete removal. Plexiform neurofibromas grow both within and outside of fascicles. Their total removal has proved very difficult.

TABLE 1.—Operative Site in 288 Benign Nerve Sheath Tumors

Operative Site	Schwannoma	NF	NF + VRD	Totals
supraclavicular brachial plexus	24 (8%)	37 (13%)	14 (5%)	75 (26%)
infraclavicular brachial plexus	13 (5%)	21 (7%)	12 (4%)	46 (16%)
median nerve	14 (5%)	13 (5%)	8 (3%)	35 (12%)
ulnar nerve	4 (1%)	16 (6%)	14 (5%)	34 (12%)
radial nerve	6 (2%)	5 (2%)	7 (2%)	18 (6%)
LS plexus	4 (1%)	7 (2%)	5 (2%)	16 (6%)
femoral complex	4 (1%)	7 (2%)	3 (1%)	14 (5%)
sciatic complex	16 (6%)	17 (6%)	17 (6%)	50 (17%)
totals	85 (30%)	123 (43%)	80 (27%)	288

Percentages are the total number of tumors.
Abbreviations: NF, neurofibroma; *VRD*, von Recklinghausen's disease; *LS*, lumbosacral.
(Courtesy of Donner TR, Voorhies RM, Kline DG: *J Neurosurg* 81:362–373, 1994.)

TABLE 2.—Status of Pain After Operation on Benign Nerve Sheath Tumors

Patients Presenting With Pain Symptoms

Tumor Type	No. of Cases	Resolved	Improved	Unchanged	Worse Pain	Patients With New Pain
schwannoma	20	15 (75%)	2 (10%)	1 (5%)	2 (10%)	4 (7%)
non-von Recklinghausen's neurofibroma	46	29 (63%)	11 (24%)	3 (7%)	3 (7%)	7 (13%)
von Recklinghausen's neurofibroma	23	10 (43%)	7 (30%)	4 (17%)	2 (9%)	4 (16%)

(Courtesy of Donner TR, Voorhies RM, Kline DG: *J Neurosurg* 81:362–373, 1994.)

▶ This is a benchmark paper that will be frequently cited in the future. The authors have compiled their data from a considerable series of primary benign tumors of the peripheral nerves, with emphasis placed on surgical treatment. They point out that neurofibromas, especially those in patients not having von Recklinghausen's disease, are frequently amenable to complete excision without complete division of the parent nerve. In general, neurosurgeons know that schwannomas can be excised from peripheral

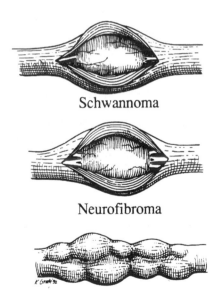

Schwannoma

Neurofibroma

Plexiform Neurofibroma

Fig 37–3.—Drawings depicting problems of removing neural sheath tumors. **Upper,** on gross dissection, the usual schwannoma requires division of one relatively small entering and exiting fascicle for removal. **Center,** removal of a neurofibroma usually requires sacrifice of more neural tissue, but these fascicles are often nonfunctional. Some of the fascicular tissue appears to enter and exit each pole of the tumor (as in this drawing), but actually enters and exits the tumor's capsule and can be dissected away and spared section. When these capsular fascicles are excluded, either 1 larger or, sometimes, 2 smaller nonfunctional fascicles must still be sectioned at both tumor poles for removal of the mass. **Lower,** plexiform tumors involve multiple fascicles within a nerve in a longitudinal, interweaving fashion. (Courtesy of Donner TR, Voorhies RM, Kline DG: *J Neurosurg* 81:362–373, 1994.)

nerves, leaving almost all of the nerve fascicles intact. However, few are aware that this is also true for many neurofibromas. This report should lead to a more aggressive approach to peripheral nerve tumors, with a more concerted effort made to excise such lesions while leaving most of the parent nerve intact.—R.H. Wilkins, M.D.

38 Cranial Nerve Disorders

Microvascular Decompression for Hemifacial Spasm
Barker FG II, Jannetta PJ, Bissonette DJ, Shields PT, Larkins MV, Jho HD
(Univ of Pittsburgh, Pa)
J Neurosurg 82:201–210, 1995   122-96-38–1

Objective.—Long-term outcome was reported for 703 patients who had undergone microvascular decompression procedures for hemifacial spasm, an uncommon disorder characterized by painless, involuntary paroxysmal movements of 1 side of the face.

Patients and Methods.—The patients were treated at the study institution between January 1, 1972 and March 1, 1992. Overall, 782 operations were done on 703 patients, 648 of whom had not had previous intracranial procedures for the hemifacial spasm. The group of 648 patients had a mean age of 52 years and a mean preoperative duration of symptoms of 7 years; 65% of the patients were women. Eight had bilateral symptoms, but only 3 required bilateral procedures. Patients were assessed for outcome at the time of hospitalization and annually thereafter by questionnaires. The results were classified as excellent, providing partial relief (75% reduction in spasm), or failure. The 57 patients who had had previous microvascular decompression elsewhere were analyzed separately.

Results.—Among patients previously untreated by microvascular decompression, 84% had excellent results at 10 years, 7% had partial relief, and 9% had treatment failure (Fig 38–1). Most of the failures occurred within 2 years of surgery. Repeat surgery for recurrent symptoms, done in 9% of patients, was less successful than the initial microvascular decompression procedure unless the second was done within 30 days of the first (Fig 38–2). Onset of the spasm had been typical in 92% of patients, with twitching starting in the upper face; 8% had an atypical hemifacial spasm, with initial twitching in the buccal muscles. Patients with typical onset had better results than those with atypical onset of symptoms, and men fared better than women after surgery. Postoperative results were not influenced by patient age, side and preoperative duration of symptoms, history of Bell's palsy, or implant material used. Complications included 1 death

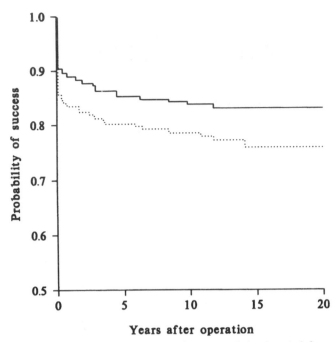

Fig 38–1.—Surgical success for all patients (men and women, typical and atypical, first surgery only). The *dotted line* represents chances of excellent relief of hemifacial spasm after first microvascular decompression; the *solid line* represents chances of a good or excellent result. (Courtesy of Barker FG II, Jannetta PJ, Bissonette DJ, et al: *J Neurosurg* 82:201–210, 1995.)

during surgery, 2 brain stem infarctions, 17 cases of total or severe permanent loss of hearing in the ipsilateral ear, and 6 instances of facial weakness. Complications were more common after repeat surgery.

Conclusion.—Microvascular decompression had a high rate of long-term success in this large series of patients with hemifacial spasm. The procedure was associated with low rates of late recurrence and death or disability, and its advantages over botulinum injections and other surgical techniques are clear.

▶ Dr. Jannetta's group has had the largest experience in the United States with the treatment of hemifacial spasm by microvascular decompression. Approximately 85% of patients achieve long-term excellent relief, and about 10% either are not relieved or they sustain a recurrence. A second microvascular decompression procedure in these patients has a significantly reduced chance of success and a significantly increased chance of injury to the lower cranial nerves. The threat of ipsilateral deafness during an initial microvascular decompression has been virtually eliminated by intraoperative monitoring of brain stem auditory evoked potentials, but it remains despite such monitoring during repeat operations.—R.H. Wilkins, M.D.

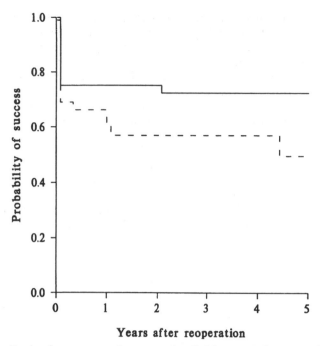

Years after reoperation

Fig 38–2.—Results of repeat surgery for recurrent hemifacial spasm. Only patients whose first microvascular decompression for hemifacial spasm was done at Presbyterian Hospital and whose second surgery occurred more than 30 days after their first are included. Results reflect all subsequent surgeries. The *disabled line* represents the chance of excellent result; the *solid line* represents the chance of good or excellent result. (Courtesy of Barker FG II, Jannetta PJ, Bissonette DJ, et al: *J Neurosurg* 82:201–210, 1995.)

Indication, Technique and Results of Facial Nerve Reconstruction
Samii M, Matthies C (Nordstadt Hosp, Hannover, West Germany)
Acta Neurochir (Wien) 130:125–139, 1994   122-96-38-2

Introduction.—Throughout this century, techniques have been refined for intracranial and extracranial reconstruction of the facial nerve and for facial nerve reanimation with a donor nerve. The indications for these 2 methods of nerve repair, the techniques, and outcomes were studied in 160 patients with facial nerve paralysis.

Methods.—During a 15-year period, 160 patients were treated with facial nerve reconstruction and were evaluated every 3–6 months for at least 2 years after surgery. The patients were divided into 6 groups based on the type of nerve reconstruction performed.

Results.—Overall, 91% of the patients achieved reliable reinnervation; 69% had good symmetry at rest, completed eye closure, and reasonable mouth innervation; and 17% achieved excellent results with movement symmetry and minimal synkinesia. Facial nerve discontinuity at the cerebellopontine angle (CPA) was caused by a large acoustic neuroma in 16 of 17 patients and was reconstructed with a sural graft. Four patients had excellent results, 8 had good symmetry at rest, and 5 had incomplete eye closure. Intracranial-intratemporal graft techniques were performed in 17 patients with discontinuity between the CPA and the mastoid segment after removal of an acoustic neuroma or facial nerve neuroma, or after a petrous bone fracture. Four patients had excellent results, 9 had symmetry at rest, and 3 had incomplete eye and mouth closure. Dott's procedure was performed in 10 patients to repair resections extending from the CPA to the mastoid caused by acoustic neuromas, meningioma, facial neurinoma, cholesteatomas, or glomus tumor. One had excellent results, 6 had good results, and 2 had fair results. Eleven intratemporal-extracranial and 6 extracranial grafts were used in the reconstruction of facial nerve discontinuity in the petrous bone or in the face caused by trauma, or by resection of hemangiomas, facial neuromas, parotid tumors, or carcinomas. Four had excellent, 6 had good, 3 had fair, and 4 had poor results. An inadequate proximal facial nerve stump in the CPA in 74 patients was caused by resections of large acoustic neuromas, meningiomas, cholesteatomas, or cavernomas, or by trauma, and was treated with reanimation procedures. There were excellent results in 12 patients, good results in 43, fair results in 17, and poor results in 2. Faciofacial anastomoses were used for 25 patients after acoustic neuroma resection or trauma and achieved excellent or good results in 52%.

Discussion.—Facial nerve lesions should be reconstructed as soon as possible. Either nerve transplantation with any established technique or reanimation with a donor nerve is effective, satisfactorily improving both cosmetic and functional results.

▶ Dr. Samii speaks with authority about facial nerve reconstruction because of his early interest and extensive work in nerve surgery and his later, even more extensive experience in surgery of the skull base and posterior cranial fossa. These results are as good as can be achieved at the present time.— R.H. Wilkins, M.D.

39 Autonomic Dysfunction

Essential Hypertension and Neurovascular Compression at the Ventro-lateral Medulla Oblongata: MR Evaluation
Akimura T, Furutani Y, Jimi Y, Saito K, Kashiwagi S, Kato S, Ito H (Konan Sentohiru Hosp, Japan; Yamaguchi Univ, Japan)
AJNR 16:401–405, 1995
122-96-39–1

Background.—Hyperactive cranial nerve dysfunction syndromes are currently treated by microvascular decompression with good results. Of the preoperative neuroradiologic examinations, MRI is one of the most important for preoperative evaluation of hyperactive cranial nerve syndromes, although surgical indications are largely determined by clinical symptoms, because examinations cannot always show the offending vessels. Since 1978, there have been various reports suggesting that neurovascular compression at the left ventrolateral medulla is a cause of essential hypertension. Neurovascular compression at the ventrolateral medulla oblongata in patients with essential hypertension was investigated using MRI.

Methods.—Thirty-two patients with essential hypertension, 6 patients with secondary hypertension, and 18 control subjects were studied (Table 1). Transaxial three-dimensional fast low-angle shot images were taken. The center of a 40-mm-thick slab was positioned at the pontomedullary

TABLE 1.—Hypertension Characteristics in 56 Cases

Characteristic	Essential Hypertension	Secondary Hypertension	Control Group
No. of cases	32	6	18
Sex, M/F	13/19	3/3	11/7
Age range, y	42–69	36–65	33–69
Average age, y	57.6 ± 7	56.6 ± 10.3	50.5 ± 11
Systolic blood pressure, mm Hg	172.9 ± 10.3	181.7 ± 11.7	128.2 ± 11
Diastolic blood pressure, mm Hg	96.8 ± 10.5	106.3 ± 8.5	70.3 ± 11
Duration of hypertension, mo	35.8 ± 31.2	92 ± 31	

Average values are expressed as mean ± SD.
(Courtesy of Akimura T, Furutani Y, Jimi Y, et al: *AJNR* 16:401–405, 1995.)

437

TABLE 2.—Findings of Neurovascular Compression in 56 MR Studies

Factor	Essential Hypertension	Secondary Hypertension	Control Group
No. of cases	32	6	18
Right side	4	0	1
Left side	22	1	2
Bilateral	3	0	1
Total	29	1	4

(Courtesy of Akimura T, Furutani Y, Jimi Y, et al: *AJNR* 16:401–405, 1995.)

junction. Relationships between upper ventrolateral medulla and vertebral arteries and branches identified by flow-related hyperintensities were evaluated in each group.

Results.—Of 32 patients with essential hypertension, 29 showed neurovascular compression. Of these 29 patients, 22 showed compression on the left side, 4 showed compression on the right side, and 3 on both sides (Table 2). In 16 patients, the medulla was apparently deformed by an artery (Fig 39–1). Of the 18 control individuals, 4 showed neurovascular compression. Of 6 patients with secondary hypertension, 1 showed neurovascular compression. Rates of neurovascular compression observed between control individuals and patients with essential hypertension were statistically significant.

Conclusions.—A close association between essential hypertension and neurovascular compression at the ventrolateral medulla oblongata on the left side was found. Magnetic resonance imaging with a 3-dimensional fast low-angle shot sequence offers acceptable spatial resolution and depicts blood vessels simultaneously by flow-related phenomena.

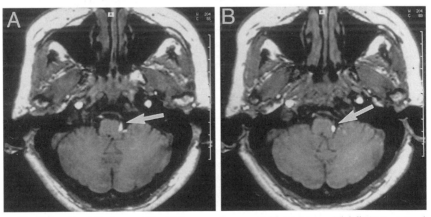

Fig 39–1.—A and B, woman, 60, with long-standing essential hypertension. Medulla is compressed and deformed by the left vertebral artery (*arrow*) at the left retro-olivery sulcus. (Courtesy of Akimura T, Furutani Y, Jimi Y, et al: *AJNR* 16:401–405, 1995.)

▶ Akimura and associates have added MRI evidence to a growing body of radiologic, intraoperative, and postmortem data that link left-sided compression of the medulla oblongata just anterior to the attachments of the ninth and tenth cranial nerves, with essential hypertension.—R.H. Wilkins, M.D.

Gustatory Facial Sweating Subsequent to Upper Thoracic Sympathectomy

Nesathurai S, Harvey DT, Schatz SW (McMaster Univ, Hamilton, Ont, Canada; Hamilton Civic Hosps, Ont, Canada)
Arch Phys Med Rehabil 76:104–107, 1995   122-96-39-2

Background.—Three patients who had reflex sympathetic dystrophy after trauma to the arm later experienced unilateral gustatory facial sweating after endoscopic thoracic ganglionectomy.

Clinical Features.—After injury to the arm, the patients experienced dysesthetic pain, vasomotor instability, swelling, and hyperhidrosis of the ipsilateral arm. Stellate ganglion blocks or guanethidine blocks were unsuccessful. An endoscopic laser ablation of the T2 and T3 ganglia was performed. Between 1 and 4 weeks after surgery, the patients experienced gustatory facial sweating. In addition to a sensory deficit consistent with the T2 dermatome ipsilateral to the ganglionectomy, 2 patients also experienced ipsilateral sensory deficit in the region of the anterior chest wall that included the nipple. Two patients experienced nipple hypersensitivity in cold environment. None of the patients had Horner's syndrome. All 3 patients were treated with amitriptyline for the chronic pain; the intensity or frequency of gustatory facial sweating did not change with amitriptyline administration.

Discussion.—Gustatory facial sweating can occur after upper thoracic sympathectomy. Other possible consequences of upper thoracic ganglionectomy include compensatory hyperhidrosis, sensory deficits, nipple hypersensitivity, and Horner's syndrome. In these patients, gustatory facial sweating may be caused by ephaptic communication from the intact sympathetic salivatory fibers to sudomotor fibers in the uppermost thoracic ganglia. This ephaptic communication may result from inadvertent collateral thermal injury during the laser sympathectomy. Consequently, gustatory stimuli would trigger facial sweating instead of salivation. The sensory deficits in the chest wall may be the consequence of collateral thermal injury to the intercostal nerves during laser ablation of the sympathetic trunk.

▶ This report calls attention to the complications that can occur with either open or endoscopic upper thoracic ganglionectomy. Among these complications, appropriate sensory alterations, Horner's syndrome, and compensatory hyperhidrosis are easy to explain anatomically and physiologically. To explain gustatory facial sweating takes more imagination.

Gustatory facial sweating actually is not uncommon after upper thoracic sympathectomy. Nesathurai and co-workers cite the reports of others. In one of these reports, gustatory facial sweating was experienced by 24 of 50 patients who had their T2, T3, and T4 sympathetic ganglia ablated with cautery by an endoscopic technique. In another, 55 of 100 patients who had bilateral T2 and T3 ganglionectomies by the supraclavicular approach had gustatory phenomena postoperatively.

In addition to their parasympathetic innervation, the salivary glands are also supplied by sympathetic fibers from the T1 and T2 ganglia. As a consequence of T2 and T3 ganglionectomy, the salivary glands may become partially denervated.

Nesathurai et al. list 5 possible mechanisms to explain gustatory facial sweating after upper thoracic sympathectomy: (1) denervation hypersensitivity to acetylcholine; (2) regrowth of preganglionic sympathetic fibers from intact upper thoracic ganglia to the superior cervical ganglion, there to synapse anomalously with sudomotor fibers that supply the face; (3) collateral sprouting of intact sympathetic fibers from the stellate ganglion to the superior cervical ganglion, there to synapse with sudomotor fibers; (4) sprouting of parasympathetic fibers that travel with the glossopharyngeal and vagus nerves to the superior cervical ganglion, there to synapse with sudomotor fibers; and (5) ephaptic communication from intact sympathetic salivatory fibers to sudomotor fibers in the upper thoracic ganglia. For reasons outlined in their discussion, Nesathurai et al. favor the last explanation to account for the gustatory facial sweating that occurred in their patients (4 instances from 61 endoscopic laser sympathectomies).—R.H. Wilkins, M.D.

Spinal Cord Stimulation for the Treatment of Progressive Systemic Sclerosis and Raynaud's Syndrome
Francaviglia N, Silvestro C, Maiello M, Bragazzi R, Bernucci C (Univ of Genoa, Italy)
Br J Neurosurg 8:567–571, 1994   122-96-39–3

Background.—Progressive systemic scleroderma (PSS) is a generalized disease that affects both the skin and other internal organs. Progressive sclerosis and loss of function or dexterity in the hands are characteristic cutaneous signs. Fifteen patients with PSS underwent spinal cord stimulation between 1987 and 1992 to determine whether this technique could improve quality of life with as few side effects as possible. Follow-up results are examined.

Patients and Findings.—Thirteen women and 2 men (average age, 55 years) were evaluated. Patients were grouped according to the Barnett type I–III classification system. Eight patients had involvement of fingers and hands to the wrist (grade I), 6 had proximal ascending sclerosis including the forearm (grade II), and 1 had the beginning of sclerosis at the trunk (grade III). Raynaud's phenomenon had also been seen in all patients for at least 10 years. Follow-up ranged from 1 to 6 years. All patients had a noticeable clinical improvement after undergoing spinal cord stimulation.

A marked reduction in the frequency of Raynaud's episodes was noted in 14 of 15 patients. Thirteen of 15 also had a reduction in edema and improved hand motility. Ulceration improvement was observed in all 4 patients, and arthralgic pain reduction was noted in 10 of 12. No major surgical complications occurred, and CSF leakage or superficial or deep wound infection was not observed. One patient required removal and replacement of the electrode because of improper initial placement. All patients have reported satisfaction with their treatment.

Conclusions.—Spinal cord stimulation is a simple and effective treatment for patients with PSS and Raynaud's phenomenon. The procedure does not involve serious trauma, can be tested and discontinued at any time, is tolerable, and is virtually complication-free. This technique may play an important role in the treatment of this chronic disorder.

▶ The authors report the beneficial effects of chronic spinal cord stimulation in treating the symptoms and signs of PSS, including Raynaud's phenomenon.—R.H. Wilkins, M.D.

The First 500 Patients With Sacral Anterior Root Stimulator Implants: General Description
Brindley GS (Royal Natl Orthopaedic Hosp, Stanmore, England)
Paraplegia 32:795–805, 1994   122-96-39–4

Introduction.—Between 1976 and 1992, sacral anterior root stimulators for bladder control were implanted in 500 patients. Total follow-up time was 2,033.5 years. Excluding periods of nonuse, the total time of use was 1,897.1 years.

Methods.—Posterior rhizotomy (within the range S2–5) was complete near root exits in 251 patients. In 477 patients, the electrodes were implanted intrathecally at the level of the fifth lumbar vertebra and last intervertebral disk. In 12 patients whose primary deafferentation was at the conus, and in 11 other patients, the electrodes were implanted extradurally in the sacrum.

Results.—Of the 479 survivors, 424 were using their stimulators between 3 months and 16.1 years (mean, 4 years) after implantation. In 45 patients, the implants were intact but not used, mainly because of inadequate implant-driven micturition. Other reasons for nonuse included pain when using the stimulator and autonomic dysreflexia. For bladder management, 15 of those patients employed intermittent self-catheterization. The total number of stimulators lost by infection was 5 (1%). Upper urinary tract function deteriorated in 12 patients, including 10 who had incomplete deafferentation or none. One patient died of renal failure, another had grade 1 ureteral reflux, and 10 had radiologic signs of upper tract deterioration (9 were in good health except for 1 with kidney stones). Ninety-five operations were performed to remedy faults in implants, including 75 for replacing blocks or rejoining broken cables and 20 for implantation of new extradural stimulators. Among 143 patients with known nondeafferentation or incomplete deafferentation, 25 subsequently underwent a secondary deafferentation at the conus medullaris. Seven of the 251 patients in whom complete deafferentation was attempted underwent a secondary deafferentation.

Summary.—Sacral anterior root stimulators provide bladder control in the majority of patients with spinal cord injury. It is usual to cut the posterior roots at the time of implantation of the electrodes, and the results of the implantation of a stimulator are much less successful without than with posterior rhizotomy. Detrusor areflexia after S2–5 posterior rhizotomy is permanent if it is achieved at all. The use of extradural electrodes is justified only in the presence of severe arachnoiditis.

▶ The sacral anterior root stimulator was developed in London between 1969 and 1977. The first human sacral anterior root stimulator was implanted in 1976, but it gave no useful micturition. This study reviewed the first 500 patients with implants of the London design. These procedures have been performed at 23 major centers and 28 minor centers around the world. Since 1981, the sacral posterior roots have usually been cut at the time of implantation of electrodes on the anterior roots, to improve continence. This detailed report documents the value of the technique in achieving bladder control in patients with major loss of spinal cord function.—R.H. Wilkins, M.D.

40 Functional Neurosurgery

Contemporaneous Bilateral Postero-Ventral Pallidotomy for Early Onset "Juvenile Type" Parkinson's Disease: Case Report
Iacono RP, Lonser RR, Yamada S (Loma Linda Univ Med Ctr, Loma Linda, Calif)
Acta Neurochir (Wien) 131:247–252, 1994   122-96--40-1

Introduction.—The occurrence of severe disabling dyskinesias of the extremities is common in patients with Narabayashi's "juvenile-type" early-onset Parkinson's disease (PD) (onset of symptoms at 45 years or younger) after 2–5 years of treatment with levodopa. The recent development of posteroventral pallidotomy (PVP) has proven more effective than thalamotomy in eliminating dyskinesias and akinetic symptoms, which are inaccessible to thalamotomy.

Case Report.—Man, 46, with juvenile-type PD and severe levedopa-induced dyskinesias had a 14-year history of Parkinson's symptomatology. The patient had good control of tremor and rigidity while taking Sinemet. In the 4th year of treatment, he experienced mild dyskinesias, precipitated by Sinemet. Akinetic symptoms worsened when "off" over the next 2 years, and the patient was not able to work. An adrenal graft implantation was done. The little relief it afforded subsided within 4 years. Before PVP, the patient experienced difficulty speaking, excessive salivation, nighttime drooling, and masklike facies. While "on," 25% to 50% of the day, he experienced violent choreoathetotic and ballistic movements that caused soft-tissue trauma to the tissues. His Unified Parkinson's Disease Rating Scale (UPDRS) score was −46 when "on" and −51 when "off."

Results.—His UPDRS score was reduced to zero after bilateral PVP. At 3 months postoperatively, his "off" states were almost eliminated while he was maintained with his previous medication regimen. The Beck Inventory for depression was reduced to zero. The patient resumed working full time.

Conclusion.—The PVP disinhibits the locomotor pedunculo-pontine nucleus, while achieving a thalamotomy effect via interruption of ansa lenticularis efferents to the ventral lateral thalamus (Fig 40–1). Unlike other surgical approaches, PVP is ideally suited for Narabayashi's "juvenile-type" PD (table).

443

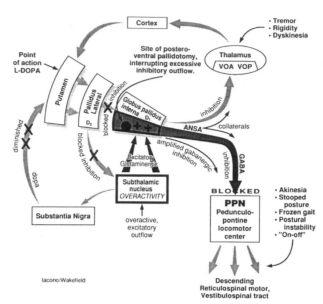

Fig 40–1.—Posteroventral pallidotomy may achieve its effects by interrupting the globus palldus interna. This results in decreased inhibition of the thalamus and pedunculopontine nucleus, explaining the apparent paradoxical improvement of both akinetic and dyskinetic symptoms. (Courtesy of Iacono RP, Lonser RR, Yamada S: *Acta Neurochir (Wien)* 131:247–252, 1994.)

▶ There has been a recent resurgence of interest in pallidotomy for the treatment of certain symptoms and signs of PD. The case reported in this study raises the possibility that posteroventral pallidotomy, with the target within the globus pallidus interna and subjacent ansa lenticularis, may be especially suitable for the treatment of the symptoms and signs of early-onset PD.—R.H. Wilkins, M.D.

Surgery in Parkinson's Disease				
	*PV-pallidotomy	Fetal graft	†A-D pallidotomy	Thalamotomy
Tremor	++	+	±	+++
Rigidity	+++	+	+++	+++
Gait freezing	+++	++	−	−
Bradykinesia	+++	++	−	−
Postural instability	+++	++	−	−
Dyskinesia	+++	+	+++	+++

* Posteroventral pallidotomy.
† Classical anterodorsal pallidotomy.
Scale: +++ excellent (complete resolution of symptoms), ++ good (exceeds response to medication), + noticeable, ± occasional minor effects, − no effect.
(Courtesy of Iacono RP, Lonser RR, Yamada S: *Acta Neurochir (Wien)* 131:247–252, 1994.)

Stereotactic Pallidotomy Results for Parkinson's Exceed Those of Fetal Graft

Iacono RP, Lonser RR, Mandybur G, Morenski JD, Yamada S, Shima F (Loma Linda Univ, Calif; Kyushu Univ, Fukuoka, Japan)
Am Surg 60:777–782, 1994   122-96-40–2

Background.—Akinetic symptoms of Parkinson's disease had previously been thought to be resistant to therapeutic surgical lesions. The use of fetal grafts and Leksell's posteroventral pallidotomy seem to show significant therapeutic effects in akinesia that was previously resistant to medication. The success of the surgical approach may even exceed that of fetal grafts, medication, or stereotactic therapy.

Patients.—A retrospective evaluation included 55 patients with Parkinson's disease who underwent pallidotomy and 5 who had fetal tissue transplantation to the caudate and putamen. All patients ranged in age from 31–73 years and had a 2- to 24-year history and Hoehn and Yahr grades of 4–5 during their period of worst akinetic symptoms. Follow-up was 24–36 months after surgery. Assessment by videotape and by the Unified Parkinson's Disease Rating Scale was done before surgery and during follow-up.

Results.—The patients who underwent pallidotomy had no visual field defects, worsened bradykinesia, or symptoms of hyperkinesia. The results were immediate and did not wane over time. The only item from the Rating Scale that was not significantly improved was memory. Patients who had the fetal graft improved during the first 6 months and reached a plateau at 18 months. Only bradykinesia and postural stability from the Rating Scale improved.

Conclusion.—The reported results of fetal graft transplants were exceeded by the immediate results of pallidotomy. There were infrequent complications of speech disturbances and hemiparesis. The relief of Parkinson's disease symptoms by pallidotomy surpasses that of conventional methods and should renew interest in the use of surgical treatment for Parkinson's disease.

▶ In recent years there has been renewed interest in the surgical treatment of Parkinson's disease. Grafting, including fetal grafting, has not yet become a widely used, practical approach. However, Laitinen's revival of Leksell's posteroventral pallidotomy (1, 2) has led to increasing use of this beneficial procedure.—R.H. Wilkins, M.D.

References

1. Laitinen LV, Hariz MI: *Movement Disorders* 5:82, 1990.
2. Laitinen LV, et al: *J Neurosurg* 76:53, 1992.

▶ The most recent studies analyzing the complex interplay between the various nuclei of the basal ganglia and subthalamic area that underlies Parkinson's disease suggest that many of the features are caused by imbalance of specific circuits and neurotransmitters. The history of neurosurgical procedures attempting to correct this imbalance goes all the way back to the initial attempts to produce a partial hemiparesis with lesions in the internal capsule. Following that, the observation was made that tremor was benefitted by contralateral thalamotomy. With the appearance of medical treatment, however, the number of such procedures decreased dramatically. As experience has proved that dopamine agonists are, unfortunately, palliative in many patients and have a limited duration of effect, attention has turned back to fetal tissue transplantation to the caudate and putamen, and to the possibility that lesions in the pallidum may correct the hypothesized imbalance between different neuronal circuits.

This study is very encouraging and is one of several recent reports that have led to a dramatic upswing in the demand for surgeons able to undertake this procedure. A number of points of caution need to be raised: the placement of lesions stereotactically still is not 100% ideal, and intraoperative electrophysiologic recording should be a part of every procedure; the long-term effect of such a "rebalancing" procedure remains to be determined. It is possible that the loss of the pallidal pathway may eventually lead to a movement disorder of its own. Hence, it is important that research continue regarding this procedure, and that the number of such treatments be limited until greater experience has been gained (see also the comment that follows Abstract 122-96-40–3).—W.G. Bradley, D.M., F.R.C.P.

Bilateral Chronic Electrostimulation of Ventroposterolateral Pallidum: A New Therapeutic Approach for Alleviating All Parkinsonian Symptoms
Siegfried J, Lippitz B (Klinik im Park, Zürich, Switzerland)
Neurosurgery 35:1126–1130, 1994   122-96-40–3

Background.—Bilateral chronic electrostimulation of the ventroposterolateral pallidum is a new therapeutic approach used to alleviate the symptoms associated with Parkinson's disease. Three patients have undergone this procedure, all of whom had severe Parkinson's disease, with akinesia and levodopa-induced dyskinesia in the foreground. The technique and outcome in a 67-year-old patient with advanced Parkinson's disease who underwent implantation of 2 electrodes (1 on each side) in the posteroventrolateral part of the pallidum were described.

Technique.—The target coordinates were 3 mm in front of the midcommissural point, 6 mm below the intercommissural line (the most ventral position of the electrode tip), and 18–22 mm lateral to the midline of the third ventricle. A monopolar electrode was introduced via a 2.5-mm diameter frontal burr hole and was checked radiographically. Electric stimulation was then applied using different parameters for testing unwanted side effects. However, the exact location of the electrode remains speculative. A watertight titanium screw was used to secure the electrode, which was then connected to a transient extension after subcutaneous tunneling. The procedure was performed bilaterally with 2 external devices. Stimulation tests were performed for several days to determine optimal stimulation parameters. Two programmable pulse generators were then implanted subcutaneously beneath the clavicles. These were connected to the intracerebral electrodes. Neuropacemakers were programmed to generate the pulse trains with the predetermined parameters.

Results.—Chronic bilateral pallidal stimulation led to an immediate postoperative improvement in this patient. Bradykinesia and gait and speech disorders were ameliorated, and the severe levodopa-induced dyskinesias were almost completely eliminated. The Webster rating scale score dropped to 8.5, and levodopa was decreased to 750 mg. At 12 months postoperatively, the patient's condition was virtually unchanged with 750 mg of benserazide. The excellent results obtained in this patient led to the same procedure being performed on 2 additional patients, both of whom demonstrated immediate global improvement after surgery.

Conclusions.—This approach is nondestructive and reversible, and it helps to avoid unwanted side effects. Further investigations using a larger patient series are warranted in light of these promising results.

▶ Dr. Siegfried has had extensive experience in the area of stereotactic and functional neurosurgery. He and his colleague report a new approach to the treatment of Parkinson's disease. Time will tell whether this approach provides results that are better than those of posteroventral pallidotomy or the other surgical procedures used to treat Parkinson's disease.—R.H. Wilkins, M.D.

▶ As indicated in the comment that follows Abstract 122-96-40–2, the clinical manifestations of Parkinson's disease may be the result of an imbalance of the complex interactive circuits of the basal ganglia and subthalamic regions. A lesion in the posteroventral pallidum appears capable of reducing the parkinsonian manifestations. The report by Siegfried and Lipitz suggests that stimulation of what they believe to be the ventral posterolateral pallidum internum is capable of producing a similar improvement. The effect in these 3 patients appears to be stimulus-related and, hence, is not caused by the production of a lesion. These are complex studies that require further research; however, the findings are intriguing.—W.G. Bradley, D.M., F.R.C.P.

Electrophrenic Respiration After Intercostal to Phrenic Nerve Anastomosis in a Patient With Anterior Spinal Artery Syndrome: Technical Case Report
Krieger AJ, Gropper MR, Adler RJ (Univ of Medicine and Dentistry, New Jersey; New Jersey Med School, Newark)
Neurosurgery 35:760–764, 1994   122-96-40–4

Background.—Electrophrenic respiration, a method of pacing the phrenic nerve to effect contraction of the paralyzed diaphragm, is an established alternative to positive pressure mechanical ventilation in patients with respiratory insufficiency caused by high cervical spine injury. Because it requires an intact phrenic nerve to act as conduit for the applied stimulus, diaphragmatic pacing is not feasible when there is damage to the spinal cord from C3 to C5, as the damage to phrenic nerve cell bodies and subsequent axonal degeneration removes the necessary conduit. Advances in microsurgical repair of peripheral nerves and nerve grafting led to research into anastomosis of a viable brachial nerve to a severed phrenic nerve in cats, with subsequent reinnervation of the diaphragm and institution of diaphragmatic pacing.

Objective.—The first successful intercostal to phrenic nerve anastomosis allowing diaphragmatic pacing was performed in a quadriplegic patient with spinal cord damage between C3 and C5.

Technique.—Via a right posterolateral thoracotomy through the seventh intercostal space, a seventh intercostal to phrenic nerve anastomosis is performed at approximately 4 cm above the diaphragm. The pacemaker is placed just distal to the anastomosis with the receiver placed in a subcutaneous pocket over the eighth and ninth ribs. Two weeks later, the phrenic nerve is directly tested through a left thoracotomy in the sixth intercostal space. A phrenic pacemaker system is inserted, and a standard pacing protocol is begun after 2 weeks. After 130 days, the anastomosis is tested for viability and diaphragmatic movement. Diaphragmatic pacing is continued.

Outcome.—A 20-year-old man with anterior spinal artery syndrome and an overall poor prognosis underwent intercostal to phrenic nerve anastomosis after 42 months of inpatient care. Phrenic nerve conduction studies demonstrated no conduction on the right and questionable response on the left that was attributed to the long thoracic nerve. Presently, the patient uses diaphragmatic pacing 24 hours a day, augmented by accessory muscle function when awake.

Discussion.—Intercostal to phrenic nerve anastomosis permits the consideration of electrophrenic respiration as a means of artificial ventilation in patients with C3–C5 or phrenic nerve injuries. Intercostal to phrenic nerve anastomosis should be considered when there is loss of conduction in the phrenic nerve of at least 3 months. Predicting an accurate time for axonal regeneration is difficult, but, given an accepted growth rate of regenerating axons of 1 mm per day, it should take about 2 months for the intercostal axons to grow 60 mm. Electrophrenic respiration after intercostal to phrenic nerve anastomosis has the potential of significantly improving the quality of life for quadriplegic ventilator-dependent patients as well as reducing the high health care cost.

▶ Dr. Krieger first developed an interest in control of respiration while analyzing the respiratory effects and complications of percutaneous upper cervical cordotomy in the late 1960s (1). He published his work on electrophrenic respiration after anastomosis of the brachial nerve with the phrenic nerve in the cat in 1983. Now, he and his colleagues report the use of electrophrenic respiration after intercostal to phrenic nerve anastomosis in a quadriplegic patient. I agree with the authors that this technique has significant potential for patient benefit and cost reduction.—R.H. Wilkins, M.D.

Reference

1. Rosomoff HL, Krieger AJ, Kuperman AS: Effects of percutaneous cervical cordotomy on pulmonary function. *J Neurosurg* 31:620–627, 1969.

41 Pain

Long-Term Results After Glycerol Rhizotomy for Multiple Sclerosis-Related Trigeminal Neuralgia

Kondziolka D, Lunsford LD, Bissonette DJ (Univ of Pittsburgh, Pa)
Can J Neurol Sci 21:137–140, 1994   122-96-41–1

Background.—Trigeminal neuralgia develops in about 2% of patients with multiple sclerosis, some of whom may be refractory to medical regimens. In such patients, percutaneous trigeminal operations including retrogasserian glycerol rhizotomy, radiofrequency thermal rhizotomy, and inflatable balloon compression have been recommended. The long-term results of patients managed via percutaneous retrogasserian glycerol rhizotomy (PRGR) were retrospectively analyzed to determine the efficacy of this procedure.

Patients and Findings.—Fifty-three patients with multiple sclerosis–related trigeminal neuralgia who underwent PRGR over an 11-year period were studied. The median patient age was 56 years. Before PRGR, all patients had been initially treated with carbamazepine. Some also required treatment with phenytoin and baclofen, either alone or in conjunction with carbamazepine. The duration of medical treatment varied, but most patients underwent therapy for more than 12 months. After PRGR, long-term follow-up ranging from 6 to 12 months was available in 49 patients. Of these patients, complete pain relief was achieved in 29, none of whom required further medication. Satisfactory pain relief necessitating occasional medication was noted in 8 patients. Twelve patients experienced unsatisfactory results with inadequate pain relief. Alternative surgical procedures were performed in 9 of these patients. Repeat PRGR was required in 16 patients to reachieve pain control. Normal trigeminal sensation was retained in 27 patients after injection. Major trigeminal sensory loss occurred in 1 patient who had undergone 4 glycerol rhizotomies over a 25-month period. Deafferentation pain was not noted in any patient.

Conclusions.—In most patients with multiple sclerosis–related trigeminal neuralgia, single or repeated PRGR is a safe, useful procedure. Marked facial hypoesthesia is uncommon following treatment and generally occurs after numerous rhizotomies. About 60% of patients refractory to medical treatment achieve long-term pain relief following PRGR.

▶ Dr. Lunsford has been a pioneer in the use of percutaneous trigeminal glycerol rhizolysis to treat trigeminal neuralgia. In this report, he and his colleagues document the value of this procedure in treating trigeminal neuralgia caused by multiple sclerosis.—R.H. Wilkins, M.D.

Microvascular Decompression for Glossopharyngeal Neuralgia
Resnick DK, Jannetta PJ, Bissonnette D, Jho HD, Lanzino G (Univ of Pittsburgh, Pa; Presbyterian Univ Hospital, Pittsburgh, Pa; Univ of Virginia, Charlottesville, Va)
Neurosurgery 36:64–69, 1995   122-96-41–2

Introduction.—In the past, glossopharyngeal neuralgia, an uncommon cause of facial pain, was treated surgically by procedures that involved destruction of the glossopharyngeal nerve or ascending sensory tracts. Microdecompression of the glossopharyngeal and vagus nerves is the first nondestructive surgical therapy for this condition. Outcomes for the 40 patients who have had this procedure since 1971 were reported.

Patients and Methods.—All patients had typical glossopharyngeal neuralgia (TGPN) and underwent decompression of either the ninth or tenth cranial nerve. The mean patient age was 55 years, and the mean duration of symptoms was 5 years; 23 patients were men and 17 were women. Neuralgia was left-sided in 25, right-sided in 14, and bilateral in 1. All patients had not responded to medical treatment. At surgery, the offending blood vessel was found to be the posterior inferior cerebellar artery in 16 cases and an artery/vein combination in 11; remaining causes were vertebral artery, a single vein, an artery/artery combination, and an unidentified artery. Patients were followed for a mean of 48 months.

Results.—Thirty-one of 39 operated sides (79%) had immediate relief of pain, and 4 patients experienced substantial improvement. Two patients died at surgery, and 3 cases of permanent ninth and tenth nerve paresis occurred. The long-term results were similar to immediate postoperative outcome, with 76% of patients having complete relief of pain without a need for medication, 15% showing substantial yet incomplete relief, and 8% failing to benefit from the procedure. The 2 deaths both occurred early in the series and were attributed to hemodynamic lability causing intracranial hemorrhage.

Conclusion.—Glossopharyngeal neuralgia has a relative incidence of 0.2% to 1.3% compared with trigeminal neuralgia. During the past 15 years, case reports and small series have supported the hypothesis that the inciting factor in TGPN is neurovascular compression. Treatment of compression of the glossopharyngeal and vagus nerves at the nerve root entry zone by microvascular decompression yields excellent results in most patients and substantial improvement in others, without sacrifice of the nerves.

▶ This paper updates known information about the treatment of glossopharyngeal neuralgia by microvascular decompression.—R.H. Wilkins, M.D.

Percutaneous Cervical Cordotomy: A Review of 181 Operations on 146 Patients With a Study on the Location of "Pain Fibers" in the C-2 Spinal Cord Segment of 29 Cases

Lahuerta J, Bowsher D, Lipton S, Buxton PH (Walton Hosp, Liverpool, England)
J Neurosurg 80:975–985, 1994   122-96-41–3

Background.—A total of 146 patients, aged 19 to 79 years, who underwent 181 percutaneous cervical cordotomies for unmanageable pain were reviewed. An anatomical-clinical correlation was also done in 29 patients. A primary aim was to report previously unpublished findings on the anatomy of the ascending fibers subserving pain sensation in the anterolateral funiculus of the human spinal cord.

Findings.—The fibers subserving pain sensation in the C-2 segment were found to lie in the anterolateral funiculus between the level of the denticulate ligament and a line drawn perpendicularly from the medial angle of the ventral gray-matter horn to the surface of the cord (Fig 41–1). Optimal analgesic results were obtained when lesions extending 5.0 mm deep to the surface of the cord were created and approximately 20% of the hemicord was destroyed. A somatotopic organization with sacral fibers running ventromedially and cervical fibers running dorsally was noted. Presumably, the ascending fibers subserving the distinct sensations of pain caused by tissue damage and pinprick are physiologically distinct from each other, although they overlap in the anterolateral funiculus of the spinal cord. As noted in previous reports, some cordotomies affect these functions differentially. However, the best pain relief appears to be obtained only when pinprick sensation is also eliminated in the affected segments.

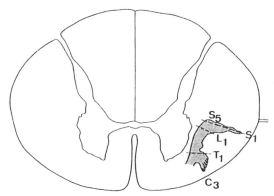

Fig 41–1.—Segmental homunculus showing the location of the "pain pathway" in the anterolateral funiculus at the C-2 spinal cord level, according to the authors' findings. (Courtesy of Lahuerta J, Bowsher D, Lipton S, et al: *J Neurosurg* 80:975–985, 1994.)

Conclusions.—Generally, ventromedial lesions of the anterolateral funiculus provide better pain relief and pinprick sensation deficit when compared with dorsolateral lesions, regardless of the segmental pain site.

▶ This benchmark article documents what can be achieved with percutaneous cervical cordotomy. Dr. Lipton and his colleagues have had extensive experience with the procedure and have analyzed their experience carefully and in detail. In doing so, they provide further information about the anatomical arrangement of the ascending fibers subserving pain sensation in the anterolateral portion of the spinal cord.—R.H. Wilkins, M.D.

Idiopathic Coccygodynia: Lateral Roentgenograms in the Sitting Position and Coccygeal Discography
Maigne J-Y, Guedj S, Straus C (Universitaire de l'Hotel-Dieu, Paris)
Spine 19:930–934, 1994   122-96-41–4

Background.—Patients with idiopathic coccygodynia have pain at the tail bone that is unrelated to any well-defined pathologic cause such as fracture, neoplasm, or infectious disease. The cause is often thought to be

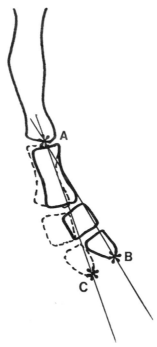

Fig 41–2.—The coccygeal range of motion is measured in degrees (angle **ABC**). *Bold line:* coccyx in the lateral decubitus position; *dotted line:* coccyx in the sitting position. A, apex of the angle located at the caudal part of the sacrum (or of the first coccygeal vertebra if the sacrococcygeal disk is ossified). (Courtesy of Maigne J-Y, Guedj S, Straus C: *Spine* 19:930–934, 1994.)

soft tissue injury or psychological disturbance. Whether a lesion of the coccygeal disk might be responsible for coccygodynia was determined.

Methods.—Fifty-one patients with coccygodynia were studied. There were 49 women and 2 men with a mean duration of pain of 7 months. The patients and a group of 51 controls with other types of symptoms underwent radiographic analysis of the coccyx in the sitting position vs. the lateral decubitus position (Fig 41–2). Coccygeal mobility was measured by superimposing graph paper with a double reading. These measurements had an accuracy of ± 2.6 degrees, an intraobserver variation of 15%, and an interobserver variation of 13%. The patients underwent coccygeal diskography at the same session.

Results.—Twenty-five of the patients demonstrated an abnormal motion of the coccyx in the sitting position that was spontaneously reduced in the lateral decubitus position (Fig 41–3). The abnormal motion consisted of a sagittal or posterior luxation in 13 cases and hypermobility in 12. None of the controls had similar findings. Coccygeal diskography was positive in 72% of patients, including all of those with abnormal coccygeal motion. Of 21 patients who had a normal dynamic study and successful diskography, the combination of provocation and anesthetization yielded a positive diskographic result in 15.

Conclusions.—About 70% of cases of "idiopathic" coccygodynia may be related to the coccygeal disk. A combination of dynamic lateral films in

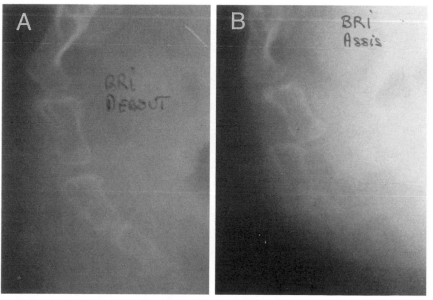

Fig 41–3.—**A**, a standard lateral ducubitus view shows the normal appearance. **B**, sitting radiograph of a subluxated coccyx. (Courtesy of Maigne J-Y, Guedj S, Straus C: *Spine* 19:930–934, 1994.)

the sitting position and diskography may reveal coccygeal subluxation, luxation, or hypermobility and is recommended in evaluating patients with coccygeal pain.

▶ Traditionally, idiopathic coccygodynia has defied etiologic explanation and satisfactory relief. Coccygectomy is sometimes performed as a last resort when nonoperative management methods have failed to provide adequate pain relief, but there has been no real rationale for the procedure, and pain relief from coccygectomy has not been predictable. This study suggests that coccygeal pain is diskogenic in many cases, which gives additional impetus and direction to the investigation of the etiology of "idiopathic" coccygodynia and its treatment.—R.H. Wilkins, M.D.

Cross-References

For further information, see also the following relevant Neurology articles:

CEREBROVASCULAR DISEASE

122-96-1–2 to 122-96-1–4
122-96-1–6
122-96-1–8 to 122-96-1–11

MOVEMENT DISORDERS

122-96-3–1 to 122-96-3–5
122-96-3–12
122-96-3–13

SEIZURE DISORDERS

122-96-6–1

PEDIATRIC NEUROLOGY

122-96-7–1 to 122-96-7–5
122-96-7–8

BEHAVIORAL NEUROLOGY

122-96-10–8

NEUROTRAUMA

122-96-11–1
122-96-11–2

NEUROLOGIC COMPLICATIONS OF GENERAL MEDICAL DISEASES

122-96-12–2
122-96-12–3

INFECTIOUS DISEASES

122-96-14–10

NEURO-OPHTHALMOLOGY

122-96-15–5

NEURO-OTOLOGY

122-96-16–4

PAIN AND HEADACHE

122-96-17–2 to 122-96-17–4
122-96-17–6

SPINAL DISORDERS

122-96-18–2
122-96-18–3

SLEEP DISORDERS

122-96-19–1

NEUROIMAGING

122-96-20–2

Subject Index*

A

Abnormal Involuntary Movement Scale
  in follow-up study of tardive dyskinesia,
    94: 46
Abscess
  brain
    otitis media and, suppurative,
      95: 175
    polymicrobial, hereditary
      hemorrhagic telangiectasia
      presenting with, 96: 342
  spinal epidural
    bacterial, review of, 95: 497
    case reports and review, 94: 383
    subperiosteal, and suppurative otitis
      media, 95: 175
Abuse
  child
    head injury in very young children
      due to, 94: 370
    retinal hemorrhage due to, 95: 435
  cocaine, long-term, cerebral perfusion
    and neuropsychological
    consequences of, 95: 190
  solvent vapor, causing
    leukoencephalopathy, comparison
    to adrenoleukodystrophy, 96: 153
Accessory
  nerve neurotization in infants with
    brachial plexus birth palsy, 96: 426
Accidents
  head injury and retinal hemorrhage due
    to, 95: 435
  motor vehicle, and Alzheimer's disease,
    95: 66
Acetazolamide
  in cerebellar ataxia, familial periodic,
    94: 183
  -enhanced regional cerebral blood flow
    measurement to predict risk to
    arteriovenous malformation
    patients, 94: 306
  in vestibulopathy, familial, 95: 275
Acetylcholine
  receptor channel openings, prolonged,
    due to mutation in M2 domain of e
    subunit causing congenital
    myasthenic syndrome, 96: 69
Acetylcholinesterase
  staining for sensory/motor-differentiated
    nerve repair in hand, 95: 526
Acetylsalicylic acid (see Aspirin)
Achievement
  school, after whole-brain radiotherapy
    for noncortical brain tumors, in
    children, 94: 364
Acidosis
  cerebral, after severe head injury, effect
    of THAM on, 94: 353

lactic
  in MELAS (see MELAS)
  pyruvate dehydrogenase deficiency
    and, 96: 116
Aciduria
  glutaric, type I, dystonia and dyskinesia
    in, 96: 112
Acoustic
  neurinoma (see Neuroma, acoustic)
  neuroma (see Neuroma, acoustic)
  schwannoma, cystic, MRI of, 95: 339
Acquired immunodeficiency syndrome (see
    AIDS)
Acromegaly
  pituitary adenoma in, GH-secreting
    adenomectomy for, transsphenoidal,
      95: 334
  surgical results, 95: 331
  sleep apnea in
    effect of octreotide on, 96: 221
    perioperative management and
      surgical outcome, 96: 281
ACTH (see Adrenocorticotropic,
    hormone)
Activity
  ordinary, for acute low back pain,
    96: 213
Acupuncture
  needles, sensory and electric stimulation
    through, effect on postural control
    after stroke, 96: 24
  in stroke patients, 95: 255
Acyclovir
  in meningitis, benign recurrent
    lymphocytic, due to herpes simplex
    virus infection, 96: 160
Acyl–coenzyme A
  dehydrogenase deficiency,
    medium-chain, clinical course of,
    96: 113
Addison's disease
  patients, screening for
    adrenoleukodystrophy/
    adrenomyeloneuropathy in,
    94: 113
Adenocarcinoma
  salivary gland, invading skull base,
    charged particle irradiation of,
    96: 276
Adenoma
  pituitary
    GH-secreting, in acromegaly,
      transsphenoidal adenomectomy for,
        95: 334
    GH-secreting, surgical results,
      95: 331
    growth hormone, invasive, SMS
      201-995 before transsphenoidal
      surgery in, 96: 280

---

* All entries refer to the year and page number(s) for data appearing in this and previous editions of the YEAR BOOK.

Inclusion body
  myopathy, hereditary, abnormal
    accumulation of prion protein
    mRNA in muscle fibers in, 96: 79
  myositis, sporadic, abnormal
    accumulation of prion protein
    mRNA in muscle fibers in, 96: 79
Incontinence
  urinary
    disability one year after first-time
      stroke and, 95: 258
    urge, cerebral etiology of, in elderly,
      96: 29
Incoordination
  in aluminum smelting plant workers,
    94: 196
  muscle, in reflex sympathetic dystrophy,
    95: 542
Indium-111
  octreotide scintigraphy for detection of
    paragangliomas, 95: 311
Indomethacin
  low-dose, in prevention of
    intraventricular hemorrhage in
    preterm neonates, 96: 102
Industrial
  painters, Japanese, neurobehavioral
    effects of chronic occupational
    exposure to organic solvents,
    95: 191
  workers, median sensory distal
    amplitude and latency in, 95: 195
Infant
  brachial plexus birth palsy in, accessory
    nerve neurotization in, 96: 426
  encephalopathy in, early myoclonic,
    95: 135
  exanthem subitum in, CNS
    complications of, 95: 128
  intracranial tumors in first year of life,
    95: 346
  muscular dystrophy in, autosomal
    recessive, fatal, hypertonic, in
    Canadian natives, 96: 72
  spasm in (see Infantile spasm below)
  torticollis in, benign paroxysmal,
    95: 138
Infantile autism
  brain in, 96: 109
Infantile spasm
  cryptogenic and symptomatic forms,
    outcome and prognostic factors,
    95: 133
  after DTP immunization, 95: 127
  vitamin B₆ in, 95: 132
Infarction
  brain (see Cerebral, infarction)
  brainstem, after microvascular
    decompression for hemifacial
    spasm, 96: 433
  capsular, functional reorganization
    patterns in cerebral cortex after,
    94: 25
  cerebellar

clinical and anatomic observations,
  94: 21
very small, distribution, causes,
  mechanisms and clinical features,
  94: 22
cerebral (see Cerebral, infarction)
medullary, small, and upbeat
  nystagmus, 95: 234
myocardial
  effect of antiplatelet therapy on,
    prolonged, 95: 20
  plasminogen activator in, tissue,
    intracranial hemorrhage after,
    94: 5
occipitotemporal, unilateral,
  hemiachromatopsia of, 96: 187
pontine, in acute posterior multifocal
  placoid pigment epitheliopathy,
  95: 238
spinal cord, due to cartilage embolus to
  anterior spinal artery, 94: 413
thalamic (see Thalamic, infarction)
vertebrobasilar, due to cervical
  manipulation, 95: 28
watershed, from vertebral dissection,
  96: 217
Infection
  shunt, reducing incidence of, in
    children, 94: 371
  ventriculostomy, relative risks of,
    96: 267
Infectious
  aneurysms, intracranial, monitoring by
    sequential CT/MRI studies,
    95: 404
  causes of optic nerve disease in AIDS,
    94: 149
  complications, daily risk of, and
    duration of intracranial pressure
    monitoring, 95: 298
Inflammation
  in reflex sympathetic dystrophy,
    95: 542
Inflammatory
  demyelination, fulminant CNS, acute
    episodes, plasmapheresis in, 95: 56
  myopathies, IV gammaglobulin in,
    96: 77
  polyneuropathy, demyelinating (see
    Polyneuropathy, demyelinating,
    inflammatory)
  polyradiculoneuropathy, chronic,
    presentation and initial clinical
    course, 95: 44
Inflicted injury
  of head in very young children, 94: 370
Infrared
  near-infrared spectroscopy, cerebral
    hypoxia detected by, 96: 353
Infratemporal
  fossa tumors, extended osteoplastic
    maxillotomy in, 94: 250
Inhalation
  aerosol paint, toluene abuse via, MRI
    findings after, 95: 162

Author Index